Z. Petrovich · L. Baert (Eds.)

Benign Prostatic Hyperplasia

Innovations in Management

With Contributions by

F. Ameye, K. Anson, M.A. Astrahan, L. Baert, K.-H. Bichler
S.D. Boyd, L.W. Brady, R.C. Bruskewitz, P. Dal Cin, P.S. Debicki
M. Devonec, C.M. Dixon, J.P. Fendler, E. Hoeben, P. Joubert, J. Keit
H. Lepor, W. Mattauch, G.B. Mieszkalski, R.H. Oyen, P. Perrin
Z. Petrovich, M.C. Pike, M. Riehmann, E. Shapiro, B. Stawarz
W.L. Strohmaier, S. Szmigielski, G. Ursin, H. Van Den Berghe
H. Vandeursen, H. Van Poppel, G. Verhoeven, G. Watson

With a Foreword by D.G. Skinner

Springer-Verlag
Berlin Heidelberg New York London Paris
Tokyo Hong Kong Barcelona Budapest

ZBIGNIEW PETROVICH, MD
Professor and Chairman
Department of Radiation Oncology
University of Southern California
Kenneth Norris Jr. Cancer Center
1441 Eastlake Avenue
Los Angeles, CA 90033
USA

LUC BAERT, MD, PhD
Professor and Chairman
Department of Urology
St. Pieter's Hospital
Catholic University of Leuven
Brusselsestraat 69
3000 Leuven
Belgium

and
Clinical Professor of Urology
and Radiation Oncology
University of Southern California
School of Medicine
Los Angeles, CA 90033
USA

With 127 Figures

ISBN 3-540-56628-7 Springer-Verlag Berlin Heidelberg New York
ISBN 0-387-56628-7 Springer-Verlag New York Berlin Heidelberg

Library of Congress Cataloging-in-Publication Data. Innovations in the management of benign prostatic hyperplasia/Z. Petrovich and L. Baert, eds.; with a foreword by D.G. Skinner; with contributions by F. Ameye . . . [et al.]. p. cm. Includes bibliographical references and index. ISBN 0-387-56628-7.—ISBN 3-540-56628-7: 1. Prostate—Hypertrophy—Congresses. I. Petrovich, Zbigniew. II. Baert, L. (Luc) III. Ameye, F. (Filip) [DNLM: 1. Prostatic Hypertrophy—therapy. 2. Prostatic Neoplasms—therapy. WJ 752 I58 1994] RC899.I56 1994 616.6′5—dc20 DNLM/DLC for Library of Congress 94-527

Typesetting: Macmillan India Ltd., Bangalore-25
SPIN: 10096605 21/3130/SPS – 5 4 3 2 1 0 – Printed on acid-free paper

This work is dedicated

to our wives

Dr. Zofia Petrovich and *Mrs. Bea Baert*

Foreword

A symposium on benign prostatic hyperplasia is appropriate at a time when new knowledge and new technology are rapidly emerging. As the age of the population has increased and diagnostic methods have improved, the incidence of diseases of the prostate has increased. Benign prostatic hyperplasia (BPH) is the most common benign tumor in men and results in urinary symptoms in the majority of men older than 50 years; furthermore it has in the past necessitated operative intervention in 20%–30% of men who live to the age of 80 years. The relief of obstruction resulting from this benign neoplasm by means of transurethral resection (TURP) or surgical enucleation represented a major advance and helped to establish urology as a major surgical science. Over the years, urologists became more and more proficient with the resectoscope, reducing the need for open surgery, and over time more procedures were done for more modest symptoms. Although unquestionably effective in the relief of bladder outlet obstruction in the majority of men treated, TURP has not been without morbidity.

In 1989, the American Urological Association (AUA) reported an 18% immediate postoperative morbidity in its cooperative study of 13 participating institutions evaluating 3885 patients (Mebust et al. 1989). Included were patients requiring transfusion, those experiencing excessive absorption of irrigating fluids ("TUR syndrome"), those experiencing myocardial arrhythmias, and a few suffering myocardial infarction. In the same group of patients, late complications of TURP included occasional bladder neck contracture or urethral stricture, a small number of cases of mild to severe urinary incontinence, and some degree of erectile or ejaculatory dysfunction. These side-effects of TURP have led to the development of new pharmacologic and minimally invasive approaches to the management of obstructive BPH that have caused the indications for treatment and the relative safety of current practices to be questioned.

From a noninvasive medical direction, the drug terazosin (Hytrin) has been advocated as an α-blocking smooth muscle relaxant with a specific action on the bladder neck and membranous urethra to facilitate voiding. In clinical trials, nearly one-half of men with modest symptoms show improvement in symptom scores and peak urinary flow rate. Hytrin is not effective in patients with prominent median lobes or those presenting in retention with a significant mechanical component of glandular hyperplasia.

Three categories of androgen suppressive agents, luteinizing hormone-releasing hormone (LHRH) agonists, antiandrogens, and 5α-reductase inhibitors, have been introduced as options in the treatment of obstruction by prostatic hyperplasia. The 5α-reductase inhibitor finasteride (Proscar) has received the greatest publicity because of its low toxicity and modest cost ($60 per month). The method of action of this drug in treating BPH is to block the conversion of testosterone to dihydrotestosterone. In North American trials, impotence and decreased libido were the only side-effects to be significantly more common in patients receiving active treatment than in those receiving placebo (they were present in 4% and 1% of the former group, respectively). However, the overall benefit of finasteride remains a modest 30% in clinical trials, similar to the efficacy of other classes of androgen suppressants. In addition, androgen suppression causes an artificial lowering of the serum prostatic specific antigen (PSA) level, which raises concerns about the ability of PSA to be an effective detector of early, potentially curable cancer of the prostate.

Technology has also evolved over the past decade, leading to the availability of more minimally invasive procedures such as transurethral incision of the prostate, laser coagulation prostatectomy, microwave hyperthermic applications, balloon dilatation, and placement of internal stents. Each of these methods has its proponents and its own associated side-effects as well as benefits. Each must be ultimately compared to the current gold standard, TURP. Some have predicted that the evolving alternative treatments for obstruction due to BPH will soon render TURP of historical interest only.

It is timely and constructive, therefore, to review the current knowledge of the etiology and pathogenesis of BPH as well as available treatment options. Ultimately, however, the success of any new approach will be appraised on the basis of the response evoked and whether it obviates the need for surgery. We are grateful to Drs. Zbigniew Petrovich and Luc Baert for organizing and assembling this material and in particular for attracting such outstanding contributors who have updated their areas of expertise.

Los Angeles, March 1994 DONALD G. SKINNER

Mebust WK, Holtgrave HG, Cockett ATK, Peters PC and Writing Committee (1989) Transurethral prostatectomy: immediate and postoperative complications. A cooperative study of 13 participating institutions evaluating 3885 patients. J Urol 141:243–247

Preface

Since the time when it was widely believed that human disease is a result of evil spirits or the improper balance of body humors, the progress of medicine has been based upon scientific research. The libraries of the world are filled with volumes containing the outcome of this research, which serves as the basis for present-day medical science.

The authors hope that, by consulting this book, the reader will increase his or her awareness of the complexities and rapid developments in the management of benign prostatic hyperplasia (BPH), which constitutes an important topic in the field of urology. This book attempts to bring into focus important issues concerning the etiology, pathogenesis, natural history, and imaging of the prostate, all of which are essential to the understanding of rationally designed treatment for BPH patients.

Prostatectomy, either as an open or endoscopic procedure, has until recently been the only effective treatment available to the countless thousands of patients who suffer from BPH. This treatment remains the gold standard against which new treatment modalities must be compared. Preliminary published data suggest that these new treatment modalities display therapeutic efficacy in selected BPH patients, but much work, including phase III prospective randomized trials, needs to be done to define the role of these new treatment modalities before they can be accepted as viable alternatives to prostatectomy. Until then, their use must remain investigational.

This book represents a review of all major treatments available to urologists in the management of BPH patients, with local prostatic hyperthermia receiving greatest emphasis. It attempts to address a wide audience which includes basic scientists, residents in training, practicing urologists, and other physicians interested in hyperthermia.

Los Angeles — Z. Petrovich
Leuven — L. Baert
March 1994

Contents

1 Etiology of Benign Prostatic Hyperplasia: Can this Disease Be Prevented?

MALCOLM C. PIKE and GISKE URSIN

CONTENTS

1.1 Introduction

The term "benign prostatic hyperplasia" (BPH) is commonly used to represent either (a) a pathologic entity, or (b) a clinical diagnosis, or (c) a treatment decision based on a clinical diagnosis. In order to discuss constructively what is known about the etiology of BPH it is essential to distinguish these different meanings of the term (ISAACS and COFFEY 1989). In this paper we will concentrate 1on discussing what is known of the etiology of the pathologic entity (which we will denote as pBPH) and of the clinical diagnosis of BPH (cBPH). Discussion of the issues involved in the decision as to whether and how to treat cBPH can be found in other chapters of this book.

1.2 Definition and Prevalence of BPH

1.2.1 Pathologic BPH

Pathologic BPH starts as a microscopic lesion involving "the development of hyperplastic changes" in the transitional zone or the periurethral region of the

MALCOLM C. PIKE, PhD, Professor and Chairman, and GISKE URSIN, MD, PhD, Post-doctoral Fellow, Department of Preventive Medicine, University of Southern California School of Medicine, 1420 San Pablo Street, Los Angeles, CA 90033-9987, USA

Petrovich/Baert (Eds.)
Benign Prostatic Hyperplasia

prostate (McNEAL 1988; ISAACS and COFFEY 1989). The transitional zone and the periurethral region are the only areas in the prostate that arise from the embryonic urogenital sinus (SHAPIRO 1990). The hyperplasia is characterized by proliferation of epithelial and stromal elements in varying proportions (McNEAL 1988). Although it is claimed that "periurethral nodules are stromal and resemble embryonic mesenchyme, whereas transitional zone nodules are glandular" (SHAPIRO 1990), documentation of this appears to be lacking. It is not clear whether the initial lesion is invariably stromal or invariably epithelial or whether this depends on the site of origin. This is critical information since it raises the issue of whether one is dealing with more than one disease entity.

Microscopic pBPH lesions can only be completely ascertained from serially sectioned prostates obtained at autopsy, and this has been done by a number of investigators. The prevalence of pBPH in these autopsy series shows a striking relationship with age (top curve in Fig. 1.1). pBPH lesions can be detected in a small proportion of autopsied men as early as age 25; by age 55 approximately

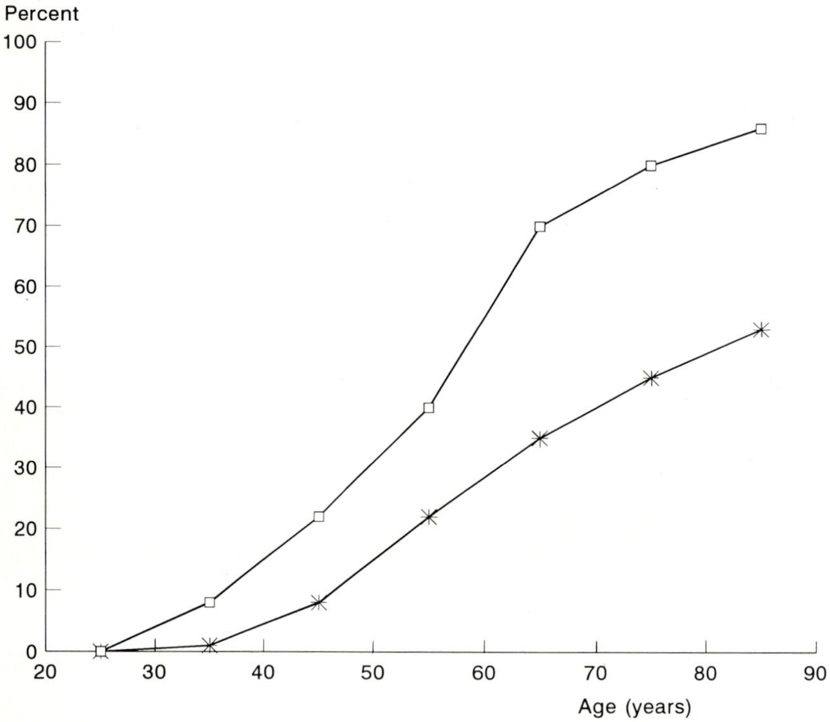

Fig. 1.1. The *top curve* shows the composite age-specific prevalence of pBPH obtained from six autopsy studies. The data were abstracted from Fig. 1 in ISAACS and COFFEY (1989). The *lower curve* shows the composite age-specific prevalence of pBPH with gross "enlargement" of the prostate obtained from two autopsy studies. The data were taken from Table I in ISAACS and COFFEY (1989)

50% of men have pBPH lesions, and by age 75 almost 80% of men have such lesions. Although an early report from China (CHANG and CHAR 1936) showed a lower prevalence of pBPH in Chinese men than in non-Chinese subjects, two other Asian studies, one from Japan and one from India, showed very similar rates to those observed in the United States and in Europe (ISAACS and COFFEY 1989).

These autopsy results strongly suggest that the etiologic factors responsible for pBPH are widespread and do not vary greatly in different countries. There are, of course, problems in interpreting such autopsy data. In particular, the selection processes involved in coming to autopsy will differ, possibly significantly, from one study or country to another. Also no allowance appears to have been made in any of these studies for autopsied persons with prostatectomies. These problems appear, however, most unlikely to alter the general conclusions one may draw from these studies.

The prevalence of pBPH lesions that are characterized by gross (macroscopic) enlargement of the prostate also increases with age (see lower curve in Fig. 1.1). Data on the volume of the prostate with pBPH lesions are only available from United States and European studies: we do not know whether there is a large international variation in the size of such lesions, and in particular whether the average size of pBPH lesions is smaller in the single studies from Japan and India. EKMAN (1989) reviewed international statistics on mortality from BPH: these data showed very low rates in Japan and North America. In our opinion, these statistics are impossible to interpret since they show evidence of extreme variation in assigning this cause of death in different countries and within a country over very short time periods. We regard these data as providing no help in estimating the prevalence of cBPH and in particular the prevalence of enlarged prostates.

It has been noted that pBPH cannot be diagnosed solely on the basis of the size of the prostate (Fig. 1.2). However, the detailed results of SWYER (1944; Fig. 1.3) show that if one excludes consideration of men under age 55, a prostate size of greater than 30 ml is almost always diagnostic of pBPH. Figure 1.3 also shows that there is some (cross-sectional) increase in prostate size with age in men with pBPH. Such data do not demonstrate the growth pattern of individual lesions, but this has been studied directly by OHNISHI et al. (1987). These investigators used transrectal ultrasonography (TRUS) to estimate the size of the prostate. They followed 16 cases of pBPH, which had been diagnosed by palpation, TRUS, and biopsy, for a period of 7 years. Only three cases showed clear evidence of a significant increase in prostate size over time (Fig. 1.4). These results suggest that most pBPH lesions increase only up to a certain size, and then remain at this size for extended periods.

In summary, one can conclude that there are at least two separate, possibly etiologically distinct, issues that need to be studied in the etiology of pBPH. The first is the etiology of microscopic pBPH, and the second is what influences the growth of the microscopic lesion.

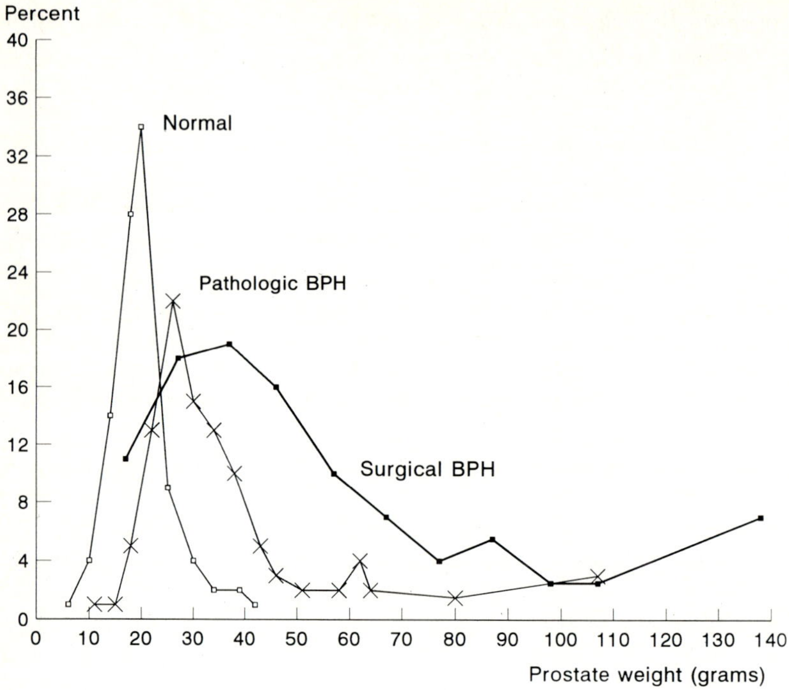

Fig. 1.2. Percent distribution of prostatic weights for normal prostates, pBPH, and surgically treated BPH. The data were abstracted from BERRY et al. (1984)

1.2.2 Clinical BPH

"Prostatic enlargement (i.e., macroscopic BPH) is a necessary but not sufficient condition for clinical dysuria (i.e., clinical BPH)" (ISAACS and COFFEY 1989). Macroscopic pBPH progresses to cPBH by causing urinary obstruction. Although cBPH is associated with larger macroscopic pBPH, a large pBPH is not equivalent to cBPH. The prevalence of cBPH has been studied by three groups of investigators (GLYNN et al. 1985; GUESS et al. 1990; GARRAWAY et al. 1991).

GLYNN et al. (1985), in a prospective study of 2063 men enrolled in the Boston Normative Aging Study, determined the incidence of cBPH over a period from 12 to 21 years. Their definition of cBPH was "a physical finding of an enlarged or abnormally firm prostate, or by a history of symptoms if the symptoms could not be attributed to another cause such as prostatitis or cancer of the prostate." Data from this study show that the prevalence of cBPH exceeded the prevalence of macroscopic pBPH (Fig. 1.1); the prevalence by age 70 was 61% compared to the macroscopic pBPH figure of less than 40% (Fig. 1.1).

GUESS et al. (1990) determined the prevalence rates of cBPH among 1057 men followed up for up to 30 years in the Baltimore Longitudinal Study of Aging. cBPH was diagnosed "on the basis of clinical judgment, taking into

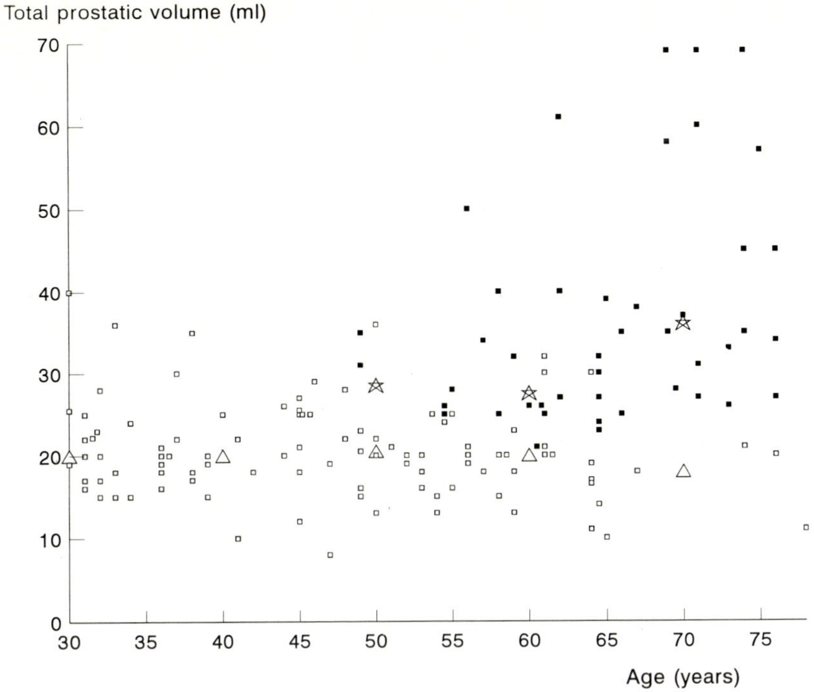

Fig. 1.3. Volume of prostate and presence (*solid squares*) or absence (*open squares*) of pBPH from autopsy series in the United Kingdom. The data were abstracted from Fig. 1 in SWYER (1944). *Open stars* show the median volume of pBPH by decade of age; *open triangles* show the median volume of normal prostates by decade of age

account the medical history and digital rectal examination". The prevalence rates from this study were much higher even than those found in the study by GLYNN et al. (1985); the rates were very similar to those of microscopic pBPH in Fig. 1.1.

In a community study in Scotland, GARRAWAY et al. (1991) determined the prevalence of cBPH in 705 men age 40–79. cBPH was defined as a prostate volume $>$ 20 ml (TRUS determined), "in the presence of symptoms of urinary dysfunction (an additive score $>$ 11), and/or Q_{max} rate $<$ 15 ml/sec." The age-specific prevalence of cBPH in this study was almost exactly the same as the prevalence of macroscopic pBPH shown in Fig. 1.1.

These results show that the prevalence rates of cBPH vary substantially depending on the criteria used, and possibly on the clinical setting in which these diagnoses are made (GLYNN et al. 1985); both of the U.S. studies relied on multiple physicians to record clinical findings. Surgical BPH (sBPH) rates are, of course, lower than cBPH rates, and depend not only on the severity of symptoms (SIDNEY et al. 1991) but also on such issues as access to health care, other (severe) health problems, and physicians' and patients' attitudes to dysuria.

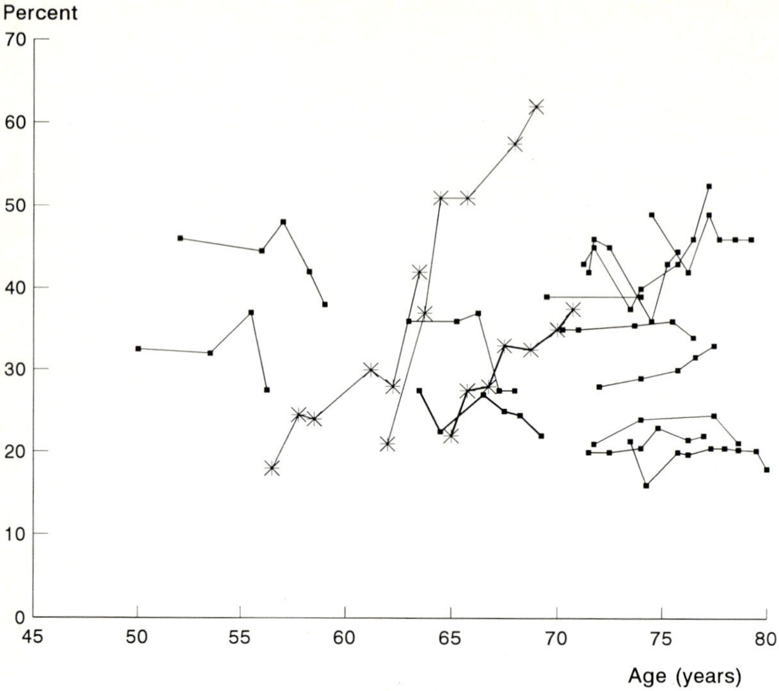

Fig. 1.4. Changes in individual volumes of prostates with pBPH as determined by TRUS. The data were abstracted from Fig. 1 in OHNISHI et al. (1987)

Surgical rates in the United States may be as high as 15% at age 70, and 30% at age 80 (GLYNN et al. 1985). Rates vary widely, even between adjacent communities, demonstrating that other issues than cBPH are major factors in determining sBPH rates (McPHERSON et al. 1982; GUESS 1992).

In summary, in addition to the issues concerning the etiology of microscopic pBPH and its growth, it may also be of value to study cBPH in order to determine the etiology of obstruction as distinct from prostate size. Because factors other than cBPH are such important determinants of which patients are surgically treated, it may not be particularly useful to study sBPH patients to understand the etiology of cBPH.

1.3 Risk Factors

Epidemiologic studies that have looked into risk factors for the development of BPH have been restricted to studies of cBPH and sBPH. The studies of cBPH have used different criteria (of varying degrees of rigidity) for defining cBPH, and, definitions of control groups are in a number of instances decidedly problematical. The control group has invariably consisted of "asymptomatic" individuals, but the definition of asymptomatic has varied from meaning nothing further than "has not been diagnosed with cBPH" to "has no symptoms of BPH". Studies using controls who have simply "not been diagnosed with cBPH," will include many men as controls with macroscopic pBPH, some with symptoms or signs that have simply not been elicited or recorded, and such studies of cBPH with a large proportion of the controls with macroscopic pBPH may have low power to detect even strong risk factors. Studies using controls "with no symptoms of BPH" will also include men with pBPH which has not resulted in gross enlargement of the prostate or any urinary obstruction. These latter studies will have increased power to detect risk factors compared to the former studies, but the results of these studies are also biased towards finding no effects. Significant results found in all such studies will, thus, underestimate the true magnitude of any effect found.

1.3.1 Hormonal Risk Factors

1.3.1.1 Testosterone and Dihydrotestosterone

"Functioning testes are required for the development of BPH" (Isaacs and Coffey 1989). BPH does not develop in men castrated prior to puberty (Wilson 1980). "In the medical literature there are careful pathologic reports, including microscopic description of the prostate of 28 eunuchs, eunuchoids or individuals with pituitary infantilism who ... lived to be over 45 years of age .... There is not a single example of benign hypertrophy in this group" (Moore 1944). This is a most striking finding considering the prevalence of pBPH found in autopsy series. It has also been consistently observed that an enlarged prostate will shrink when testosterone is reduced to castrate levels by actual castration or by use of gonadotropin releasing hormone analogues (Peters and Walsh 1987). It is important to note that this latter shrinkage is only about 25%. In experimental studies it has been reported that castration affects primarily the secretory rather than the basal epithelium or stromal elements (Evans and Chandler 1987; Serio and Fiorelli 1991). This latter finding is consistent with the finding that gross prostate shrinkage is not invariably found in all castrated patients (Steiner 1993). There is some evidence that the prostatic stroma in men with BPH does not regress after castration treatment, but this evidence does not exclude the possibility that the stroma simply requires more than a few months to respond (McConnel 1990).

Testosterone (T) is converted irreversibly to dihydrotestosterone (DHT) in the prostate via 5α-reductase. DHT is the main intraprostatic androgen, and the importance of this conversion was strikingly demonstrated by Imperato-McGinley and his colleagues (Imperato-McGinley 1984) in their studies of a particular form of pseudohermaphroditism. The affected males are deficient in the main form of prostatic 5α-reductase and are born with ambiguous genitalia, but at the time of puberty develop normal T levels, spermatogenesis, and external genitalia. The prostate, however, remains small, and BPH is reported not to develop. Further evidence for the importance of DHT comes from studies of the effects of finasteride, a 5α-reductase inhibitor. Finasteride administration reduces intraprostatic DHT concentration by 85% or more, without affecting serum T levels (MCCONNELL 1990), and reduces the volume of enlarged prostates to a similar extent as does castration, although it appears to take somewhat longer to do so (STONER and GROUP 1992). Thus, "normal" levels of androgens are required for the development and maintenance (at least of the epithelial elements) of BPH.

There have been seven epidemiologic studies that have compared serum levels of T and DHT in patients with BPH and in controls (Table 1.1). These studies have consistently found that serum levels of DHT are on average approximately 30% greater in cases than in controls. The results for T are inconsistent, and none of them are statistically significant. However, the three studies that collected serum from cases before surgery all showed elevated T in the cases, and this may be an important variable to control for in future studies.

DE JONG et al. (1991) found an 11% decrease in serum DHT levels in Japanese men compared to men in the Netherlands. DHT is mainly converted locally to 3α-, 17β-androstanediol (A-diol), which circulates as the glucuronide conjugate (A-diol-g). ROSS et al. (1992) studied A-diol-g in Japanese and American men and showed that the conversion of T to DHT in the prostate may be as much as 30% lower in the Japanese men. LOOKINGBILL et al. (1991) have reported similar results comparing Chinese to American men. Thus, if the level of DHT in the prostate is important in determining the risk of BPH, or its rate of growth, then cBPH should be much lower in Japan and China than in the United States. The data on this are sparse and contradictory (CHANG and CHAR 1936; KARUBE 1961). The rates should also be lower in Japanese and Chinese-Americans than in Caucasians living in the United States. We know of no comparative data on these different immigrant groups.

It may be that the elevated serum DHT levels in BPH cases are the result of the increased size of their prostates, not the cause of the increased size. This distinction could possibly be addressed by expressing the serum DHT levels in terms of the prostate weight, but this has not been done. An alternative approach is to compare the concentration of DHT in BPH tissue to that in normal prostatic tissue. Early reports consistently found higher tissue levels of DHT in BPH tissue, but this was shown by WALSH et al. (1983) to be an artifact of comparing fresh BPH tissue to normal prostatic tissue obtained at autopsy. They found no difference between BPH and normal prostatic tissue when care was taken to use comparably collected tissue. This suggests that the elevated serum DHT levels may be no more than an effect of the enlarged prostate of BPH patients.

1.3.1.2 Estrogen

There has been much interest in the possible synergistic action between estrogens and androgens in inducing BPH, an effect observed in experimental

Table 1.1. Serum testosterone (T), dihydrotestosterone (DHT) and estradiol (E_2) levels in men with BPH and controls

References	Cases	Controls	Elevation in cases			Remarks
			T	DHT	E_2	
VERMEULEN and DE SY (1976)	$n = 27$ sBPH Before surgery Age 60–80	$n = 36$ No evidence of cBPH Ambulatory, good health Similar age to cases	29%	49% ($P < 0.03$)	14%	
GHANADIAN et al. (1977)	$n = 25$ sBPH ?Before/after surgery Av. age = 66	$n = 24$ No evidence of cBPH Screening program Av. age = 68	– 8%	21% ($P < 0.02$)	ND	
SKOLDEFORS et al. (1978)	$n = 20$ sBPH Before surgery Av. age = 70	$n = 49$ No evidence of cBPH Minor surgery Av. age = 64	11%	ND	39%* ($P < 0.05$)	*E_1, not E_2
HAMMOND et al. (1978)	$n = 40$ sBPH ?Before/after surgery	$n = 25$ No evidence of cBPH Screening Program	20%	25% ($P < 0.01$)	0%	Adjusted for age
BROCHU and BELANGER (1987)	$n = 10$ sBPH Before surgery Av. age = 69	$n = 16$ No evidence of cBPH ?source Av. age = 72	18%	60% ($P < 0.05$)	20%	15 days after urological examination
HULKA et al. (1987)	$n = 41$ cBPH ?Before/after surgery Av. age = 69	$n = 161$ General medical outpatients Av. age = 66	6%	ND	– 36% ($P < 0.05$)	QI: 8% lower in cases (> 50% missing data for controls)

Table 1.1. (*Contd.*)

References	Cases	Controls	Elevation in cases			Remarks
			T	DHT	E_2	
de Jong et al. (1991) (Netherlands)	$n = 119$ sBPH Majority after surgery Av. age = 67	$n = 123$ Minor surgery Av. age = 63	− 9%	7%	0%	Results not affected by adjustment for age
de Jong et al. (1991) (Japan)	$n = 89$ sBPH Majority after surgery Av. age = 70	$n = 91$ Minor surgery Av. age = 70	− 4%	19% ($P = 0.06$)	− 3%	Results not affected by adjustment for age

studies (WALSH and WILSON 1976; HO et al. 1992). The results from the epidemiologic studies of serum estrogen in BPH cases and controls are shown in Table 1.1. The results are inconsistent. However, as with the results of serum T level measurement, the three studies where the serum was collected before surgery show higher estrogen levels in the cases.

1.3.2 Other Risk Factors

1.3.2.1 Body Weight

There are some data suggesting that elevated body weight is associated with a decreased risk of cBPH. GLYNN et al. (1985) found that the incidence of cBPH as approximately half in men with a Quetelet Index (QI, weight/height^2) $\geq 28\,kg/m^2$ compared to those with a QI $< 23\,kg/m^2$. The effect was stronger in the older age groups; in fact, there was no evidence of an effect in men below the age of 50. Although HULKA et al. (1987) also observed a lower mean QI in cases diagnosed as cBPH, information on QI was missing from more than half of the controls in their study, making interpretation of the result problematical. Both of these studies used men simply with no diagnosis of cBPH as controls. The main possible problem with these studies is, however, in the selection of the cases. Cases in these studies were not found by any systematic study of a population of men. It is thus possible that this result is an artifact of possible relative difficulty of diagnosis of cBPH in obese men in a normal clinical setting with no special protocol for diagnosis of the condition (BARRY 1990).

Increased body weight is associated with lower serum T and DHT levels, as has been reviewed by ELDRUP et al. (1987). It is difficult to judge whether this reduction in DHT would be sufficient to account for the lower prevalence of cBPH with increasing weight.

1.3.2.2 Cirrhosis

There have been five autopsy studies of the relationship between cirrhosis (almost always alcoholic cirrhosis) and BPH. They have consistently shown a decrease in the frequency of BPH in severely cirrhotic patients (GUESS 1992). STUMPF and WILENS (1953) found the effect to be most pronounced in men under age 70; in such men the BPH frequency was less than half of that in "normal" men. This may be regarded as supportive evidence for a role of T and DHT in cBPH since men with alcoholic cirrhosis have serum T and DHT levels that are less than half those of "normal" men (CHOPRA et al. 1973).

SIDNEY et al. (1991) found a 25% reduction in risk of sBPH in men who consumed three or more drinks per day, but no reduction in risk was found for cBPH or sBPH by GLYNN et al. (1985), and no dose response was found for sBPH by MORRISON (1992). Alcohol consumption has been associated with reduced T levels in an experiment in which men were given large amounts (15 drinks/day) of alcohol over a few months (GORDON et al. 1976), but the applicability of this result to "normal" drinking is not clear.

1.3.2.3 Smoking and Other Risk Factors.

There is no evidence of a strong effect of smoking on the prevalence of cBPH. SIDNEY et al. (1991), MORRISON (1992), and ROSS et al. (1992) found some evidence of a slight (10%) reduction of sBPH in smokers, while GLYNN et al. (1985) found no effect of smoking in their large study of cBPH. Smoking has been found to be associated with increased T levels independent of body weight (DAI et al. 1988), so this may be considered weak evidence against T and DHT serum levels being of etiologic significance.

1.3.2.4 Vasectomy and Other Risk Factors

Vasectomy has been found to influence the risk of BPH (SIDNEY 1987; JAKOBSEN et al. 1988a). No evidence of a relation between sexual activity and BPH has been found. No other risk factors have been established. A further discussion of epidemiologic risk factors can be found in recent reviews by GUESS (1992) and ISAACS and COFFEY (1989).

1.4 Conclusions and Suggestions for Future Research

At relatively young ages (< 45 years, say) most men do not show any evidence of pBPH, and the lesions that are present will presumably have been present for only a relatively short period. Comparative studies of such young men with and without pBPH should therefore have the greatest chance of being etiologically informatives as regards the origin of microscopic lesions. In older men many of the pBPH lesions will have been present for years and etiologic studies may be uninformative as regards the origin of microscopic lesions. It would, however, appear reasonable to study the determinants of growth of pBPH lesions in men at any age.

Use of TRUS is generally accepted as a noninvasive method of determining prostatic volume (HASTAK et al. 1982; OKAFOR et al. 1983). Another possibly very important use of TRUS for etiologic research has been suggested by JAKOBSEN et al. (1988b). pBPH was previously often referred to as benign nodular hyperplasia (BNH) (FRANKS 1954; KARUBE 1961), and JAKOBSEN et al. (1988b) maintain that macroscopic BNH can be recognized by TRUS (trusBNH) through an echo pattern distinct from the recognition of prostate size (TORP-PEDERSEN et al. 1988; POLLACK 1991). Early lesions cannot be completely satisfactorily studied with

TRUS since to detect trusBPH the lesion has already to be large enough to be visible on TRUS, but TRUS would appear to permit one to get reasonably close both to the early identification of pBPH and to its development into an enlarged lesion.

JAKOBSEN et al. (1988b) performed TRUS on volunteers who either presented for vasectomy or were recruited from the general population in Denmark, and found a high prevalence of trusBNH (Fig. 1.5). As in the autopsy studies of pBPH, the prevalence of trusBNH increased with age; however, the prevalence of trusBNH was higher than that seen in autopsy studies of pBPH. This raises the question of whether some of the trusBNH lesions in this study may have been artifactual (overdiagnosis) or may have represented entities other than pBPH. Studies of the validity of this work need to be carried out, since such a technique would permit the study of early BPH lesions.

The etiology of an enlarged prostate due to BPH must be distinguished from the clinical entity of cBPH, which depends not only on prostate size but also on the precise location of the lesion and other factors. In order to further our understanding of BPH, etiologic studies of BPH need, for the immediate future, to be restricted to microscopic and macroscopic pBPH.

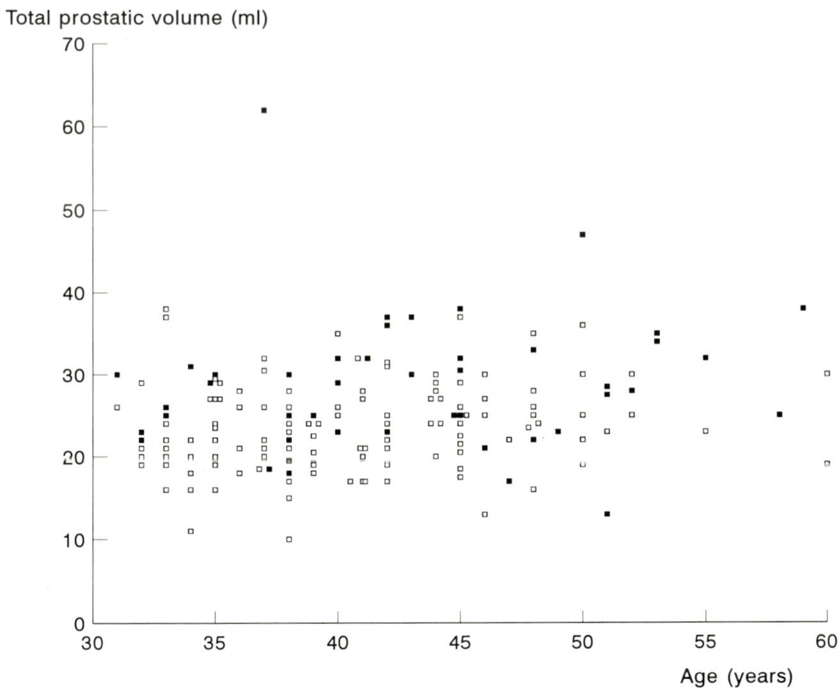

Fig. 1.5. Volume of prostate and presence (*solid squares*) or absence (*open squares*) of BPH as detected by transrectal ultrasonography (trusBPH). The data were abstracted from Fig. 1 in JAKOBSEN et al. (1988b)

"Normal" testicular function, i.e., "normal" T production, is clearly essential for the development of BPH. However, the evidence that elevated serum T levels in the physiologic range increase the risk of BPH is weak (Table 1.1).

The conversion of T to DHT within the prostate is also essential for the development of BPH. cBPH is strongly associated with elevated serum DHT levels (Table 1.1), but this does not definitely imply that elevated T to DHT conversion (within the physiologic range) in the prostate is associated with an increased risk of BPH, since it is possible that the elevated serum DHT levels merely reflect the increased volume of prostatic tissue in BPH.

Japanese and Chinese men have (on average) reduced serum levels of DHT and metabolites of DHT reflecting reduced levels of DHT in the prostate. If the prostatic concentration of DHT is important in the etiology of pBPH, i.e., if an increased prostatic DHT concentration within the physiologic range increases the prevalence of pBPH, then Japanese and Chinese men in their homelands, and Japanese- and Chinese-Americans, should have a lower prevalence of BPH. The data on this are sparse. Further comparative data are needed on the prevalence of microscopic and macroscopic pBPH in these groups and in U.S. whites and blacks. Such data collected over the age range 40–74 would permit study of the possible effects of DHT on the formation of microscopic pBPH and on the growth of microscopic pBPH to macroscopic BPH (enlarged prostate size). Data on serum DHT (as well as T and estradiol) in Japanese- and Chinese-American men need to be collected to confirm that these men do have lower levels of DHT.

If a cohort of men with blood collected before age 25, i.e., before the age at which microscopic pBPH has ever been found in autopsy series, can be identified (e.g., from college student populations), then measurement of serum DHT and its relation to prostate size at age 45 or older would complement the above studies of Japanese and Chinese men.

Increased body weight has been consistently found to be associated with a markedly reduced risk of cBPH. This may be because increased body weight is associated with decreased T and DHT levels as well as with other metabolic differences, but it may be that cBPH is simply more difficult to diagnose with increasing weight. This needs to be elucidated by a study in which macroscopic pBPH is measured by a method not affected by body size. If increased body weight is truly a protective factor, then the reason for this needs to be sought.

Can BPH be prevented? We know too little about this disease at the moment to make any recommendations for its prevention. Hopefully when we understand more about the etiology of pBPH, especially the relationship with DHT and body weight, we will be able to develop preventive measures.

References

Barry MJ (1990) Epidemiology and natural history of benign prostatic hyperplasia. Urol Clin North Am 17:495–507

Berry SJ, Coffey DS, Walsh PC, Ewing LL (1984) The development of human benign prostatic hyperplasia with age. J Urol 132:474–479

Brochu M, Belanger A (1987) Comparative study of plasma steriod and steriod glucuronide levels in normal men and in men with benign prostatic hyperplasia. Prostate 11:33–40

Chang HL, Char GY (1936) Benign hypertrophy of prostate. Chin Med J 50:1707–1722

Chopra IJ, Tulchinsky D, Greenway FL (1973) Estrogen-androgen imbalance in hepatic cirrohsis, Ann Intern Med 79:198–203

Dai WS, Gutai JP, Kuller LH, Cauley JA (1988) Cigarette smoking and serum sex hormones in men. Am J Epidemiol 128:796–805

de Jong FH, Oishi K, Hayes RB, et al. (1991) Peripheral hormone levels in controls and patients with prostatic cancer or benign prostatic hyperplasia: results from the Dutch-Japanese case-control study. Cancer Res 51:3445–3450

Ekman P (1989) BPH epidemiology and risk factors. Prostate Suppl 2:23–31

Eldrup E, Lindholm J, Winkel P (1987) Plasma sex hormones and ischemic heart disease. Clin Biochem 20:105–112

Evans GS, Chandler JA (1987) Cell proliferation studies in the rat prostate. II. The effects of castration and androgen-induced regeneration upon basal and secretory cell proliferation. Prostate 11:339–351

Franks LM (1954) Benign nodular hyperplasia of the prostate: a review. Ann R Coll Surg Engl 14:92–106

Garraway WM, Collins GN, Lee RJ (1991) High prevalence of benign prostatic hypertrophy in the community. Lancet 338:469–471

Ghanadian R, Lewis JG, Chisholm GD, Donoghue EPN (1977) Serum dihydrotestosterone in patients with benign prostatic hypertrophy. Br J Urol 49:541–544

Glynn RJ, Campion EW, Bouchard GR, Silbert JE (1985) The development of benign prostatic hyperplasia among volunteers in the normative aging study. Am J Epidemiol 121:78–90

Gordon GG, Altman K, Southren AL, Rubin E, Lieber CS (1976) Effect of alcohol (ethanol) administration on sex-hormone metabolism in normal men. N Engl J Med 295:793–797

Guess HA (1992) Benign prostatic hyperplasia: antecedents and natural history. Epidemiol Rev 14:131–153

Guess HA, Arrighi HM, Metter EJ, Fozard JL (1990) Cumulative prevalence of prostatism matches the autopsy prevalence of benign prostatic hyperplasia. Prostate 17:241–246

Hammond GL, Kontturi M, Vihko P, Vihko R (1978) Serum steroids in normal males and patients with prostatic diseases. Clin Endocrinol 9:113–121

Hastak SM, Gammelgaard J, Holm HH (1982) Transrectal ultrasonic volume determination of the prostate–a preoperative and postoperative study. J Urol 127:1115–1118

Ho S-M, Yu M, Leav I, Viccione T (1992) The conjoint actions of androgens and estrogens in the induction of proliferative lesions in the rat prostate. In: Li J (ed) Hormonal carcinogenesis. Springer, Berlin Heidelberg New York, pp 18–26

Hulka BS, Hammond JE, DiFerdinando G, et al. (1987) Serum hormone levels among patients with prostatic carcinoma or benign prostatic hyperplasia and clinic controls. Prostate 11:171–182

Imperato-McGinley J (1984) 5α reductase deficiency in man. Prog Cancer Res Ther 31:491–495

Isaacs JT, Coffey DS (1989) Etiology and disease process of benign prostatic hyperplasia. Prostate Suppl 2:33–50

Jakobsen H, Torp-Pedersen S, Hald T (1988a) The long-term influence of vasectomy on prostatic volume and morphology in man. Prostate 13:57–67

Jakobsen H, Torp-Pedersen S, Juul N (1988b) Ultrasonic evaluation of age-related human prostatic growth and development of benign prostatic hyperplasia. Scand J Urol Nephrol 107:26–31

Karube K (1961) Study of latent carcinoma of the prostate in the Japanese based on necropsy material. Tohoku J Exp Med 74:265–285

Lookingbill DP, Demers LM, Wang C, Leung A, Rittmaster RS, Santen RJ (1991) Clinical and biochemical parameters of androgen action in normal healthy Caucasian versus Chinese subjects. J Clin Endocrinol Metab 72:1242–1248

McConnell JD (1990) Androgen ablation and blockade in the treatment of benign prostatic hyperplasia. Urol Clin North Am 17:661–670

McNeal JE (1988) Normal histology of the prostate. Am J Surg Pathol 12:619–633

McPherson K, Wennberg JE, Hovind OB, Clifford P (1982) Small-area variations in the use of common surgical procedures: an international comparison of New England and Norway. N Engl J Med 307:1310–1314

Moore RA (1994) Benign hypertrophy and carcinoma of the prostate. Surgery 16:152–167

Morrison AS (1992) Risk factors for surgery for prostatic hypertrophy. Am J Epidemiol 135:974–980

Ohnishi K, Watanabe H, Ohe H (1987) Development of benign prostatic hypertrophy estimated from ultrasonic measurement with long-term follow up. Tohoku J Exp Med 151:51–56

Okafor PIS, Wild SR, Beynon LL, Chisholm GD (1983) Progress in transrectal ultrasonography for prostatic disease. Br J Urol 55:721–725

Peters CA, Walsh PC (1987) The effect of nafarelin acetate, a luteinzing-hormone-releasing-hormone agonist, on benign prostatic hyperplasia. N Engl J Med 317:599–604

Pollack HM (1991) Imaging of the prostate gland. Eur Urol 20 (Suppl):50–58

Ross R, Bernstein L, Lobo R, et al. (1992) 5-alpha-reductase activity and risk of prostate cancer among Japanese and US white and black males. Lancet 339:887–889

Serio M, Fiorelli G (1991) Dual control by androgen and peptide growth factors of prostatic growth in human benign prostatic hyperplasia. Mol Cell Endrocrinol 78:C77–C81

Shapiro E (1990) Embryologic development of the prostate. Urol Clin North Am 17:487–493

Sidney S (1987) Vasectomy and the risk of prostatic cancer and benign prostatic hypertrophy. J Urol 138:795–797

Sidney S, Quesenberry C Jr, Sadler MC, Lydick EG, Guess HA, Cattolica EV (1991) Risk factors for surgically treated benign prostatic hyperplasia in a prepaid health care plan. Urology 38:13–19

Skoldefors H, Blomstedt B, Carlstrom K (1978) Serum hormone levels in benign prostatic hyperplasia. Scand J Urol Nephrol 12:111–114

Steiner JF (1993) Finasteride: a 5α-reductase inhibitor. Clin Pharm 12:15–23

Stoner E, Group TFS (1992) The clinical effects of a 5α-reductase inhibitor, finasteride, on benign prostatic hyperplasia. J Urol 147:1298–1302

Stumpf HH, Wilens SL (1953) Inhibitory effects of portal cirrhosis of liver on prostatic enlargement. Arch Intern Med 91:304–309

Swyer GIM (1944) Post-natal growth changes in the human prostate. J Anat 78:130–145

Torp-Pedersen S, Juul N, Jakobsen H (1988) Transrectal prostatic ultrasonography: equipment, normal findings, benign hyperplasia and cancer. Scand J Urol Nephrol 107:19–25

Vermeulen A, de Sy W (1976) Androgens in patients with benign prostatic hyperplasia before and after prostatectomy. J Clin Endocrinol Metab 43:1250–1254

Walsh PC, Wilson JD (1976) The induction of prostatic hypertrophy in the dog with androstanediol. J Clin Invest 57:1093–1097

Walsh PC, Hutchins GM, Ewing LL (1983) Tissue content of dihydrotestosterone in human prostatic hyperplasia is not supranormal. J. Clin Invest 72:1772–1777

Wilson J (1980) The pathogenesis of benign prostatic hyperplasia. Am J Med 68:745–756

2 Pathogenesis of Benign Prostatic Hyperplasia: Potential Role of Mesenchymal – Epithelial Interactions

GUIDO VERHOEVEN and EEF HOEBEN

CONTENTS

2.1 Introduction

Benign prostatic hyperplasia (BPH) is the most common nonmalignant proliferative abnormality observed in any internal organ in men. The primary cause of the disease remains elusive but age and androgens unequivocally play a major role in its evolution. Autopsy studies have revealed that microscopic disease may be present as early as 25–30 years of age. At this age, however, the prevalence of the disease is below 10%. With increasing age the prevalence of microscopic BPH rapidly increases to reach approximately 80% in the eighth decade (for review: OESTERLING 1991a). BPH does not occur in men castrated before puberty and it is extremely rare in men who have undergone castration before the age of 40 years (WALSH 1984). Moreover, chemical castration using luteinizing hormone-releasing hormone agonists (OESTERLING 1991b) or interference with androgen action by administration of androgen antagonists (STONE and CLEJAN 1991) or 5α-reductase inhibitors (GORMLEY et al. 1991) reduces the volume of the prostate in patients with BPH.

GUIDO VERHOEVEN, PhD, Professor of Pathophysiology, and EEF HOEBEN, Doctorate Student, Department of Developmental Biology, Laboratory for Experimental Medicine and Endocrinology, Catholic University of Leuven, 3000 Leuven, Belgium

Petrovich/Baert (Eds.)
Benign Prostatic Hyperplasia

The present review focuses on the mechanisms by which androgens may influence the evolution of prostatic hyperplasia and particularly on the role of cell–cell interactions in the pathogenesis of this disease.

Androgens are steroid hormones and accordingly they are generally assumed to act on their target tissues via specific intracellular receptors. The androgen receptor is a member of a large superfamily of nuclear receptors with significant structural homology which act as ligand-responsive transcription factors to activate or to repress the expression of selective genes (for review: BRINKMAN et al. 1992). There are a number of factors, however, which make the interplay of androgens with their target cells more difficult to interpret than this simple scheme suggests. Firstly, in several (but not all) androgen target tissues the major circulating androgen, testosterone, is converted into an active metabolite 5α-dihydrotestosterone (DHT) (WILSON and GLOYNA 1970). This metabolite has a higher biologic activity and a higher affinity for the receptor than testosterone (LIAO et al. 1973; VERHOEVEN et al. 1975). The enzyme responsible for this conversion is known as the 5α-reductase and, as illustrated most convincingly in patients with congenital 5α-reductase deficiency (IMPERATO-MCGINLEY et al. 1974), for some androgen effects DHT formation is an absolute requirement. Testosterone may also be converted in other active metabolites such as 17β-estradiol and in this case it may act via another receptor, the estradiol receptor (SIITERI and MACDONALD 1973). Secondly, several circulating steroids with limited inherent biologic activities, such as dehydroepiandrosterone, androstenedione, and 3α-androstanediol, may be converted in target tissues into active metabolites (FARNSWORTH 1973; HARPER et al. 1974). The ability to catalyze these reactions and accordingly the ability to respond to these precursors varies from target tissue to target tissue and may be influenced by a number of physiologic or pathologic factors. Finally, of all hormones androgens may well be the ones with the most impressive effects on the morphogenesis and differentiation of their own target tissues. In the absence of androgens or androgen action during critical sensitive periods the development of target tissues such as the prostate is irreversibly disturbed (WILSON et al. 1981). Morphogenesis and differentiation are processes which typically involve complex interactions between various cell types. Accordingly, it is not surprising that cell interactions represent a cardinal element in androgen action in general and more particularly in the pathogenesis of BPH.

2.2 Epithelium, Stroma, and Androgen Action in the Normal Prostate and in BPH

Theoretically androgens may influence the development of BPH in at least three different ways. One possibility is that their role in the pathogenesis of this disease is merely a permissive one. Alternatively changes in circulating hormone levels might result in excessive stimulation of the prostate. Finally it is conceivable that changes in responsiveness to androgens might result in disordered growth. A comprehensive overview of the subject has recently been published by KRIEG and TUNN (1990) and we will limit the present discussion to some of the main points.

There is increasing evidence that with increasing age the endocrine status of the male changes. Age correlates negatively with serum total and free testosterone concentration while estradiol concentration remains stable (NASS et al. 1990; VERMEULEN 1991; VELDHUIS et al. 1992). This results in an altered androgen–estrogen balance. Whether and how this altered sex hormone balance influences the development of BPH remains unknown.

A large body of evidence suggests that the prostate itself largely determines the concentration of androgens and active metabolites to which it is exposed. The observation that DHT is the major metabolite of testosterone in BPH tissue (FARNSWORTH and BROWN 1963) and that in several accessory organs of reproduction DHT rather than testosterone is the active androgen (WILSON and GLOYNA 1970) rapidly led to the suggestion that excessive production or accumulation of DHT might play a major role in the pathogenesis of BPH (WILSON 1980). Several studies have confirmed that the levels of DHT in the human prostate are nearly ten times higher than circulating levels whereas the opposite is observed for testosterone (KRIEG 1984). Moreover, most of this DHT is found in prostatic nuclei, the expected site of androgen action (GHANADIAN et al. 1976; VERDONCK et al. 1980; BARTSCH et al. 1982). Furthermore, it has been demonstrated that in the dog prolonged administration of DHT or 3α-androstanediol results in prostatic hyperplasia, an effect which can be markedly enhanced by simultaneous treatment with 17β-estradiol (GLOYNA et al. 1970; WALSH and WILSON 1976). A number of early studies suggested that DHT levels are considerably higher in BPH than in normal prostatic tissue (SIITERI and WILSON 1970; HAMMOND 1978; MEIKLE et al. 1980). These claims have been challenged and attenuated, however, by more recent studies demonstrating that the difference in DHT concentration between normal prostatic tissue and BPH largely disappears when metabolism after removal of the tissues (particularly the normal prostate) is minimized (WALSH et al. 1983; VOIGT and BARTSCH 1986; BRUCHOVSKY et al. 1988).

Since, during embryonic development, the stroma rather than the epithelium is the primary site of androgen action and since prostatic stroma may play a major role in the pathogenesis of BPH (see below), several investigators have examined whether, in the adult prostate, androgens act primarily on the stroma or on the epithelium and which of these two sites of action may be the most important one with respect to the development of BPH. The available data are equivocal, in part because of differences in experimental design and expression of results. The concentration of DHT in stroma is probably equal to (SIRETT et al. 1980; BRUCHOVSKY et al. 1988) or slightly higher than (BOLTON et al. 1981; BARTSCH et al. 1982) that in epithelium. In both tissue compartments DHT is mainly localized in the nuclei (BARTSCH et al. 1982). Furthermore, both in stroma and in epithelium from patients with BPH there seems to be a trend to higher DHT concentrations than in tissues derived from normal patients (BARTSCH et al.

1982; BRUCHOVSKY et al. 1988). Interestingly, recent data suggest that different 5α-reductase isoenzymes prevail in the stroma and in the epithelium. The stromal enzyme displays a higher V_{max} value than its epithelial counterpart. Excessive accumulation of DHT in the stroma may be prevented, however, by a lower affinity (K_m value) of this enzyme for its substrate, testosterone (BRUCHOVSKY et al. 1988). As a function of age and independent from the development of BPH the mean K_m values increase in stroma as well as in epithelium whereas V_{max} values correlate with age only in stroma (TUNN et al. 1988). The reason for these changes in kinetic parameters and the implications for the accumulation of DHT in the different compartments of the prostate certainly merit further investigation.

Androgen receptors are found in stroma and epithelium. Using conventional ligand exchange techniques, levels have been reported to be similar (KRIEG et al. 1981; ROBEL et al. 1984) or to be slightly higher in stroma (SIRETT et al. 1980; LAHTONEN et al. 1983). Recent immunohistochemical studies with antibodies directed against the androgen receptor demonstrate comparable patterns of nuclear staining in epithelial and stromal cells (HUSMANN et al. 1990). In BPH samples with a predominance of epithelial hyperplasia, stromal cells were only weakly immunostained. In samples characterized by fibromuscular hyperplasia, however, more intense staining was observed in the stroma (SAR et al. 1990). In the ventral prostate of adult rats staining was pronounced in nuclei from epithelial cells and only rare stromal cells reacted positively (HUSMANN et al. 1990; SAR et al. 1990; PRINS et al. 1991); nonetheless, periacinar smooth muscle cells were strongly positive (PRINS et al. 1991).

Estrogens have also been implicated in the pathogenesis of BPH. As already mentioned, 17β-estradiol coadministered with 3α-androstanediol strongly potentiates the induction of prostatic hyperplasia in beagles (WALSH and WILSON 1976). Moreover, induction of prostatic growth in adult castrated beagles by administration of androstenedione, an aromatizable androgen, is antagonized by an aromatase inhibitor. Similarly, administration of an aromatase inhibitor prevents stimulation of the smooth muscular component of prostatic stroma in intact adult cynomolgus monkeys treated for 3 months with androstenedione (HABENICHT and EL ETREBY 1991). In the beagle model estrogens may increase prostatic androgen receptor concentration (MOORE et al. 1979). Interestingly, estrogen receptors are present in the human prostate and seem to be located mainly in prostatic stroma (BASHIRELAHI et al. 1976; KRIEG et al. 1981; EKMAN et al. 1983; SCHULZE and CLAUS 1990).

It may be concluded that in the adult prostate both the epithelium and the stroma dispose of the necessary equipment to act as androgen target tissues. At the moment there is no convincing evidence to favor one of these compartments as the primary site of androgen action. Equally, there is no firm evidence of major alterations in androgen action in stroma or epithelium of patients with BPH. A tendency to a higher accumulation of DHT remains possible. Estrogens may act on the stroma and may directly or indirectly potentiate the effects of androgens. Again, however, their exact role in human BPH remains elusive.

2.3 Stromal–Epithelial Interactions and the Pathogenesis of BPH

Although circulating androgens are undoubtedly required both for the development of the prostate and for maintenance of its adult function, it is obvious that local control systems are at least equally important to control prostate growth and to guarantee normal epithelial function. For example, in explant cultures of undissociated prostatic tissue, epithelial cells can survive for months. When these cells are mechanically dissociated from the stroma, however, they completely lose their growth capacity (FRANKS et al. 1970). Prostatic epithelial cells may be maintained in serum-free medium supplemented with cholera toxin, epidermal growth factor, pituitary extract, and hydrocortisone, but such cells do not respond to androgens and little is known on their differentiated functions (PEEHL and STAMEY 1986).

The idea that stromal–epithelial interactions are essential for normal prostatic function and that disturbed interactions between these tissue compartments may form an essential element in the pathogenesis of BPH actually dates from the beginning of this century (for review: OESTERLING 1991a; MCNEAL 1978). Rigorous studies on the exact anatomic and histologic origin of BPH and on its evolution as a function of age (MCNEAL 1978), and animal experiments on the role of stroma and epithelium during embryonic development of the prostate (CUNHA et al. 1983) have set the stage for our present thinking on the pathogenesis of BPH.

Using precise quantitative analysis, MCNEAL (1978, 1990) studied the location, the characteristics, and the evolution of BPH nodules in 63 autopsy prostates. He demonstrated that nodules originate selectively from a very small region situated proximal to the verumontanum and near to the upper urethral sphincter that emanates from the neck of the bladder. Most nodules arise from the glands and stroma of the so-called transition zone, a small wedge of tissue lying immediately lateral to the lower and distal end of the sphincter. In this zone the earliest stage of nodule formation is characterized by a cluster of new gland branches budding from the wall of one or possibly more adjacent prostatic ducts. Nodule formation is also observed in the periurethral tissue enclosed inside the urethral sphincter. The latter nodules are fewer in number, however, and smaller in size. Moreover, initially they are almost always purely fibroblastic. Only during later stages does eccentric budding of duct-derived glands become common.

These observations strongly suggest that in its initial stages BPH is not a *diffuse* disease – as would be expected if an endocrine imbalance were the primary pathogenic factor – but a *focal* disease. It remains possible that changes in endocrine status contribute to later stages of BPH development. In fact, between the seventh and eighth decades a general and marked enlargement of the nodules is observed in a large portion of patients with BPH (MCNEAL 1978).

The nature of the primary focal disturbance remains poorly understood. The characteristic eccentric duct budding suggests stromal inductive effects resembling those observed during embryonic development and accordingly the hypothesis has been advanced that the initial lesion of BPH may be due to a reawakening of the embryonic inductive interaction between responsive prostatic glands and an aberrant inappropriate stroma. One possibility, suggested by MCNEAL (1990), is that the mingling of the tissue of the transitional zone with a "foreign" sphincteric stroma derived from the bladder neck may render this region more susceptible to disturbances of stromal–epithelial interactions.

2.4 Mesenchymal–Epithelial Interactions and the Embryonic Development of the Prostate

Organogenesis is critically dependent on inductive interactions between tissues. These interactions are usually reciprocal, they display at least some degree of specificity, and they are often limited to a particular sensitive period (GROBSTEIN 1976). Some of the most commonly observed interactions are those between mesenchymal and epithelial cells. A typical and distinguishing feature of the developing urogenital tract is that these mesenchymal–epithelial interactions are controlled by androgens.

In the human fetus prostatic development begins around the 10th week of gestation. At this time small epithelial buds start invading the large mass of mesenchyme which surrounds the endodermal urogenital sinus. During the initial stages of development the amount of mesenchyme vastly exceeds the prostatic epithelium. As a result of ductal morphogenesis, branching, and growth, first during the prenatal period and later also during puberty, the mesenchyme becomes progressively filled by invading epithelial ducts and ultimately the mesenchymal–epithelial ratio approximates 1:1.

It has been shown convincingly that reciprocal interactions between mesenchymal and epithelial cells are critically important for both the morphogenesis and the secretory cytodifferentiation of the prostate (CUNHA et al. 1987). Moreover, the changing ratio of stromal versus epithelial tissue may be the ultimate determinant of prostatic size. In a series of experiments in which homotypic recombinants containing variable amounts of mouse urogenital epithelium (UGE) and urogenital mesenchyme (UGM) were grown in intact male hosts, CHUNG and CUNHA (1983) clearly demonstrated that the final prostatic tissue mass obtained increases in proportion to the amount of UGM utilized. In a similar experimental set up it could be shown that adult prostatic epithelium maintains its ability to respond with increased growth when recombined with fetal UGM (NORMAN et al. 1986). Along the same lines, implantation of intact fetal urogenital sinus(es) in the ventral prostate of adult athymic mice results in a 10- to 20-fold overgrowth of the chimeric lobe of the ventral prostate, depending on the number of sinuses implanted (CHUNG et al. 1984). These data suggest that the growth arrest in the normal adult prostate may be related to a lack of inductive influences from the normal adult stroma. In addition they support the hypothesis that the development of BPH might be related to a reawakening of the embryonic inductive potential of the prostatic stroma.

It has been known for a long time that normal male development of the wolffian ducts and of the urogenital sinus depends on androgens secreted during fetal life (JOST 1965). More recent data show that, in the developing prostate, as in many other developing androgen target tissues, the mesenchyme is the actual target of androgen action and that this mesenchyme functions as an obligatory mediator of the effects of androgens upon the epithelium (CUNHA et al. 1983, 1987). In fact, LASNITZKI and MIZUNO (1979) demonstrated that, in organ culture, urogenital sinus mesenchyme is essential for the initiation of the fetal rat prostate and that this mesenchyme may mediate or complement the effects of androgens on the epithelium. This concept gained further support from chimeric tissue recombination experiments using epithelium and mesenchyme derived from the urogenital tract of wild-type and testicular feminized (Tfm) mice (CUNHA and LUNG 1978; CUNHA et al. 1987). Tfm mice are androgen insensitive due to a frameshift mutation in their androgen receptor (CHAREST et al. 1991). When UGE and UGM from wild-type and Tfm mice are recombined and implanted in intact male hosts, it appears that prostatic morphogenesis and epithelial cytodifferentiation occur only in the presence of a mesenchyme capable of androgen response (wild-type) whereas androgen responsiveness of the epithelium itself is not required (CUNHA and LUNG 1978; CUNHA et al. 1987). Full development of the secretory potential of the epithelium, however, may depend on the presence of androgen receptors in the epithelium (CUNHA and YOUNG 1991).

In accordance with these observations, autoradiographic studies on the localization of androgen-binding sites suggest that prenatally nuclear labeling in the developing urogenital sinus is restricted to the mesenchyme (SHANNON and CUNHA 1983; TAKEDA et al. 1985; COOKE et al. 1991). Postnatally nuclear labeling in the prostatic epithelium increases progressively from approximately day 10, and concordantly mesenchymal labeling decreases (TAKEDA et al. 1985; COOKE et al. 1991). Recent immunohistochemical studies and in situ hybridization analysis suggest that, despite the absence of ligand binding observed by autoradiographic analysis, fetal epithelium may express the same amount of receptor protein and mRNA as fetal mesenchyme. This would imply that for some unknown reason the androgen receptor in fetal epithelium may not be able to bind androgens until postnatally (TAKEDA and CHANG 1991). The factors which govern the appearance of functional epithelial androgen receptors postnatally in the prostate remain to be defined. Postnatal androgen action seems not to be required (HUSMANN et al. 1991). It is conceivable that, once more, mediators produced by the mesenchyme are involved. The nature of these putative mediators, however, remains unknown.

2.5 Growth Factors with Known Biochemical Identity and Stromal–Epithelial Interactions in the Prostate

The notion that local control systems such as mesenchymal (or stromal)–epithelial interactions may be instrumental for normal prostatic development and function and that disregulation of these interactions may play a role in the pathogenesis of nonmalignant diseases such as BPH and conceivably even in the development of malignant diseases such as prostatic carcinoma has elicited numerous studies on the mechanisms controlling cell–cell interactions in the prostate and on the mechanisms by which androgens may modulate such interactions. It may be worthwhile mentioning that disordered stromal–epithelial interactions are attracting more and more interest not only in the context of prostatic disease but also in the context of breast pathology (see, e.g., KANAZAWA and HOSICK 1992).

Stromal and epithelial cells can interact in at least two different ways. Very often these cells cooperate in the deposition of a specific extracellular matrix which in turn may influence the function of the depositing cells. Alternatively, stromal and epithelial cells may communicate by diffusible mediators that act in a paracrine fashion. Little is known on specific matrix formation in the human prostate; by contrast, in recent years remarkable efforts have been made to clarify the role of growth factors in the control of prostatic growth and function (for review: DAVIES and EATON 1991; SERIO and FIORELLI 1991; STORY 1991). The present discussion will be limited to those growth factors which may play a role in stromal–epithelial interactions or which may act as mediators of androgen action.

The prostate is a rich source of growth factors. These growth factors comprise members of at least six different families: the heparin-binding growth factor (HBGF) family with basic fibroblast growth factor (bFGF; STORY et al. 1987), the epidermal growth factor family (EGF; JACOBS et al. 1988 KISHI et al. 1988), the transforming growth factor-β family (TGF-β; MORI et al. 1990), the insulin-like growth factors (IGF; COHEN et al. 1991; FIORELLI et al. 1991a), platelet-derived growth factor (PDGF; SITARAS et al. 1988), and nerve growth factor (NGF; HARPER et al. 1979; DJAKIEW et al. 1991).

Both the human prostate (STORY 1991) and the rat prostate (JACOBS et al. 1988) contain a high concentration of bFGF. Moreover, the concentration of immunoreactive bFGF (STORY 1991) and the concentration of the corresponding mRNA (MORI et al. 1990) are significantly increased in BPH. The available data suggest that the stroma is the main source of bFGF although some bFGF may also be produced by the epithelium. Cultured human prostate fibroblasts produce a factor with the characteristics of bFGF which stimulates their own proliferation (STORY et al. 1989). Immunohistochemical staining also localizes bFGF in the stromal compartment. There are indications, however, that bFGF may stimulate not only stromal cell proliferation (STORY et al. 1989; LEVINE et al. 1992) but also proliferation of normal (MCKEEHAN and ADAMS 1988) or transformed (GLEAVE et al. 1991) prostatic epithelial cells. Recent data indicate that an androgen-induced FGF-like protein acting in an autocrine fashion may be responsible for the androgen-dependent growth of the mouse mammary epithelial carcinoma cell-line SC-3 (TANAKA et al. 1992). The production of bFGF by prostate fibroblasts seems not to be affected by androgens but it may be decreased by TGF-β (STORY et al. 1990). Another member of the HBGF family, namely keratinocyte growth factor (KGF or FGF-7), has recently been shown to be produced by rat stromal cells under the influence of androgens and to be mitogenic for prostatic epithelial cells (YAN et al. 1992). The role of this peptide in the human prostate remains to be defined.

Growth-stimulating peptides related to EGF have been detected in rodent (HARPER et al. 1979; JACOBS et al. 1988) and human prostate (ELSON et al. 1984). Moreover, of all body fluids, prostatic fluid is one of the richest sources of EGF (for review: HABIB 1990). The relative contribution of stroma and epithelium to the production of EGF-related factors remains unknown. Significantly higher levels of EGF have been reported in BPH than in prostatic cancer (HABIB 1990; SHAIKH et al. 1990). EGF-specific receptors have also been demonstrated in the human prostate and in BPH (MADDY et al. 1987; DAVIES and EATON 1989; FIORELLI et al. 1989; LUBRANO et al. 1989). These receptors seem to be located mainly in the basal layer of the epithelium. In the rodent as well as in the human prostate (FIORELLI et al. 1989; LUBRANO et al. 1989) androgens may negatively affect EGF receptor expression. In the androgen-dependent prostatic carcinoma cell line LNCaP, however, androgens stimulate EGF binding (SCHUURMANS et al. 1988). Cell culture experiments suggest that EGF may be required for the proliferation of both prostatic fibroblasts (LEVINE et al. 1992) and prostatic epithelium (PEEHL and STAMEY 1986).

Members of the extremely complex TGF-β family undoubtedly also play an important role in the control of prostate growth. TGF-β transcripts have been demonstrated in human (MORI et al. 1990) and rat (KYPRIANOU and ISAACS 1989) prostate. Moreover, several human prostate tumor cell lines such as DU-145 and PC-3 secrete TGF-β and display high-affinity binding sites for this growth factor (WILDING et al. 1989; WILDING 1991). In patients with BPH the level of TGF-β2 transcripts is significantly increased as compared to the normal prostate whereas the level of TGF-β1 transcripts remains unaffected (MORI et al. 1990). The contribution of epithelial and stromal cells to the prostatic production of TGF-βs remains to be explored. TGF-βs have a wide spectrum of activities. In general they promote the growth of fibroblasts and inhibit the growth of epithelial cells. In addition, however, they are important regulators of the synthesis of extracellular matrix components. TGF-β1 inhibits proliferation and activates death of the glandular cells of the rat ventral prostate (MARTIKAINEN et al. 1990). Similarly, primary cultures of epithelial cells derived from normal, hyperplastic, and cancerous human prostates are very sensitive to the inhibitory effects of TGF-β whereas considerably higher concentrations of TGF-β are required to inhibit established tumor cell lines such as PC-3 and DU-145 (WILDING 1991). TGF-β may well be a physiologic intermediate in the activation of castration-induced cell death in the rat ventral prostate. In fact, castration increases both the level of TGF-β mRNA and TGF-β receptor binding (KYPRIANOU and ISAACS 1988, 1989). A similar increase in TGF-β transcripts is observed after androgen ablation in xenografts of the human prostatic adenocarcinoma PC-82 (KYPRIANOU et al. 1990).

As already mentioned, the prostate is a rich source of NGF (HARPER et al. 1979). During recent years there has been renewed interest in the role of this growth factor as a mediator of paracrine interactions in the prostate. NGF-like substances with a high M_r (61 000 and 42 000) were identified by bioassay experiments in conditioned media from neoplastic epithelial cell lines and from stromal cell cultures of the human prostate (DJAKIEW et al. 1991; DJAKIEW 1992). These conditioned media mediate paracrine interactive growth of both cell types and their effects are markedly reduced by immunoneutralization with an antibody against NGF. Immunocytochemical studies localize the NGF-like protein predominantly in the stromal compartment of normal prostatic tissue, BPH, and adenocarcinoma. Conversely, the NGF receptor localizes predominantly in the epithelial cells of these tissues (GRAHAM et al. 1992). Interestingly, expression of the receptor seems to decrease in BPH and in adenocarcinoma and to disappear in metastatic tumor lines, suggesting an inverse association of NGF receptor expression with neoplastic progression (PFLUG et al. 1992). The effects of androgens on NGF production and NGF receptor concentration in the human prostate remain to be explored. It may be mentioned that in rat Sertoli cells expression of NGF receptor mRNA is downregulated by testosterone (PERSSON et al. 1990).

Relatively little is known on insulin-related growth factors and prostatic growth. Both epithelial and mesenchymal cell proliferation seem to be supported preferentially by IGF-I (COHEN et al. 1991; MCKEEHAN 1991). Androgen treatment of castrated rats results in elevated levels of IGF-I expression and this effect is mainly observed in the mesenchymal cells (MCKEEHAN 1991). The effects of IGF-I are apparently mediated by type 1 receptors (COHEN et al. 1991; FIORELLI et al. 1991a). Under basal conditions these receptors are mainly located in the basal layer of the glandular epithelium. After testicular suppression with gonadotropin-releasing hormone analogues, the number of type 1 receptors increases and positive staining also becomes apparent in the secretory cells (FIORELLI et al. 1991a). Both in the normal prostate and in patients with BPH the action of IGF-I may be modulated by specific IGF-I binding proteins. Two of these binding proteins are secreted by the epithelial cells: IGFBP-2 and IGFBP-4 (COHEN et al. 1991; FIORELLI et al. 1991b). Both of these proteins are also found in seminal plasma. Prostate fibroblasts seem to be able to secrete IGFBP-3. The effect of these binding proteins on IGF-I action in the prostate as well as the factors governing their secretion remain to be determined (COHEN et al. 1991). Interestingly, recent data suggest that prostate-specific antigen (PSA) may act as an IGFBP-3 protease and may modulate IGF action in the reproductive system by altering the interaction of IGF with this binding protein (COHEN et al. 1992).

It may be concluded that many growth factors are produced in the prostate and that they undoubtedly represent important elements in the control of prostatic growth and function. Moreover, there obviously are complex interactions between androgens and this local regulatory system. Finally, disturbances in prostatic development are accompanied by disturbances in the production or activity of several growth factors. Our present knowledge is too fragmentary, however, to permit a coherent picture of the changes that may play a role in the pathogenesis of BPH. Furthermore, the present overview has been limited to the main known growth factors and there are several indications that other, still unidentified, local regulatory molecules may be involved.

2.6 Growth Factors with Unknown Biochemical Identity and Mesenchymal–Epithelial Interactions

It is evident that apart from the biochemically identified growth factors described above, other still unidentified factors may play a role in mesenchymal–epithelial interactions in the prostate. In vitro studies indicate that prostate fibroblasts produce both factors which stimulate (Kabalin et al. 1989) and factors which inhibit (König et al. 1987) the growth of epithelial cells and these factors are not related to known growth factors. Similar conclusions may be derived from in vivo experiments. Human bone fibroblasts, embryonic rat urogenital sinus mesenchyme, and rat prostate fibroblasts coïnoculated with human LNCaP cells (epithelial prostate tumor cells) promote carcinoma formation in athymic mice. The effect is most marked in male hosts and is not observed with 3T3 cells. bFGF may play a role, but again, it is apparently not the only factor involved.

During recent years, considerable interest in androgen-regulated mediators of mesenchymal–epithelial interactions has been generated by studies on another androgen target tissue, namely the testis. The testis is a typical target tissue in which the major part of the effects of androgens may be indirect. In fact, although androgens are the main factors responsible for the maintenance of spermatogenesis, germ cells apparently do not contain classical androgen receptors (Sanborn et al. 1975; Grootegoed et al. 1977). Accordingly, it is generally assumed that germ cell development is controlled indirectly by androgen action on Sertoli cells. Studies on isolated and cultured testicular cells, however, have revealed that the effects of androgens on isolated Sertoli cells are disappointingly small (Louis and Fritz 1977; Swinnen et al. 1990) and that a number of interstitial cells such as peritubular myoid cells contain concentrations of androgen receptor that are at least equal to those observed in Sertoli cells (Verhoeven 1980; Isomaa et al. 1985; Verhoeven and Cailleau 1988). Moreover, if Sertoli cells are cocultured with peritubular cells, a number of androgen effects on Sertoli cells [e.g., secretion of androgen-binding protein (ABP), secretion of transferrin, secretion of inhibin, inhibition of aromatase activity] are enhanced (TUNG and FRITZ 1980; HUTSON and STOCCO 1981; HOLMES et al. 1984; SKINNER and FRITZ 1985a; VERHOEVEN and CAILLEAU 1988). Interestingly, this type of mesenchymal (peritubular)–epithelial (Sertoli) interaction seems to be mediated at least in part by one or more paracrine mediators produced by the peritubular cells (SKINNER and FRITZ 1985b; VERHOEVEN and CAILLEAU 1988; NORTON and SKINNER 1989; SWINNEN et al. 1990). These putative mediators are conveniently referred to as P-Mod-S (peritubular factors which modulate Sertoli cell function) and two potentially related P-Mod-S factors have been purified from peritubular cell-conditioned medium (SKINNER et al. 1988). These factors seem not to be related to known growth factors but amino-acid or nucleotide sequences are not yet available. Moreover, many questions remain as to their exact origin, control, role, and mechanism of action.

Using cultured Sertoli cells as a bioassay system we have addressed the question of whether these P-Mod-S factors are testis-specific or whether they might be more universal mediators of androgen action in other target tissues such as the prostate. To this end we have compared the characteristics of cultured testicular peritubular cells and prostatic stromal cells and the characteristics of the respective conditioned media (SWINNEN et al. 1990, 1991; VERHOEVEN et al. 1992). Striking morphologic and functional similarities are observed between both types of cells. After 6-9 days of culture both cell populations react virtually 100% positive upon immunostaining for α-smooth muscle isoactin. Immunostaining of the original tissues locates the reactive cells in the peritubular region in the testis, in a slightly broader periacinar region in the prostate, and in the vessel walls. Furthermore, when cocultured with Sertoli cells both cell types induce the formation of tubular structures and "balls" and both cell types stimulate the production of an extracellular matrix that enhances Sertoli cell transferrin secretion. Finally and most importantly, both peritubular cells and stromal cells secrete into the medium one or more mediators that are androgen responsive and that have the same effects on Sertoli cells as those described for P-Mod-S. Secretion of ABP, transferrin, inhibin, and cGMP are increased and follicle-stimulating hormone (FSH)-induced aromatase activity is inhibited (Fig. 2.1). Characterization and purification of these factors has proven difficult but the available data suggest a large number of similarities with the factors described by SKINNER et al. (1988). The molecular weight of the mediators studied in our laboratory, however, may be slightly lower. None of the studied growth factors (IGF-I, EGF, bFGF, TGF-β, activin, NGF) mimics the effects of these mesenchymal mediators in the Sertoli cell system (HOEBEN and VERHOEVEN, unpublished results). Interestingly, up to now we have not observed any physicochemical difference between the putative mediators produced by prostatic stromal cells and those produced by testicular peritubular cells, suggesting that these factors might act as more universal mediators of androgen action. Apart from the fact that they may be more universal mediators of androgen action, P-Mod-S-like agonists display a number of other interesting features. In contrast with most of the other known and unknown growth factors

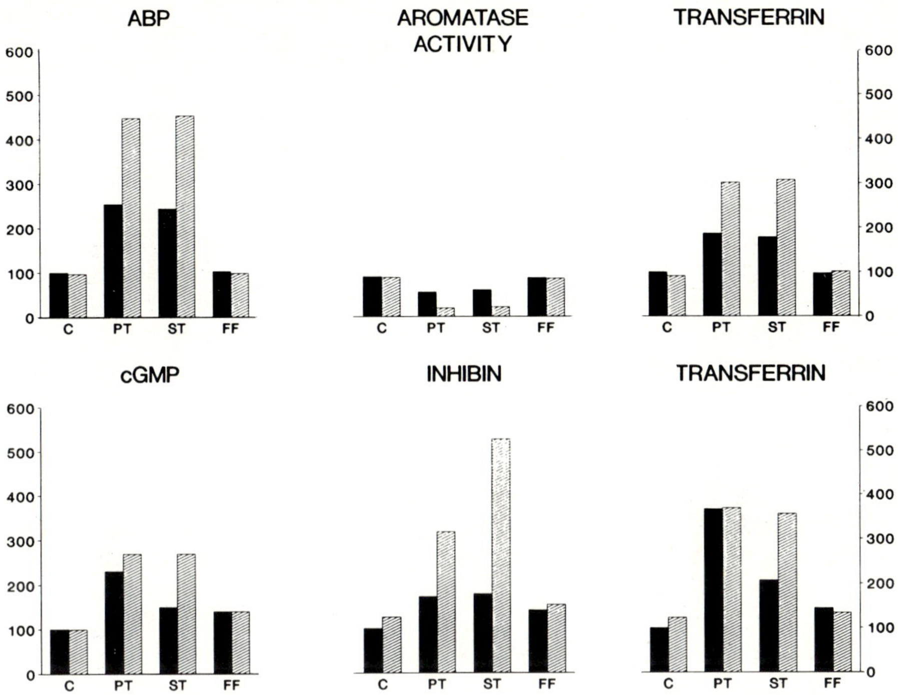

Fig 2.1. Influence of peritubular and stromal cell conditioned medium on various parameters of Sertoli cell function. Spent media were collected from peritubular cells (*PT*), stromal cells (*ST*), and footsole fibroblasts (*FF*) treated (*hatched bars*) or not (*black bars*) with 10^{-7} *M* testosterone. The media were extensively dialyzed and their influence on various parameters of Sertoli cell function was compared with control medium (*C*). In the *upper panel*, 2×10^6 Sertoli cells were seeded in 2 ml dialyzed spent medium in six-well multidishes. In the *lower panel*, 2×10^5 Sertoli cells were resuspended in 1 ml dialyzed spent medium and seeded in 24-well multidishes. ABP, transferrin, inhibin, and cGMP were measured in the media collected from day 4 to day 7. On day 7 aromatase activity was measured by incubating the Sertoli cell monolayers for 24 h in the presence of FSH (100 ng/ml), testosterone (0.5 μ*M*), MIX (0.1 m*M*). Values are expressed as a percentage of the activity observed with control medium. (From VERHOEVEN et al. 1992)

discussed, they affect differentiated functions rather than proliferation, suggesting that they may be instrumental for androgen action not only during development but also during adult function. Moreover, they are produced by cells with characteristics of smooth muscle cells and, as outlined in the preceding paragraphs, such cells have been related to the pathogenesis of BPH. Accordingly, the question of whether P-Mod-S-like factors affect human prostatic epithelium and whether such factors are produced in the human prostate certainly deserves further investigation.

2.7 Conclusion

It is obvious that the growth and function of the prostate depend not only on circulating androgens and other endocrine factors, but also on a local and complex network of intercellular communications. This network comprises autocrine and paracrine interactions within and between the stromal and the epithelial compartments. Only some of the growth factors involved have been fully characterized. Some of these growth factors and/or their receptors are controlled by androgens. The available evidence suggests that both the endocrine system and the local control system play a role in the pathogenesis of BPH. The relative contributions of these control systems, however, as well as the exact pathogenetic mechanisms involved, remain far from understood. The interpretation of many studies on the pathogenesis of BPH is hampered by two important features inherent to the disease itself:

1. In its initial stages BPH is a focal disease limited to a small and defined region of the prostate. Most of our biochemical knowledge on the mechanisms responsible for the control of prostatic growth (androgen metabolism, receptor concentration, growth factor production), however, does not differentiate between this region and the remainder of the prostate.
2. BPH is an extremely slow disease. This implies not only that a minor imbalance in growth control mechanisms may cause the disease, but also that changes noted during later stages may be related to secondary phenomena such as changes in the cellular composition of the diseased prostate. In addition, it is quite possible that the factors involved in the initiation of BPH are not the same as those responsible for its progression.

Within the context of what we know at the present time about growth control in the prostate, several pathogenetic mechanisms should be considered (Fig. 2.2). One possibility is that the initial lesion results from an imbalance in the secretion of one or more growth regulators, the secretion of which is not affected by androgens. In this case androgens could still act as permissive factors allowing survival and growth of the disregulated cell population. Alternatively androgens or disturbed androgen action could play a more active role in the pathogenesis of BPH. Increased androgen sensitivity (e.g., as a result of increased production of active metabolites or increased receptor activity) could directly stimulate the proliferation of stromal and or epithelial cells or could do so by androgen-stimulated production of autocrine or paracrine growth factors. Similarly, a loss of androgen sensitivity could result in an uncontrolled production or activity of local regulatory molecules normally suppressed by androgens. The hypothesis that BPH may be due to a reawakening of the embryonic androgen-dependent inductive potential of prostatic stroma certainly is a very attractive one which might account for the focal nature of the initial lesions. As long as we do not understand the exact nature of these embryonic

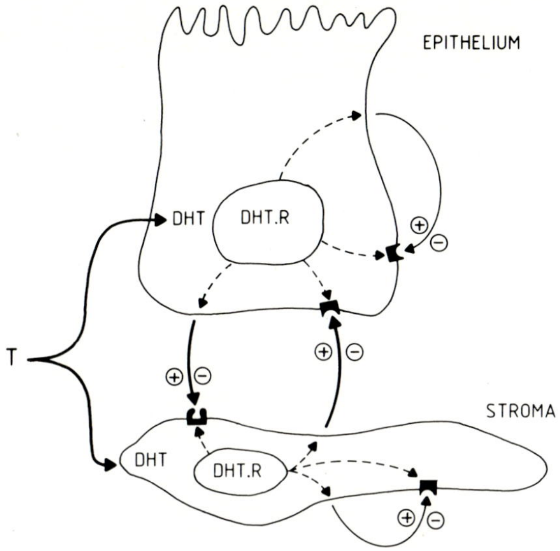

Fig 2.2. Androgens, growth factors, and the control of prostatic growth and function. Proliferation and function of prostatic epithelium and stroma are controlled by androgens and by autocrine and paracrine growth factors. Bilateral interactions between stroma and epithelium are essential both for normal development and for adult function. Androgens may affect stromal cells, epithelial cells, and the interaction between both cell types either by acting directly on stromal and/or epithelial cells or by controlling the production of autocrine or paracrine growth factors and their respective receptors (*broken arrows*). Disordered growth may result either from a primary disregulation in growth factor secretion and activity or from a primary disregulation in androgen action. *T*, testosterone; *DHT*, dihydrotestosterone; *R*, androgen receptor

mediators of androgen action, however, as well as the mechanisms responsible for their inappropriate secretion, every alternative explanation remains to be considered.

Acknowledgements. This research was supported in part by a grant from the National Fund for Scientific Investigation (NFWO) and by a grant from the Vereniging voor Kankerbestrijding.

References

Bartsch W, Krieg M, Becker H, Mohrmann J, Voigt KD (1982) Endogenous androgen levels in epithelium and stroma of human benign prostatic hyperplasia and normal prostate. Acta Endocrinol (Copenh) 100:634–640

Bashirelahi N, O'Toole JH, Young JD (1976) A specific 17β-estradiol receptor in human benign hypertrophic prostate. Biochem Med 15:254–261

Bolton NJ, Lahtonen R, Hammond GL, Vihko R (1981) Distribution and concentrations of androgens in epithelial and stromal compartments of the human benign hypertrophic prostate. J Endocrinol 90:125–131

Brinkman AO, Jenster G, Kuiper GGJM, Ris-Stalpers C, van Laar JM, Faber PW, Trapman J (1992) Structure and function of the human androgen receptor. In: Nieschlag E, Habenicht U-F (eds) Spermatogenesis, fertilization, contraception. Schering Foundation Workshop 4. Springer, Berlin Heidelberg New York

Bruchovsky N, Rennie PS, Batzold FH, Goldenberg SL, Fletcher T, McLoughlin MG (1988) Kinetic parameters of 5α-reductase activity in epithelium and stroma of normal, hyperplastic and carcinomatous human prostates. J Clin Endocrinol Metab 67:806–816

Charest N, Zhou Z, Lubahn DB, Olsen KL, Wilson EM, French FS (1991) A frameshift mutation destabilizes androgen receptor messenger RNA in the Tfm mouse. Mol Endocrinol 5:573–581

Chung LWK, Cunha GR (1983) Stromal-epithelial interactions. II. Regulation of prostatic growth by embryonic urogenital sinus mesenchyme. Prostate 4:503–511

Chung LWK, Matsuura J, Rocco AK, Thompson TC, Miller GJ, Runner MN (1984) Tissue interactions and prostatic growth: a new mouse model for prostatic hyperplasia. Ann NY Acad Sci 438:394–404

Cohen P, Peehl DM, Lamson G, Rosenfeld RG (1991) Insulin-like growth factors (IGFs), IGF receptors, and IGF-binding proteins in primary cultures of prostate epithelial cells. J Clin Endocrinol Metab 73:401–407

Cohen P, Graves HCB, Peehl DM, Kamarei M, Giudice LC, Rosenfeld RG (1992) Prostate-specific antigen (PSA) in an insulin-like growth factor binding protein-3 protease found in seminal plasma. J Clin Endocrinol Metab 75:1046–1053

Cooke PS, Young P, Cunha GR (1991) Androgen receptor expression in developing male reproductive organs. Endocrinology 128:2867–2873

Cunha GR, Lung B (1978) The possible influences of temporal factors in androgenic responsiveness of urogenital tissue recombinants from wild-type and androgen-insensitive (Tfm) mice. J Exp Zool 205:181–194

Cunha GR, Young P (1991) Inability of Tfm (testicular feminization) epithelial cells to express androgen-dependent seminal vesicle secretory proteins in chimeric tissue recombinants. Endocrinology 128:3293–3298

Cunha GR, Chung LWK, Shannon JM, Taguchi O, Fuji H (1983) Hormone-induced morphogenesis and growth: role of mesenchymal-epithelial interactions. Recent Prog Horm Res 39:559–598

Cunha GR, Donjacour AA, Cooke PS, Mee S, Bigsby RM, Higgins SJ, Sugimura Y (1987) The endocrinology and developmental biology of the prostate. Endocr Rev 8:338–362

Davies P, Eaton CL (1989) Binding of epidermal growth factor by human normal, hypertrophic and carcinomatous prostate. Prostate 14:123–132

Davies P, Eaton CL (1991) Regulation of prostate growth. J Endocrinol 131:5–17

Djakiew D (1992) Role of nerve growth factor-like protein in the paracrine regulation of prostate growth. J Androl 13:476–487

Djakiew D, Delsite R, Pflug B, Wrathall J, Lynch JH, Onoda M (1991) Regulation of growth by a nerve growth factor-like protein which modulates paracrine interactions between a neoplastic epithelial cell line and stromal cells of the human prostate. Cancer Res 51:3304–3310

Ekman P, Barrack ER, Greene GL, Jensen EV, Walsh PC (1983) Estrogen receptors in human prostate: evidence for multiple binding sites. J Clin Endocrinol Metab 57:166–176

Elson SD, Browne CA, Thorburn GD (1984) Identification of epidermal growth factor-like activity in human male reproductive tissues and fluids. J Clin Endocrinol Metab 58:589–594

Farnsworth WE (1973) Human prostatic dehydroepiandrosterone sulfate sulfatase. Steroids 21:647–664

Farnsworth WE, Brown JR (1963) Metabolism of testosterone by the human prostate. JAMA 183:140–143

Fiorelli G, De Bellis A, Longe A, Natali A, Constantini A, Serio M (1989) Epidermal growth factor receptors in human hyperplastic prostate and their modulation by chronic treatment with a gonadotropin-releasing hormone analog. J Clin Endocrinol Metab 68:740–743

Fiorelli G, De Bellis A, Longo A, et al. (1991a) Insulin-like growth factor-I receptors in human hyperplastic prostate tissue: characterization, tissue localization, and their modulation by chronic treatment with a gonadotropin-releasing hormone analog. J Clin Endocrinol Metab 72:740–746

Fiorelli G, De Bellis A, Longo A, et al. (1991b) Growth factors in the human prostate. J Steroid Biochem Mol Endocrinol 40:199–205

Franks LM, Riddle PN, Carbonell AW, Gey GO (1970) A comparative study of the ultrastructure and lack of growth capacity of adult human prostate epithelium mechanically separated from its stroma. J Pathol 100:113–119

Ghanadian R, Chisholm GD, Fotherby K (1976) Intracellular localization of 5α-dihydrotestosterone in human benign prostatic hyperplasia. Clin Chim Acta 73:521–526

Gleave M, Hsieh J-T, Gao C, von Eschenbach AC, Chung LWK (1991) Acceleration of human prostate cancer growth in vivo by factors produced by prostate and bone fibroblasts. Cancer Res 51:3753–3761

Gloyna RE, Siiteri PK, Wilson JD (1970) Dihydrotestosterone in prostatic hypertrophy. II. The formation and content of dihydrotestosterone in the hypertrophic canine prostate and the effect of dihydrotestosterone on prostatic growth in the dog. J Clin Invest 49:1746–1753

Gormley G, MK-906 Study Group (1991) One-year experience in the treatment of benign prostatic hyperplasia with finasteride. J Androl 12:372–375

Graham CW, Lynch JH, Djakiew D (1992) Distribution of nerve growth factor-like protein and nerve growth factor receptor in human benign prostatic hyperplasia and prostatic adenocarcinoma. J Urol 147:1444–1447

Grobstein C (1967) Mechanisms of organogenetic tissue interaction. Natl Cancer Inst Monogr 26:279–299

Grootegoed JA, Peters MJ, Mulder E, Rommerts FFG, Van Der Molen HJ (1977) Absence of a nuclear androgen receptor in isolated germinal cells of rat testis. Mol Cell Endocrinol 9:159–167

Habenicht UF, El Etreby MF (1991) Rationale for using aromatase inhibitors to manage benign prostatic hyperplasia. J Androl 12:395–402

Habib FK (1990) Peptide growth factors: a new frontier in prostate cancer. In: EORTC Genitourinary Group Monograph 7: prostate cancer and testicular cancer. Wiley-Liss, New York, pp 107–115

Hammond GL (1978) Endogenous steroid levels in the human prostate from birth to old age. A comparison of normal and diseased tissues. J Endocrinol 78:7–19

Harper GP, Barde YA, Burnstock YA, Carstairs JR, Dennison ME, Suda K, Vernon CA (1979) Guinea pig prostate is a rich source of nerve growth factor. Nature 279:160–162

Harper ME, Pike A, Peeling WB, Griffiths K (1974) Steroids of adrenal origin metabolized by human prostatic tissue both in vivo and in vitro. J Endocrinol 60:117–125

Holmes SD, Lipshultz LI, Smith RG (1984) Regulation of transferrin secretion by human Sertoli cells cultured in the presence or absence of human peritubular cells. J Clin Endocrinol Metab 59:1058–1062

Husmann DA, Wilson CM, McPhaul MJ, Tilley WD, Wilson JD (1990) Antipeptide antibodies to two distinct regions of the androgen receptor localize the receptor protein to the nuclei of target cells in the rat and human prostate. Endocrinology 126:2359–2368

Husmann DA, McPhaul MJ, Wilson JD (1991) Androgen receptor expression in the developing rat prostate is not altered by castration, flutamide or suppression of the adrenal axis. Endocrinology 128:1902–1906

Hutson JC, Stocco DM (1981) Peritubular cell influence on the efficiency of androgen-binding protein secretion by Sertoli cells in culture. Endocrinology 108:1362–1368

Imperato-McGinley J, Guerrero L, Gauti (1974) reductase deficiency in man: an inherited form of male pseudohermaphroditism. Science 186:1213–1215

Isomaa V, Parvinen M, Jänne OA, Bardin CW (1985) Nuclear androgen receptors in different stages of the seminiferous epithelial cycle and the interstitial tissue of rat testis. Endocrinology 116:132–137

Jacobs SC, Story MT, Sasse J, Lawson RK (1988) Characterization of growth factors derived from the rat ventral prostate. J Urol 139:1106–1110

Jost A (1965) Gonadal hormones in the sex differentiation of the mammalian fetus. In: Haan RL, Ursprung H (eds) Organogenesis. Holt, Rinehart and Wilson, New York, pp 611–628

Kabalin JN, Peehl DM, Stamey TA (1989) Clonal growth of human prostatic epithelial cells is stimulated by fibroblasts. Prostate 14:251–263

Kanazawa T, Hosick HL (1992) Transformed growth phenotype of mouse mammary epithelium in primary culture induced by specific fetal mesenchymes. J Cell Physiol 153:381–391

Kishi H, Ishibe T, Usui T, Miyachi Y (1988) Epidermal growth factor (EGF) in seminal plasma and prostatic gland: a radioreceptor assay. Arch Androl 20:243–249

König JJ, Romijn JC, Schröder FH (1987) Prostatic epithelium inhibiting factor (PETF): organ specificity and production by prostatic fibroblasts. Urol Res 15:145–149

Krieg M (1984) Biochemical endocrinology of human prostatic tumors. Prog Cancer Res Ther 31:425–440

Krieg M, Tunn S (1990) Androgens and human benign prostatic hyperplasia. In: Nieschlag E, Behre HM (eds) Testosterone. Action, deficiency, substitution. Springer, Berlin Heidelberg New York, pp 219–244

Krieg M, Klötzl G, Kaufmann J, Voigt KD (1981) Stroma of human benign prostatic hyperoplasia: preferential tissue for androgen metabolism and oestrogen binding. Acta Endocrinol (Copenh) 96:422–432

Kyprianou N, Isaacs JT (1988) Identification of a cellular receptor for transforming growth factor beta in rat ventral prostate and its negative regulation by androgens. Endocrinology 123:2124–2131

Kyprianou N, Isaacs JT (1989) Expression of transforming growth factor beta in the rat ventral prostate during castration-induced programmed cell death. Mol Endocrinol 3:1515–1522

Kyprianou N, English HF, Isaacs JT (1990) Programmed cell death during regression of PC-82 human prostate cancer following androgen ablation. Cancer Res 50:3748–3753

Lahtonen R, Bolton NJ, Konturri M, Vihko R (1983) Nuclear androgen receptors in the epithelium and stroma of human benign prostatic hypertrophic glands. Prostate 4:129–139

Lasnitzki I, Mizuno T (1979) Role of the mesenchyme in the induction of the rat prostate gland by androgens in organ culture. J Endocrinol 82:171–178

Levine AC, Ren M, Huber GK, Kirschenbaum A (1992) The effect of androgen, estrogen and growth factors on the proliferation of cultured fibroblasts derived from human fetal and adult prostates. Endocrinology 130:2413–2419

Liao S, Liang T, Fang S, Castaneda E, Shao TC (1973) Steroid structure and androgenic activity. J Biol Chem 248:6154–6162

Louis BG, Fritz IB (1977) Stimulation by androgens of the production of androgen binding protein by cultured Sertoli cells. Mol Cell Endocrinol 7:9–16

Lubrano C, Petrangli E, Catizone A, et al. (1989) Epidermal growth factor binding and steroid receptor content in human benign prostatic hyperplasia. J Steroid Biochem 34:499–504

Maddy SQ, Chisholm GD, Hawkins RA, Habib FK (1987) Localization of epidermal growth factor receptors in the human prostate by biochemical and immunocytochemical methods. J Endocrinol 113:147–153

Martikainen P, Kyprianou N, Isaacs JT (1990) Effect of transforming growth factor-β1 on proliferation and death of rat prostatic cells. Endocrinology 127:2963–2968

McKeehan WL (1991) Growth factor receptors and prostate cell growth. In: Isaacs JT (ed) Prostate cancer. Cell and molecular mechanisms in diagnosis and treatment. Cancer surveys, Cold Spring Harbor Laboratory Press, pp 165–175

McKeehan WL, Adams PS (1988) Heparin-binding growth factor/prostatropin attenuates inhibition of rat prostate tumor epithelial cell growth by transforming growth factor type beta. In Vitro 24:243–246

McNeal JE (1978) Origin and evolution of benign prostatic enlargement. Invest Urol 15:340–345

McNeal JE (1990) Pathology of benign prostatic hyperplasia. Insight into etiology. Urol Clin North Am 17:477–486

Meikle AW, Collis ES, Middleton RG, Fang SM (1980) Supranormal nuclear content of 5α-dihydrotestosterone in benign hyperplastic prostates of humans. J Clin Endocrinol Metab 51:945–947

Moore RJ, Gazak JM, Wilson JD (1979) Regulation of cytoplasmic dihydrotestosterone binding in dog prostate by 17β-estradiol. J Clin Invest 63:351–357

Mori H, Maki H, Oishi K, Jaye M, Igarashi K, Yoshida O, Hatanaka M (1990) Increased expression of genes for basic fibroblast growth factor and transforming growth factor type β2 in human benign prostatic hyperplasia. Prostate 16:71–80

Nass R, Tunn S, Braun BE, Krieg M (1990) Age dependent steroid levels in epithelium and stroma of human benign prostatic hyperplasia. Acta Endocrinol (Copenh) 79:157

Norman JT, Cunha GR, Sugimura Y (1986) The induction of new ductal growth in adult prostatic epithelium in response to an embryonic inductor. Prostate 8:209–220

Norton JN, Skinner MK (1989) Regulation of Sertoli cell function and differentiation through the actions of a testicular paracrine factor P-Mod-S. Endocrinology 124:2711–2719

Oesterling JE (1991a) The origin and development of benign prostatic hyperplasia: an age-dependent process. J Androl 12:346–355

Oesterling JE (1991b) LHRH agonists. A nonsurgical treatment for benign prostatic hyperplasia. J Androl 12:381–388

Peehl DM, Stamey TA (1986) Serum-free growth of adult human prostatic epithelial cells. In Vitro 22:82–90

Persson H, Ayer-Lievre C, Sodez O, et al. (1990) Expression of beta nerve growth factor receptor mRNA in Sertoli cells downregulated by testosterone. Science 247:704–707

Pflug BR, Onoda M, Lynch JM, Djakiew D (1992) Reduced expression of the low affinity nerve growth factor receptor in benign and malignant human prostate tissue and loss of expression in four human metastatic prostate tumor cell lines. Cancer Res 52:5403–5406

Prins GS, Birch L, Greene GL (1991) Androgen receptor localization in different cell types of the adult rat prostate. Endocrinology 129:3187–3199

Robel P, Eychenne B, Blondeau JP, Picard-Groyer MT, Baulieu EE, Bruner-Lorand J, Hechter O (1984) Characteristics of separated epithelial and stromal subfractions of prostate. II. Human prostate. Prostate 5:255–268

Sanborn BM, Steinberger A, Meistrich HL, Steinberger E (1975) Androgen binding sites in testis cell fractions as measured by a nuclear exchange assay. J Steroid Biochem 6:1459–1465

Sar H, Lubahn DB, French FS, Wilson EM (1990) Immunohistochemical localization of the androgen receptor in rat and human tissues. Endocrinology 127:3180–3186

Schulze H, Claus S (1990) Histological localization of estrogen receptors in normal and diseased human prostates by immunocytochemistry. Prostate 16:331–343

Schuurmans ALG, Bolt J, Mulder E (1988) Androgens stimulate both growth rate and epidermal growth factor receptor activity of the human prostate tumor cell LNCaP. Prostate 12:55–63

Serio M, Fiorelli G (1991) Dual control by androgens and peptide growth factors of prostatic growth in human benign prostatic hyperplasia. Mol Cell Endocrinol 78:C77–C81

Shaikh N, Lai L, McLaughlin J, Clark D, Williams G (1990) Quantitative analysis of epidermal growth factor in human benign prostatic hyperplasia and prostatic carcinoma and its prognostic significance. Anticancer Res 10:873–874

Shannon JM, Cunha GR (1983) Autoradiographic localization of androgen binding in the developing mouse prostate. Prostate 4:367–373

Siiteri PK, MacDonald PC (1973) Role of extraglandular estrogen in human endocrinology. In: Greep RO, Astwood ED (eds) Ect 7: endocrinology, female reproductive system. American Physiol Soc, vol II, Washington DC, pp 491–508

Siiteri PK, Wilson JD (1970) Dihydrotestosterone in prostatic hypertrophy. I. The formation and content of dihydrotestosterone in the hypertrophic prostate of man. J Clin Invest 49:1737–1745

Sirett DAN, Corvan SK, Janecko AE, Grant JK, Glen ES (1980) Prostatic tissue distribution of 17β-hydroxy-5α-androstan-3-one and of androgen receptors in benign hyperplasia. J Steroid Biochem 13:723–728

Sitaras NM, Sariban E, Bravo M, Pantazin P, Antoniades HN (1988) Constitutive production of platelet-derived growth factor-like proteins by human prostatic carcinoma cell lines. Cancer Res 48:1930–1935

Skinner MK, Fritz IB (1985a) Androgen stimulation of Sertoli cell function is enhanced by peritubular cells. Mol Cell Endocrinol 40:115–122

Skinner MK, Fritz IB (1958b) Testicular peritubular cells secrete a protein under androgen control that modulates Sertoli cell functions. Proc Natl Acad Sci USA 82:114–118

Skinner MK, Fetterolf PM, Anthony CT (1988) Purification of a paracrine factor, P-Mod-S, produced by testicular peritubular cells that modulates Sertoli cell function. J Biol Chem 263:2884–2890

Stone NE, Clejan SJ (1991) Response of prostate volume, prostate-specific antigen, and testosterone to flutamide in men with benign prostatic hyperplasia. J Androl 12:376–380

Story MT (1991) Polypeptide modulators of prostatic growth and development. In: Isaacs JT (ed) Prostate cancer. Cell and molecular mechanisms in diagnosis and treatment. Cancer Surveys, Cold Spring Harbor Laboratory Press, pp 123–146

Story MT, Sasse J, Jacobs SC, Lawson RK (1987) Prostatic growth factor: purification and structural relationship to basic fibroblast growth factor. Biochemistry 26:3843–3849

Story MT, Livingston B, Baeten L, Swartz SJ, Jacobs SC, Begun FP, Lawson RK (1989) Cultured human prostate-derived fibroblasts produce a factor that stimulates their growth with properties indistinguishable from basic fibroblast growth factor. Prostate 15:355–365

Story MT, Baeten LA, Molter MA, Lawson RK (1990) Influence of androgen and transforming growth factor beta on basic fibroblast growth factor levels in human prostate-derived fibroblast cell cultures. J Urol 143:241A

Swinnen K, Cailleau J, Heyns W, Verhoeven G (1990) Prostatic stromal cells and testicular peritubular cells produce similar paracrine mediators of androgen action. Endocrinology 126:142–150

Swinnen K, Deboel L, Cailleau J, Heyns W, Verhoeven G (1991) Morphological and functional similarities between cultured prostatic stromal cells and testicular peritubular myoid cells. Prostate 19:99–112

Takeda H, Chang C (1991) Immunohistochemical and in-situ hybridization analysis of androgen receptor expression during the development of the mouse prostate gland. J Endocrinol 129:83–89

Takeda H, Mizuno T, Lasnitzki I (1985) Autoradiographic studies of androgen-binding sites in the rat urogenital sinus and postnatal prostate. J Endocrinol 104:87–92

Tanaka A, Miyamoto K, Minamino N, Takeda M, Sato B, Matsuo H, Matsumoto K (1992) Cloning and characterization of and androgen-induced growth factor essential for the androgen-dependent growth of mouse mammary carcinoma cells. Proc Natl Acad Sci USA 89:8928–8932

Tung PS, Fritz IB (1980) Interactions of Sertoli cells with myoid cells in vitro. Biol Reprod 23:207

Tunn S, Hochstrate H, Grunwald I, Flüchter SH, Krieg M (1988) Effect of aging on kinetic parameters of 5α-reductase in epithelium and stroma of normal and hyperplastic human prostate. J Clin Endocrinol Metab 67:979–985

Veldhuis JD, Urban RJ, Lizarraldi G, Johnson ML, Iranmanesh A (1992) Attenuation of luteinizing hormone secretory burst amplitude as a proximate basis for the hypoandrogenism of healthy aging in men. J Clin Endocrinol Metab 75:707–713

Verdonck L, Deslypere JP, Sayed MA, Van Sande M, Van Kamp K, Vermeulen A (1980) Subcellular distribution of androgens is hyperplastic human prostate. J Steroid Biochem 13:607–611

Verhoeven G (1980) Androgen receptor in cultured interstitial cells derived from immature rat testis. J Steroid Biochem 13:469–474

Verhoeven G, Cailleau J (1988) Testicular peritubular cells secrete a protein under androgen control that inhibits induction of aromatase activity in Sertoli cells. Endocrinology 123:2100–2110

Verhoeven G, Heyns W, De Moor P (1975) Testosterone receptors in the prostate and other tissues. Vitam Horm 33:265–281

Verhoeven G, Swinnen K, Cailleau J, Deboel L, Rombauts L, Heyns W (1992) The role of cell-cell interactions in androgen action. J Steroid Biochem Mol Biol 41:487–494

Vermeulen A (1991) Clinical review 24: androgens in the aging male. J Clin Endocrinol Metab 73:221–224

Voigt KD, Bartsch W (1986) Intratissular androgens in benign prostatic hyperplasia and prostatic cancer. J Steroid Biochem 25:749–757

Walsh PC (1984) Human benign prostatic hyperplasia: etiological considerations. Prog Clin Biol Res 145:1–25

Walsh PC, Wilson JD (1976) The induction of prostatic hypertrophy in the dog with androstanediol. J Clin Invest 57:1093–1097

Walsh PC, Hutchings GM, Ewing L (1983) Tissue content of dihydrotestosterone in human prostatic hyperplasia is not supranormal. J Clin Invest 72:1772–1777

Wilding G (1991) Response of prostate cancer cells to peptide growth factors: transforming growth factor-β. In: Isaacs JT (ed) Prostate cancer cell and molecular mechanisms in diagnosis and treatment. Cancer Surveys, Cold Spring Harbor Laboratory Press, pp 147–163

Wilding G, Knabbe C, Zugmaier G, Flanders K, Gelmann EP (1989) Differential effects of TGFβ on human prostate cancer cells in vitro. Mol Cell Endocrinol 62:79–87

Wilson JD (1980) The pathogenesis of benign prostatic hyperplasia. Am J Med 68:745–756

Wilson JD, Gloyna RE (1970) The intranuclear metabolism of testosterone in the accessory organs of reproduction. Recent Prog Horm Res 26:309–336

Wilson JD, George FW, Griffin JE (1981) The hormonal control of sexual development. Science 211:1278–1284

Yan G, Fukabori Y, Nikolaropoulos S, Wang F, McKeehan WL (1992) Heparin-binding keratinocyte growth factor is a candidate stromal to epithelial cell andromedin. Mol Endocrinol 6:2123–2128

3 The Natural History of Benign Prostatic Hyperplasia

GLENN B. MIESZKALSKI, JOAN KEIT, and LUTHER W. BRADY

CONTENTS

3.1 Introduction

Benign prostatic hyperplasia (BPH) is a very common but poorly understood disorder. The first description of BPH dates back several thousand years, and in spite of our best efforts, BPH remains a significant problem throughout the world today. An estimated \$3–4 billion health care dollars are spent on the surgical correction of this problem each year in the United States alone (COTTON 1991). As the elderly population continues to expand, it is likely that the scope of this problem will continue to increase.

The natural history of a disease process refers to its untreated course. An understanding of the natural history of BPH is vital to establishing treatment strategies for this disorder. Surprisingly, little is known about the natural history of BPH. This paper will review the available literature in an attempt to describe the natural history of this common problem.

Many theories have been proposed as to the origin of BPH but the exact etiology remains unclear. Only two factors have definitely been established as necessary for the development of BPH: the presence of testosterone and aging

GLENN B. MIESZKALSKI, MD, Chief Resident, JOAN KEIT, MD, Chief Resident, and LUTHER W. BRADY, MD, Professor and Chairman, Department of Radiation Oncology and Nuclear Medicine, Hahnemann University, Broad and Vine Streets, Philadelphia, PA 19102, USA

Petrovich/Baert (Eds.)
Benign Prostatic Hyperplasia

(see Chap. 1). No association has been found with socioeconomic status, sexual activity, specific blood groups, tobacco use, alcohol use, or medical problems such as coronary artery disease, cerebral vascular disease, hypertension, diabetes, or cirrhosis (ROTKIN 1983).

3.2 Phases of Development of BPH

ISAACS (1989) has suggested that the natural history of BPH is composed of two sequential phases, a pathologic and a clinical phase. Changes which occur in the prostate during the asymptomatic pathologic phase may lead to the symptomatic clinical phase. Any discussion on the natural history of BPH must first distinguish between anatomic or pathologic BPH and clinical BPH. BARRY (1990) has noted that these conditions differ in both prevalence and incidence, with anatomic BPH being far more common than clinical BPH.

The changes that occur in the prostate with the development of BPH have been described by MCNEAL (1978, 1990), who differentiates two distinct stages in the pathologic development of BPH. First, there is the development of nodules in the glandular tissue of the transition zone and in the periurethral region of the prostate. This can be seen as early as the fourth decade of life, and the number of nodules increases linearly with age, while the size of the individual nodules increases slowly. The second stage of BPH generally occurs between the late seventh and the mid-eighth decade of life. This stage is characterized by an abrupt increase in the mass of the individual nodules, which may result in clinically significant BPH. As the age of onset of this stage is quite variable, and as it does not always occur, clinically significant BPH will not necessarily develop in all men with hyperplastic nodules in the prostate.

3.3 Histologic Changes

Microscopically, nodular hyperplasia involves both glandular and stromal elements to varying degrees. It is usually accompanied by some degree of atrophy and involution. Glandular hyperplasia may involve ducts or acini. Ductal changes usually present as papillary projections of a two-cell layered epithelium into the lumen of the duct. Acinar hyperplasia expands a lobule and may appear as an aggregation of crowded small glands within the stroma. This is sometimes difficult to distinguish from adenocarcinoma. Corpora amylacea, which represents inspissated secretions that react with periodic acid Schiff reagent, PSA, and PAP, are prominent in the glands of nodular hyperplasia but can also be found in the glands of young men. Ultrastructurally, the hyperplastic glands do not differ significantly from normal glands. The cells exhibit no evidence of mitoses, abnormal nuclei, or abnormal cytoplasm (Murphy and Gaeta 1989).

Stromal hyperplasia may be diffuse or nodular. It is rich in smooth muscle and can resemble leiomyomas of the uterus. Isolated skeletal muscle fibers may be present. Elastic tissue is scanty or absent. Stromal hyperplasia may contain elements of lymphocytic infiltration. Areas of atrophy and involution are also common (Murphy and Gaesta 1989).

Much of the information regarding the histologic prevalence of BPH comes from autopsy studies. Berry et al. (1984) combined five different autopsy studies (Swyer 1944; Moore 1943; Franks 1954; Horbitz and Haugen 1972; Pradhan and Chandra 1975) containing a total of 1075 autopsy specimens to determine the prevalence of BPH. The pathologic changes of BPH were found to be increasingly prevalent with age (Table 3.1). The first pathologic evidence of BPH was observed between the ages of 31 and 40, but this was seen in only 8% of the men in this age group. Prevalence then increased rapidly, and by the seventh decade, the prevalence was 71%. By the ninth decade, the prevalence of BPH approached 90%.

In this same paper, Berry et al. (1984) also reviewed prostate size in 925 specimens from five autopsy studies (Swyer 1944; Pradhan and Chandra 1975; Lowsley 1915; Tornblom 1946; Haugen and Morbitz 1972). They found that the weight of the prostate increased with advancing age. The first growth spurt occurred during puberty, when prostatic weight increased by an average of 1.6 g per year. The growth rate then markedly decreased to 0.4 g per year from age 31 to over age 90. Berry et al. (1984) then used data from two of the studies (Berry et al. 1984; Tornblom 1946) containing 236 patients and determined that the weight of the normal prostate plateaus at 20 ± 6 g during the third decade. The development of BPH is associated with a continued increase in prostatic weight beginning in the fifth decade.

In addition, Berry ct al. (1984) were able to calculate the doubling time of BPH lesions for different age groups. Subjects between 31 and 50 years of age had a doubling time of 4.5 years. Subjects between 51 and 70 years of age had

Table 3.1. Prevalence of pathologic BPH with age in 1075 human prostates collected at autopsy (data from Berry et al. 1984)

Age range	No. of men with BPH/total no. of men	% men with BPH
1–10	0/27	0
11–20	0/35	0
21–30	0/86	0
31–40	8/105	8
41–50	22/94	23
51–60	81/191	42
61–70	171/242	71
71–80	181/221	82
≥ 80	65/74	88

a doubling time of 10 years, and subjects over age 70 had a doubling time of more than 100 years. Using these data, the authors estimated that it would take 10–20 years for hyperplastic changes in the prostate to develop into a pathologic nodule.

3.4 Symptoms of BPH

The symptoms which define the clinical phase of BPH have been termed "prostatism", which encompasses all symptoms related to prostatic enlargement secondary to BPH. These symptoms are classified as obstructive or irritative. Obstructive symptoms include decreased force and caliber of the urinary stream, urinary hesitancy, intermittence, terminal dribbling, and urinary retention. Irritative symptoms include nocturia, frequency, and dysuria. Although these symptoms are frequently seen in BPH, they are not specific for BPH and can be seen in unrelated conditions such as urinary tract infection, neurogenic bladder, and urethral stricture.

SCHROEDER and BLOM (1989) have described a staging system which is commonly used in Europe to classify the symptomatology of BPH according to its severity. In stage I, symptoms which may be present include slow stream, frequency, urgency, and hesitancy. These are associated with a residual urine volume less than 50 ml. In stage II, symptoms are the same as in stage I, but the residual volume is greater than 50 ml. Stage III is characterized by chronic retention and upper urinary tract damage, with or without uremia. Other symptoms include urge incontinence, paradoxic incontinence, and acute urinary retention.

3.5 Incidence

Although the incidence of pathologic BPH has been well documented (BERRY et al. 1984; SWYER 1944; MOORE 1943; FRANKS 1954; HORBITZ and HAUGEN 1972; PRADHAN and CHANDRA 1975; LOWSLEY 1915; TORNBLOM 1946; HAUGEN and HORBITZ 1972), little is known about the incidence and importance of clinical BPH. Two prospective studies have provided information on the incidence and prevalence of clinical BPH. GLYNN et al. (1980) described the occurrence of BPH in prospectively followed men in the Normative Aging Study. Two thousand and forty-nine men were routinely assessed for the development of BPH. This diagnosis was made by the finding of an enlarged prostate on digital examination or by the development of urinary symptoms not attributed to another cause. This study also recorded all prostatectomies. The incidence of both clinical BPH and of surgery for BPH increased with age. Age was noted to be the most important predictor of prostatectomy and of a new diagnosis of BPH. A prior history of BPH was found to be a strong predictor of prostatectomy, but there were many patients with clinically diagnosed BPH at entry into the study who did not have surgery during the 15-year follow-up period. Glynn estimated that a 40-year-old man who lived to be 80 years old had a 78% chance of developing BPH and a 29% chance of undergoing surgery for BPH. In assessing these results, one must note that the incidence of BPH may have been overestimated by including patients with an enlarged prostate but with no symptoms of clinical BPH. Also, the rates of surgery for BPH reflect statistics from the Boston area and may differ from other areas of the country.

A second prospective study was performed by ARRIGHI et al. (1991) in the Baltimore Longitudinal Study of Aging. This study analyzed 1057 men with respect to the development of obstructive symptoms and the possibility of surgery for BPH. Prostatic size and the diagnosis of BPH both increased with age. By the seventh decade, nearly 60% of all men had clinical evidence of BPH, and by the eighth decade this figure increased to greater than 80%. Symptoms in both men with an enlarged prostate and in men with a diagnosis of BPH increased with age. In addition, the probability of prostatectomy increased greatly in men with an enlarged prostate and symptoms of BPH (Table 3.2).

It is clear that the incidence of BPH (both histologic and clinical) increases with age. Unfortunately, there is a paucity of literature which describes the progression of this disorder after the diagnosis is established. Most of the available literature seems to indicate that the course of BPH is quite variable. CLARKE (1937) retrospectively reviewed 36 cases of uncomplicated BPH followed for a mean of 3.4 years without surgical intervention. Twenty-five of these patients improved symptomatically and were stable for at least some part of the follow-up period.

In 1969, CRAIGEN et al. reported on 212 patients presenting to general practitioners with urinary symptoms and no evidence of prostatic carcinoma. Eighty-nine of these patients presented with acute urinary retention, and 123 presented with other urinary symptoms. At 5 years, 48% of the patients had required prostatectomy. Of the patients who required prostatectomy, approximately 70% were in the first year of follow-up. It is important to note that the high percentage of men presenting with acute retention indicates that many of

Table 3.2. Probability of BPH surgery among men in the Baltimore Longitudinal Study of Aging (data from ARRIGHI et al. 1991)

	Percentage of men with an enlarged prostate and symptoms		Percentage of men without an enlarged prostate and no symptoms	
Age range	10 years	20 years	10 years	20 years
40–49	3	13	2	4
50–59	7	24	2	9
60–69	16	39	9	22
≥ 70	34	41	13	–

these men were presenting with advanced stages of BPH. In addition, the fact that the percentage of men who deteriorated symptomatically (45%) closely matched the percentage who underwent surgery (48%) indicates that surgical intervention is often based on subjective criteria.

3.6 Clinical Course of Untreated Patients

BIRKHOFF et al. (1976) reviewed 26 patients with untreated BPH who were followed by objective and subjective measures. Patients with both large and small prostates were found to deteriorate subjectively and objectively at similar rates. Although the overall trend was toward progression of the disease, there was considerable variation in the natural history of individual patients. Both subjective and objective improvement were noted for periods of up to 5 years. During the study, ten episodes of acute urinary retention developed. This event was not predictable as it did not necessarily occur in the patients who were most symptomatic.

BALL et al. (1981) reported on 107 men with clinical symptoms of BPH. After a period of 5 years, ten patients had undergone surgery for worsening of BPH. Sixty-four patients returned for repeat measurement of urinary flow. Thirty-nine (61%) had a fall in peak flow while 25 (39%) had no change or an improvement in peak flow. Only six of the patients had a change in urinary flow that was ≥ 1.2 SD, and three of them complained of worsening symptoms. No association was found with the original parameters of urinary obstruction and subsequent deterioration. This study did suggest that urinary flow was a reasonable screening procedure, as no patient with a peak flow within 2 SD of normal required surgery. USON et al. (1991) have also noted that although it is impossible to predict which patients will develop clinically significant BPH, urinary flow rate is a good and minimally invasive test to identify and follow up patients with BPH (see Chap. 6).

Additional information on the natural history of BPH can be obtained from the placebo arms of drug trials. ISAACS (1990) reviewed response rates from the placebo arms of 12 drug trials (DAMRAU 1962; RANGNO et al. 1971; CASTRO et al. 1971; CAINE et al. 1975, 1978; ABRAMS 1977; GELLER et al. 1979; ABRAMS et al. 1982; BROOKS et al. 1983; HEDLUND et al. 1983; RAMSAY et al. 1985; KIRBY et al. 1987). Subjective improvement was noted in 15%–70% of patients on placebo. Four of the studies (ABRAMS 1977; CAINE et al. 1978; HEDLUND et al. 1983; KIRBY et al. 1987) also reported objective improvement with a range of 17%–80%. In interpreting these data, one must realize that follow-up in these studies was short, with a range of 2 weeks to 6 months. It is also impossible to distinguish a symptomatic response to placebo from a natural remission of symptoms. ISAACS (1990) has suggested that the percentage of patients who improved on placebo was essentially the same as the percentage of BPH patients who are followed up without treatment.

3.7 Complications in Untreated BPH

Complications of long-standing BPH include acute urinary retention, chronic renal failure, repeated urinary tract infection, and irreversible bladder decompensation. Unfortunately, little is known about the incidence of these complications. In CRAIGEN et al.'s (1969) report of 123 patients with varying degrees of prostatism, approximately 10% were expected to develop acute urinary retention during a 7-year follow-up period. BIRKHOFF et al. (1976) observed ten episodes of acute retention in nine patients (out of 26 followed up) during a period of 3 years. In BALL et al.'s (1981) analysis of untreated patients, 2 of 97 developed acute retention. None of these studies were able to predict the occurrence of retention on the basis of clinical symptoms. Patients who developed acute retention were often not the patients who were the most symptomatic. This may indicate that acute retention is not a result of progressive BPH, but may be due to another event such as prostatic infarction (SPIRO et al. 1974).

Chronic renal failure may occur in patients with minimal symptoms, and once it occurs, it may not be reversible (BECK 1970; DOWD and EWERT 1961; SARMINA and RESNICK 1989). Azotemia has been reported to be the single most significant finding influencing morbidity and mortality in patients with BPH (MELCHIOR et al. 1974). The available data relative to the frequency of this feared complication are inadequate to make any estimation of the incidence of chronic renal failure due to BPH.

Urinary tract infection is another potential serious complication of untreated BPH. MEBUST et al. (1989) reported that approximately 12% of patients undergoing prostatectomy had repeated urinary tract infections. HASNER (1962) observed that 8.6% of patients with prostatic obstruction and ≥ 50 ml of residual urine presented with infection. This correlation of urinary tract infection with residual urine volume was not confirmed by BRUSKEWITZ et al. (1982).

Bladder decompensation may also occur with bladder obstruction due to BPH. ANDERSEN et al. (1979) reported that the irritative symptoms of prostatism correlated with cystometric evidence of uninhibited detrusor contractions. During long-standing obstruction, trabeculation and diverticula formation may be seen in the bladder (ISAACS 1989). Histologically, fibrosis in the muscle of the obstructed bladder may be noted (GILPIN et al. 1985). The frequency with which these changes occur, and whether or not they may be prevented by early therapeutic intervention, has yet to be determined.

3.8 Conclusion

In spite of the fact that BPH is an extremely common disorder, reports of the natural history of this problem are few and far between. Clearly, this disease process involves two phases, an asymptomatic histologic phase and a symptomatic clinical phase. Although the incidence and prevalence of histologic and clinical BPH increase with age, not all men with histologic evidence of hyperplastic changes will develop clinical BPH. Untreated, BPH may lead to acute urinary retention, recurrent urinary tract infection, chronic renal failure, and bladder decompensation. Unfortunately, the incidence of these complications is not predictable on the basis of symptoms. This makes the selection of patients for treatment rather difficult. Certainly, the presence of one of the above complications is an indication for treatment. In the absence of one of these indications, it would seem that careful observation is appropriate as spontaneous improvement, both subjective and objective, is fairly common. Hopefully, an ongoing Veterans Administration randomized trial comparing the results of early transurethral prostatic resection with "watchful waiting" will reveal whether delayed intervention results in inferior clinical outcomes. Finally, one must not overlook the importance of patient preference in selecting patients for treatment.

Currently, there are many options for the treatment of BPH. These include transurethral prostatic resection, balloon dilatation, urethral stents, pharmacologic agents, and microwave hyperthermia. As the natural history of BPH is quite variable, any clinical trial evaluating the efficacy of these treatments must include a placebo or no-treatment arm. The American Urological Association is currently conducting a randomized prospective clinical trial in the treatment of BPH (HOLTGREW 1992). This study will include a watch and wait arm for patients with prostates < 80 g. The patients in these arms may be able to provide us with additional information regarding the natural history of BPH.

An understanding of the natural history of BPH is vital to establishing treatment strategies to prevent its complications and relieve its symptoms. As the population continues to age, it is likely that BPH and its complications will become an increasing problem. Presently, the natural history of BPH is poorly understood. Therefore, further studies are needed to better define the natural history of this common problem.

References

Abrams PH (1977) A double-blind trial of the effects of candicidin on patients with benign prostatic hyperplasia. Br J Urol 49:67–71

Abrams PH, Shah PJR, Stone R, Choa RG (1982) Bladder outflow obstruction treated with phenoxybenzamine. Br J Urol 54:527–530

Andersen JT, Nordling J, Walter S (1979) Prostatism I. The correlation between symptoms, cystometric, and urodynamic findings. Scand J Urol Nephrol 13:(3) 229–236

Arrighi HM, Metter EJ, Guess HA, Fozzard JL (1991) Natural history of benign prostatic hyperplasia and risk of prostatectomy. The Baltimore Longitudinal Study of Aging. Urology 38:4–8

Ball AJ, Feneley RC, Abrams PH (1981) The natural history of untreated "prostatism". Br J Urol 53:613–616

Barry MJ (1990) Epidemiology and natural history of benign prostatic hyperplasia. Urol Clin North Am 17:495–507

Beck AD (1970) Benign prostatic hypertrophy and uraemia: a review of 315 cases. Br J Surg 57:561–565

Berry SJ, Coffey DS, Walsh PC, Ewing LL (1984) The development of human benign prostatic hyperplasia with age. J Urol 132:474–479

Birkhoff JD (1976) The natural history of prostatic hyperplasia and acute urinary retention. Urology 7:48–52

Brooks ME, Sidi AA, Hanami Y, Braf ZF (1983) Ineffectiveness of phenoxybenzamine in treatment of benign prostatic hypertrophy: a controlled study. Urology 21:474–478

Bruskewitz RC, Iversen P, Madisen PO (1982) Value of postvoid residual urine determination in evaluation of prostatism. Urology 20:602–604

Caine M, Perlberg S, Gordon R (1975) The treatment of benign prostatic hypertrophy with flutamide (SCH 13521): a placebo-controlled study. J Urol 114:564–568

Caine M, Perlberg S, Meretyk S (1978) A placebo-controlled double-blind study of the effect of phenoxybenzamine in benign prostatic obstruction. Br J Urol 50:551–554

Castro JE, Griffiths HJL, Edwards DE (1971) A double-blind, controlled, clinical trial of spironolactone for benign prostatic hypertrophy. Br J 58:485–489

Clarke R (1937) The prostate and the endocrines. A control series. Br J Urol 9:254–271

Cotton P (1991) Case for prostate therapy wanes despite more treatment options. JAMA 266:459–460

Craigen AA, Hickling TB, Saunders CR, et al. (1969) Natural history of prostatic obstruction. J R Coll Gen Pract 18:226–232

Damrau F (1962) Benign prostatic hypertrophy: Amino acid therapy for symptomatic relief. J Am Geriatr Soc 10:426–430

Dowd JB, Ewert EE (1961) Silent prostatism (unrecognized bladder neck obstruction). JAMA 178:296–300

Franks LM (1954) Benign nodular hyperplasia of the prostate: a review. Ann R Coll Surg 14:92–106

Geller J, Nelson CG, Albert JD, Pratt C (1979) Effect of megestrol acetate on uroflow rates in patients with benign prostatic hypertrophy: double-blind study. Urology 14:467–474

Gilpin SA, Gosling JA, Barnard RJ (1985) Morphologic and morphometric studies of the human obstructed trabeculated bladder. Br J Urol 57:525–529

Glynn RJ, Campion EW, Bourchard GR, et al. (1980) The development of benign prostatic hyperplasia among volunteers in the Normative Aging Study. Am J Epidemiol 121:78–90

Hasner E (1962) Prostatic urinary infection. Acta Chir Scand (Suppl) 285:1–40

Haugen TB, Morbitz TB (1972) Prostatic weight in elderly men. An analysis in an autopsy series. Acta Pathol Microbiol Scand [A] 80:759–777

Hedlund H, Anderson KE, Ek A (1983) Effects of prazosin in patients with benign prostatic obstruction. J Urol 130:275–278

Holtgrew HL (1992) An American Urological Association prospective randomized clinical trial in the treatment of benign prostatic hyperplasia. Cancer (Suppl) 70:351–354

Horbitz TB, Haugen OA (1972) Histology of the prostate in elderly men. A study in an autopsy series. Acta Pathol Microbiol Scand [A] 80:756–768

Isaacs JT (1989) Etiology and disease process of benign prostatic hyperplasia. Prostate Suppl 2:35–50

Isaacs JT (1990) Importance of the natural history of benign prostatic hyperplasia in the evaluation of pharmacologic intervention. Prostate Suppl 3:1–7

Kirby RS, Coppinger SWC, Corcoran MQ, et al. (1987) Prazosin in the treatment of prostatic obstruction: a placebo-controlled study. Br J Urol 60:136–142

Lowsley OS (1915) The gross anatomy of the human prostate gland and contiguous structures. Surg Gynecol Obstet 20:183–192

McNeal J (1978) Origin and evaluation of benign prostatic enlargement. Invest Urol 15:340–345

McNeal J (1990) Pathology of benign prostatic hyperplasia. Insight into etiology. Urol Clin North Am 17:477–486

Mebust WK, Holtgrew HL, Cockett AT, et al. (1989) Transurethral prostatectomy: immediate and postoperative complications: a cooperative study of 13 participating institutions evaluating 3,885 patients. J Urol 141:243–247

Melchior J, Valk Wl, Foret WL, Mebust WK (1974) Transurethral prostatectomy: computerized analysis of 2,223 consecutive cases. J Urol 112:634–642

Moore RA (1943) Benign hypertrophy of the prostate. A morphological study. J Urol 50:680–710

Murphy WM, Gaeta JF (1989) Diseases of the prostate gland and seminal vesicles. In: Murphy, WM (eds) Urological pathology. W.B. Saunders, Philadelphia, pp 147–218

Pradhan BK, Chandra K (1975) Morphogenesis of nodular hyperplasia prostate. J Urol 113:210–213

Ramsay JWA, Scott Gi, Whitfield HN (1985) A double-blind controlled trial of a new alpha-blocking drug in the treatment of bladder outflow obstruction. Br J Urol 57:657–659

Rangno RE, McLeod PJ, Ruedy J, Ogilvie RI (1971) Treatment of benign prostatic hypertrophy with medrogestrone. Clin Pharmacol Ther 12:658–665

Rotkin ID (1983) Origins, distribution, and risk of benign prostatic hypertrophy. In: Hinman F (ed) Benign prostatic hypertrophy. Springer, New York Berlin Heidelberg, p 10

Sarmina L, Resnick MI (1989) Obstructive uropathy in patients with benign prostatic hyperplasia. J Urol 141:868–869

Schroeder FH, Blom JHM (1989) Natural history of benign prostatic hyperplasia (BPH). Prostate Suppl 2:17–22

Spiro LH, Labay G, Orkin LA (1974) Prostatic infaction: role in acute urinary retention. Urology 57:561–565

Swyer GLM (1944) Post-natal growth changes in the human prostate. J Anat 78:130–145

Tornblom N (1946) Contribution to the discussion on the etiology of prostatic hyperplasia in man. I. The weight of the prostate and seminal vesicles in men of different ages. Acta Med Scand (Suppl) 170:1–9

Uson AC, Paez AB, Uson-Jaeger J (1991) The natural history and course of untreated benign prostatic hyperplasia. Eur Urol (Suppl 2) 3:1–7

4 Chromosome Abnormalities in Benign Prostatic Hyperplasia*

PAOLA DAL CIN and HERMAN VAN DEN BERGHE

CONTENTS

4.1 Introduction

Advances in the cytogenetics of solid tumors have been and still are at the mercy of methodology. However, improvements of cytogenetic techniques, better collaboration with surgeons and pathologists to obtain appropriate tumor samples, and careful examination of the karyotypes of a number of tumors with the same histologic picture have led to the description of a number of specific chromosome changes in solid tumors (Table 4.1). Cytogenetic abnormalities have been reported in about 1000 epithelial tumors and a small number of characteristic changes have been identified in these tumors, particularly in those of common occurrence such as tumors of the breast, lung, large bowel, ovary, and prostate (MITELMAN 1991).

* This text presents research results of the Belgian programme on Interuniversity Poles of Attraction initiated by the Belgian State, Prime Minister's Office, Science Policy Programming. The scientific responsibility is assumed by its authors.

PAOLA DAL CIN, PhD, Center for Human Genetics, University of Leuven, Herestraat 49, 3000 Leuven, Belgium
HERMAN VAN DEN BERGHE, PhD, Professor and Chairman, Department of Human Genetics, and Head of Center for Human Genetics, University of Leuven, Herestraat 49, 3000 Leuven, Belgium

Petrovich/Baert (Eds.)
Benign Prostatic Hyperplasia

Table 4.1 Specific (primary) chromosome changes in solid tumors

Tumors	Chromosome changes[a]
Benign	
Meningioma	− 22/22q −
Pleiomorphic adenoma of the salivary gland	t(3;8)(p21;q12)/t with 12q14 − 15
Lipoma	t with 12q14/t with 6p22 − 23/13q − / + r
Leiomyoma (uterine)	t with 12q14 − 15/7q − / + 12/13q − /t(1;2)(p36;p24)/t with 6p22 − 23
Colonic adenoma	12q − / + 8
Endometrial polyp	t with 6p22 − 23/t with 12q14 − 15
Follicular thyroid	t with 19q13/t(2;3)(q21;p24)
Cystadenomalymphoma (Warthin's tumor)	t(11;19)(q21;p13)
Fibroma (ovary)	+ 12
Renal cell adenoma	− Y, + 7, + 7, + 17
Oncocytoma	− Y, − 1
Pulmonary chondroid hamartoma	t with 6p21/t with 12q14 − 15
Carcinoma	
Bladder	i(5p)/ + 7/ − 9 or 9q − /11p −
Prostate	del(10)(q24)[c]
Lung (SCLC)[b]	del(3)(p14p23)
Colon	12q − [c]/ + 7[c]/ + 8[c]/ + 12[c]/17(q11)[c]/ − 18[c]
Kidney	del(3)(p11 − p21)/t(X;1)(p11.2;q21.1)
Uterus	1q − [c]
Ovary	6q − [c]
Papillary thyroid	10q11 − q26
Sarcoma	
Liposarcoma (myxoid)	t(12;16)(q13;p11)
Synovial sarcoma	t(X;18)(p11.2;q11.2)
Rhabdomyosarcoma (alveolar)	t(2;13)(q37;q14)/t(1;13)(p36;q14)
Extraskeletal myxoid chondrosarcoma	t(9;22)(q31;q12.2)
Leiomyosarcoma (small bowel)	t or del(1)(p12-13)
Fibrosarcoma (congenital)	Combination of trisomies[c]
Dermatofibrosarcoma protuberans	+ r
Endometrial stromal sarcoma	t(7;17)(p15 − 21;q12-21)
Clear cell sarcoma	t(12;22)(q13;q12)
Embryonal and other	
Germ cell tumors (gonadal and extragonadal)	i(12p)
Retinoblastoma	del(13)(q14)[d]/i(6p)[c]
Wilms' tumor	del(11)(p13)[d]
neuroblastoma	del(1)(p32p36)
Medulloblastoma	i(17q)
Malignant melanoma	del(6)(q11q27)[c]/i(6p)[c]/del91)(p11p22)[c]/t(1;19)(q12;q13)
mesothelioma	del(3)(p13 − p23)
Ewing's sarcoma, PNET	t(11;22)(q24;q12)

[a]/: divides subgroups in the same entity
[b]SCLC, small cell lung cancer; PNET; peripheral neuroendocrine tumor
[c]Not yet proven to be primary
[d]Associated with a constitutional chromosome change

4.2 Chromosomes in Benign and Malignant Tumors of the Prostate

Tumors of the prostate are among the more difficult neoplasms to examine cytogenetically because of the low in vitro mitotic index which leads to preferential growth of normal cells at the expense of the tumor cells. However, progress has been made in some respects. Growth of prostatic epithelium has been achieved using media supplemented with mitogens such as epidermal growth factor, hydrocortisone, insulin, or serum free media with cholera toxin (PEEHL and STAMEY 1984, 1986). Nevertheless, even with these improvements in tissue culturing, 75% of cytogenetically investigated prostatic tumors, almost exclusively adenocarcinomas, have shown a normal male karyotype (46, XY) and no consistent chromosome change has so far been associated with this malignancy (LIMON et al. 1990; LUNDGREN et al. 1992). However, a survey of all available cytogenetic data on human prostatic carcinomas (primary and metastatic tumors as well as cell lines) indicates that (a) chromosomes 1, 2, 5, and Y are frequently lost, (b) chromosomes 7, 14, 20, and 22 are gained, and (c) recurrent rearrangements of 2p, 7q, and 10q are observed (for review see SANDBERG 1992)

A variety of specific chromosome changes have been identified in several benign neoplasms (Table 4.1), indicating that the concept of chromosome abnormality being related to a malignant status versus normality related to

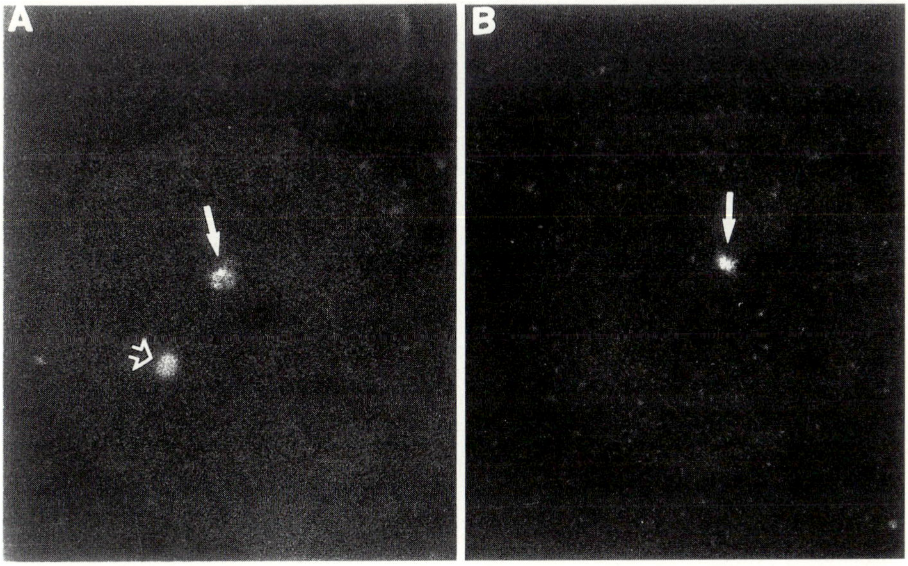

Fig 4.1A, B. Loss of the Y chromosome in BPH using double FISH. **A** Positive signal for pBAMX5 (*arrow*) (X chromosome) and for pHY2.1 (*Open head-arrow*) (Y chromosome). **B** Positive signal only for pBAMX5 (*arrow*). No Y chromosome present

a benign status may have to be revised. Moreover, certain chromosome regions seem to be nonrandomly affected (12q13-15, 6p21).

Benign prostatic hyperplasia (BPH) does not occur uniformly through the gland but develops mostly in a small region, the transition zone, close to the urethra (MCNEAL 1988). Cytogenetic investigations on seven specimens of BPH have been reported: six showed a normal male karyotype, whereas loss of the Y chromosome was found in the remaining one (JELLINGHAUS et al 1976; BROTHMAN et al. 1989). We have performed conventional cytogenetic analysis, using PFMR-4 medium modified for prostatic cell culturing as described by PEEHL and STAMEY (1984), combined with fluorescence in situ hybridization

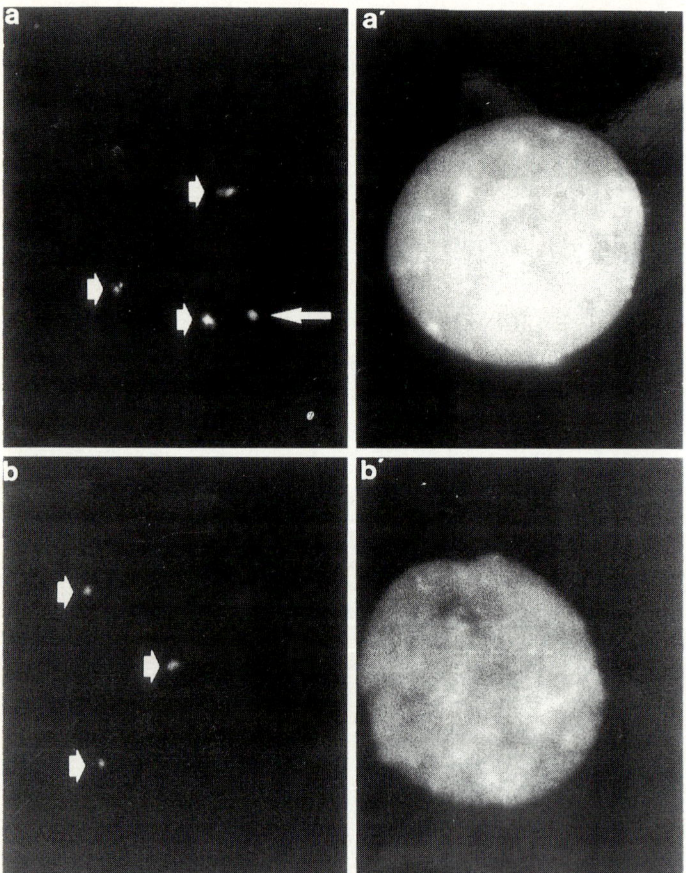

Fig 4.2a, b. Trisomy 7 in BPH using double FISH. **a** Three positive signals for p7t1 (*head-arrow*) (chromosome 7) and one for pHY2.1 (*arrow*) (Y chromosome). **a′** DAPI counterstain, **b** only 3 positive signals for chromosome 7 (*head-arrows*) and no signal for Y-chromosome **b′** DAPI counterstrain

(FISH) on 20 specimens of BPH from adenomectomies and transurethral resections. The FISH technique allows one to obtain cytogenetic information on interphase nuclei of nondividing cells using chromosome-specific probes (PINKEL et al. 1986). Combining both techniques we found that the loss of the Y chromosome and trisomy 7 were frequent chromosome changes in BPH (Figs. 4.1, 4.2) (ALY et al. 1993a).

4.3 Loss of the Y Chromosome

The missing Y chromosome is a common finding in many malignant disorders. It is usually observed in conjunction with other karyotypic changes but also occurs as the sole abnormality (MITELMAN 1991). Assessment of significance of the loss of the Y chromosome in neoplastic conditions is complicated by the fact that this chromosome anomaly is known to occur in bone marrow cells of healthy elderly males, where it is thought to be a normal aging phenomenon (PIERRE and HOAGLAND 1971, 1972). In malignancies, however, Y chromosome loss is not related to patient age, and the possibility remains that, at least in an occasional patient, the cells with a missing Y as the only abnormality may be neoplastic (ALY et al. 1993b).

4.4 Trisomy 7

Trisomy 7, as the only chromosome change, is a frequent chromosome abnormality in renal cell carcinomas (for review see SANDBERG 1990), but it has also been found in other malignant and non-malignant tumors (for review see MITELMAN 1991). It is less frequently observed in lymphomas, and very infrequently in leukemias. The finding of trisomy 7 in nonneoplastic tissues from patients with lung, kidney, or brain tumors by conventional cytogenetic analyses on short-term cultures, raised the question of whether these cells carrying an extra chromosome 7 reflect a normal in vivo organ specific mosaicism, a culture-induced artifact, or the presence of (pre)malignant cells (LEE et al. 1987; KOVACS and BRUSA 1989; HEIM et al. 1989; ELFVING et al. 1990). Moreover, ARNOLDUS and co-workers (1991), using the FISH technique, which allows the identification of trisomy 7 without culturing the cells, did not find trisomy 7 in normal brain samples from autopsies. In short-term cultures of colorectal adenocarcinomas BARDI et al. (1991) found trisomy 7 in fibroblast-like cells whereas other abnormalities were present in epithelial-like cells.

We have recently identified trisomy 7 (and trisomy 10) in a substantial number of mononuclear inflammatory cells infiltrating kidney tumors and surrounding tissue. The predominant cell population with an abnormal chromosome 7 complement was characterized as T-helper/inducer lymphocytes, while trisomy 10 was highest in cells characterized as T-suppressor/cytotoxic lymphocytes. These findings were confirmed by combined immunohistochemistry and in situ hybridization on isolated tumor-infiltrating inflammatory cells as well as in sections of frozen kidney tissue. Trisomy 7, however, was found only in the presence of a tumor in the kidney, and not in nonneoplastic conditions. In an attempt to explain the origin of these trisomies, we found the same aneuploidy for chromosomes 7 and 10 in a considerable percentage of fetal thymocytes, and not in other fetal tissues, which suggests that these subpopulations could be the precursors of the trisomy 7 and trisomy 10 cells detected in 5%–6% and 5%, respectively, of isolated T cells from the peripheral blood of normal adults and of patients with kidney cancer (Dal Cin et al. 1992).

It is tempting to speculate that the presence of tumor-infiltrating lymphocytes is responsible for trisomy 7 and 10 observed in a range of other tumors. We studied a series of cancers which includes epithelial tumors originating in the lung, breast, thyroid, prostate, colon, and bladder and mesenchymal tumors such as lipoma, myxoid liposarcoma, synovial sarcoma, neurofibrosarcoma, leiomyosarcoma, malignant fibrous histiocytoma, and uterine leiomyoma, and found that trisomy 7 is almost exclusively found in connection with tumors of epithelial origin.

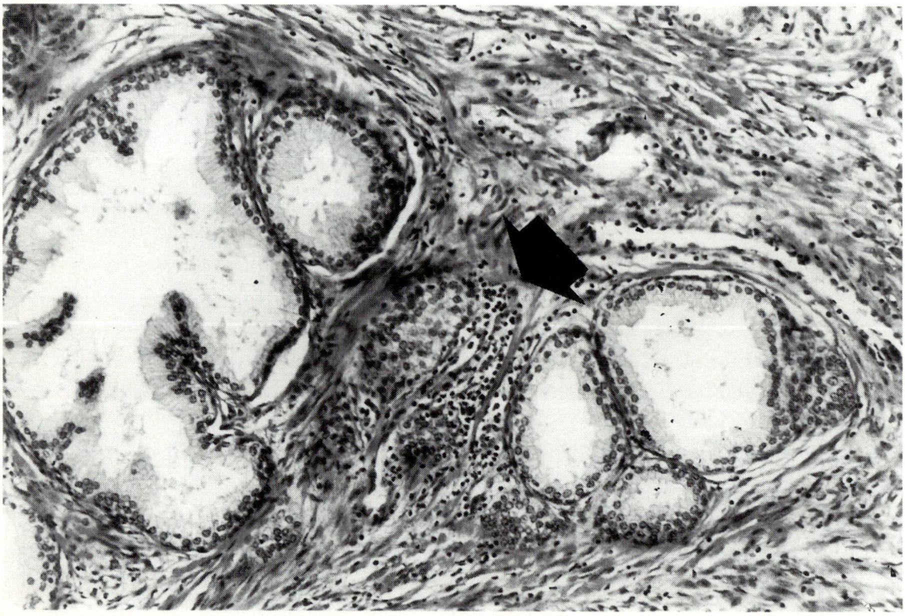

Fig 4.3. Detail of glandular hyperplasia with associated stromal lymphocytic infiltration (lymphocytic aggregate →). Original magnification ×100

4.5 Chromosome Abnormalities in BPH

Nodular hyperplasia of the prostate is always associated with a slight to moderate dense lymphocytic interstitial infiltrate and some periglandular lymphocytic aggregates (Fig. 4.3). These lymphocytic infiltrations vary from sample to sample without a rim pattern, as in kidney carrying a tumor where inflammatory cells are not only present in the tumor but are even more numerous in the tumor pseudocapsule and the surrounding nonneoplastic kidney tissue (DAL CIN et al. 1992). This variation of tumor-infiltrating lymphocytes can perhaps explain the wide range in the percentage of trisomy 7 cells in the cases of BPH investigated by us, especially with the FISH technique.

4.6 Conclusion

We conclude that in BPH trisomy 7 is probably unrelated to the tumor cells, in which the only and not very specific change seems to be loss of the Y chromosome.

References

Aly MS, Dal Cin P, Ameye F, Van Poppel H, Baert L, Van den Berghe H (1993a) Abstract. Chromosome abnormalities in adenomas of prostate. 5th International Workshop on Chromosomes in Solid Tumors. Tucson, 10–12 January 1993

Aly MS, Dal Cin P, Moerman P, et al. (1993b) Loss of the Y-chromosome in a malignant Sertoli tumor. Cancer Genet Cytogenet 65:104–106

Arnoldus EPJ, Noordermeer IA, Peters ACB, Raap A, Van der Ploeg M (1991) Interphase cytogenetics reveals somatic pairing of chromosome 17 centromeres in normal human brain tissue, but no trisomy 7 or sex-chromosome loss. Cytogenet Cell Genet 56:214–216

Bardi G, Johansson B, Pandis N, et al. (1991) Trisomy 7 in short-term cultures of colorectal adenocarcinomas. Genes Chrom Cancer 3:149–152

Brothman AR, Lesho LJ, Somers KD, Schellhammer PF, Ladaga LE, Merchant DJ (1989) Cytogenetic analysis of four primary prostatic cultures. Cancer Genet Cytogenet 37:241–248

Dal Cin P, Aly MS, Delabie J, et al. (1992) Trisomy 7 and trisomy 10 characterize subpopulations of tumor-infiltrating lymphocytes in kidney tumors and in the surrounding kidney tissue. Proc Natl Acad Sci USA 89:9744–9748

Elfving P, Cigudosa JC, Lundgren R, et al. (1990) Trisomy 7, trisomy 10, and loss of the Y chromosome in short-term cultures of normal kidney tissue. Cytogenet Cell Genet 53:123–125

Heim S, Mandahl N, Jin Y, Strömblad S, Lindström E, Salford LG, Mitelman F (1989) Trisomy 7 and sex chromosome loss in human brain tissue. Cytogenet Cell Genet 52:136–138

Jellinghaus W, Okada W, Ragg C, Gerhard H, Schroder FH (1976) Chromosomal studies of human prostatic tumors in vitro. Invest Urol 14:16–19

Kovacs G, Brusa P (1989) Clonal chromosome aberrations in normal kidney tissue from patients with renal cell carcinoma. Cancer Genet Cytogenet 37:289–290

Lee JS, Pathak S, Hopwood V, et al. (1987) Involvement of chromosome 7 in primary lung tumor and nonmalignant normal lung tissue. Cancer Res 47:6349–6352

Limon J, Lundgren R, Elfving P, Heim S, Kristoffersson U, Mandahl N, Mitelman F, (1990) An improved technique for short term culturing of human prostatic adenocarcinoma tissue for cytogenetic analysis. Cancer Genet Cytogenet 39:191–194

Lundgren R, Mandahl N, Heim S, Limon J, Henrikson H, Mitelman F, (1992) Cytogenetic analysis of 57 primary prostatic adenocarcinomas. Genes Chrom Cancer 4:16–24

McNeal JE (1988) Normal histology of the prostate. Am J Surg Pathol 12:619

Mitelman F (1991) Catalog of chromosome aberrations in cancer, 4th edn. Wiley-Liss, New York

Peehl DM, Stamey TA (1984) Serial propagation of adult human prostatic epithelial cells with cholera toxin. In Vitro 20:981–986

Peehl DM, Stamey TA (1986) Serum-free growth of adult human prostatic epithelial cells. In Vitro Cell Dev Biol 22:82–90

Pierre RV, Hoagland HC (1971) 45, X cell lines in adult men: loss of Y chromosome, a normal aging phenomenon? Mayo Clin Proc 46:52–55

Pierre RV, Hoagland HC (1972) Age-associated aneuploidy: loss of Y chromosome from human bone marrow cells with aging. Cancer 30:889–894

Pinkel D, Straume T, Gray JW (1986) Cytogenetic analysis using quantitative, high-sensitivity, fluorescence hybridization. Proc Natl Acad Sci USA 83:2934–2938

Sandberg AA (1990) The chromosomes in human cancer and leukemia, 2nd edn. Elsevier, New York

Sandberg AA (1992) Chromosomal abnormalities and related events in prostate cancer. Hum Pathol 23:368–380

5 Quantifying the Smooth Muscle Content of the Prostate Using Double Immunoenzymatic Staining and Color-Assisted Image Analysis

ELLEN SHAPIRO and HERBERT LEPOR

CONTENTS

5.1 Introduction

Benign prostatic hyperplasia (BPH) describes a hyperplastic process of the stromal and epithelial elements of the prostate (FRANKS 1975). The clinical manifestations of BPH are related primarily to symptoms of bladder outlet obstruction (BARRY 1990). The specific histologic features of the prostate which lead to the development of bladder outlet obstruction are unknown.

5.2 Morphometric Analysis

In order to determine whether the cellular composition of the hyperplasia is related to the development of symptomatic BPH, we have applied a technique of morphometric analysis which permits quantification of the histologic elements of the prostate. Morphometrics is a method that provides a quantitative histologic analysis of fixed tissue sections (WEIBEL et al. 1966; WEIBEL and

ELLEN SHAPIRO, MD, FACS, FAAP, and HERBERT LEPOR, MD, FACS, Professor of Urology, Department of Urology, New York University, School of Medicine, New York, New York 10016, USA

Petrovich/Baert (Eds.)
Benign Prostatic Hyperplasia

BOLENDER 1973) Stereologic analysis allows measurements to be taken from a representative number of two-dimensional samples (tissue sections). These measurements are used to quantify the internal structure of a three-dimensional object (prostate). Stereologic results are expressed as densities that relate a volume, a surface area, or a number of tissue or cellular components to a unit or reference volume. Quantitative morphometry complements qualitative descriptions obtained from light microscopy and yields objective and reproducible values for morphologic structures that allow statistically defined comparisons.

5.3 Stereologic Techniques

In 1977, BARTSCH applied stereologic techniques to light microscopic prostatic tissue sections. He examined hematoxylin and eosin-stained paraffin sections of normal prostate glands from six men (< 30 years old) and seven patients undergoing suprapubic prostatectomy for bladder outlet obstruction due to BPH. The tissue was divided into morphologically defined compartments: the inner and the outer dimensions as described by FRANKS (1975). The normal gland was subdivided into the acinar parenchyma and the interstitial fibromuscular (stromal) tissue. The BPH acinar component of the tissue was further subdivided into the lumina and glandular cells. Stereologic analysis involves superimposing an ocular grid on a microscopic field and counting points of intersection of the grid with the various components of the tissue. This method provides the percentage distribution of each tissue component within the area of interest and this can be converted into percent of section volume.

An extension of this methodology termed "biomorphometrics" has been reported by DEKLERK and COFFEY (1978) in a study of rat ventral prostate. This technique determines the ratio of various cellular types determined by standard morphometric analysis and the total number of cells in the gland obtained by knowledge of the total DNA content in the gland and DNA per cell nucleus. This method eliminates the differential effects of fixation, dehydrating, and embedding of sections on the volume and shapes of different tissue components. This type of analysis is useful as an index of hyperplastic growth and can be performed in animal studies where the whole gland is available for DNA analysis.

5.4 Cellular Composition of Normal Prostate and in BPH

BARTSCH et al. (1979) performed an elegant stereologic analysis using the point counting method. They showed that in normal human prostate, the volume density of the stroma, glandular cells, and acinar lumina was 0.45, 0.21, and 0.34, respectively. In BPH, these values were 0.6, 0.12 and 0.28, respectively. The ratio of stroma to epithelium in BPH and normal prostates was 5:1 and 2:1, respectively. These studies suggest that BPH is predominantly stromal hyperplasia.

Siegel et al. (1990) recently utilized a point counting stereology method to determine the cellular composition of human prostate. Prostate specimens were obtained from nine males undergoing prostatectomy for BPH. The tissue sections were stained with hematoxylin and eosin. The percent area densities of prostatic connective tissue, smooth muscle, vascular elements, and epithelium were 47%, 7%, 3% and 18%, respectively. Twenty-five percent of the adenoma was edema, leukocytes, nerve, lymphatics, and other poorly defined tissues. The relative proportion of stroma to epithelium was 4.6:1, which is consistent with Bartsch's observation. Although these studies have provided the foundation of our knowledge about normal and pathologic morphogenesis, application of this point counting technique is cumbersome.

5.5 Application of Computer Image Analysis in Quantifying Cellular Elements in BPH

Shapiro et al. (1992a) recently reported the application of computer image analysis that adapts Weibels's multipurpose test grid and line intersect stereologic analysis to quantify the relative amounts of stroma and epithelium in BPH. Prostatic adenoma specimens were obtained from 12 subjects undergoing transurethral resection of the prostate (TURP), 12 subjects undergoing open prostatectomy, and six subjects undergoing cystoprostatectomy. Prostatic biopsies were performed on nine additional subjects prior to receiving medical therapy for clinical BPH. Uroflowmetry and symptom scores were determined on all patients prior to undergoing surgery or biopsy. The baseline clinical data demonstrated that the subjects undergoing TURP, open prostatectomy, and pharmacotherapy had clinical BPH (symptomatic BPH) whereas the subjects undergoing cystoprostatectomy had no clinical evidence of BPH (asymptomatic BPH). The age and prostate size of the TURP/pharmacotherapy versus cystoprostatectomy groups were similar.

The prostatic specimens were fixed in 10% phosphate-buffered formalin for 8-36 h before paraffin embedding. The fixed tissues were processed through xylene, embedded in paraffin, and sectioned at 6 μm for hematoxylin and eosin staining. The stained sections were used for determination of stromal, epithelial, and glanular luminal area densities. For each slide examined, coordinates were determined with a micrometer on the microscopic stage and areas were selected by randomized coordinate mapping. A total of 20 fields was examined for each histologic section representing 5%–25% of the cross-sectional area on the slide. Prior to performing the morphometric analysis, a staff pathologist confirmed the histologic diagnosis of BPH in all specimens.

The instrument that was used for the quantitative image analysis in this study was the R & M Biometrics Bioquant MEG IV-M8 System (Nashville, Tenn.). Video images were captured from Wild-Leitz Diaplan Research Light Microscope using a 6.3X plan fluotar objective and a variolum adapter with filters for control of light intensity, color temperature, and color contrasting. The microscope is fitted with a Dage Model 70 video camera fit with a high-resolution Newvicon tube. The captured video images are displayed on a Sony RGB 12-inch color monitor and simultaneously digitized by an AT & T M-8 Targa board in a Dell System 200 personal computer. The automated analysis will be done on a Bioquant Image Analysis System (MEG IV-M8) as well as the initial statistical analysis. The volume densities for various tissue components were determined with gray-scale analysis with 256 shades of gray on digitized images with 256 lines of resolution. All of the determined values were expressed in mm^2.

The mean stroma–epithelial ratio in the TURP, open prostatectomy, pharmacotherapy and cystoprostatectomy groups were 5.1 ± 0.4, 3.2 ± 0.1, 5.7 ± 0.8, and 2.7 ± 0.1, respectively (SHAPIRO et al. 1992b). The gray density computer image analysis confirmed previous observations that BPH is primarily a stromal process. The mean stroma–epithelial ratios in the TURP/pharmacotherapy versus cystoprostatectomy groups were 5.5 versus 2.7, respectively. The morphometry study suggested that the development of clinical BPH is related to the stroma–epithelial ratio of the prostate adenoma. The age and severity of clinical BPH in the subjects undergoing TURP/pharmacotherapy versus open prostatectomy groups were similar. The mean stroma–epithelial ratio in the TURP/pharmacotherapy versus open prostatectomy groups were 5.7 and 3.2, respectively. This morphometric study suggested that the histologic composition of large prostates ultimately requiring enucleation prostatectomy and smaller prostates obtained from males with asymptomatic BPH are similar. The large prostates presumably did not cause obstruction at an earlier stage in the hyperplastic process since the histology did not predispose to obstruction.

5.6 Immunoenzymatic Staining Techniques

We have recently developed a technique for quantifying the cellular elements of the prostate (SHAPIRO et al. 1992a). The technique involves double immunoenzymatic staining and color-assisted computer image analysis. There are many immunoenzymatic staining techniques which can be used to localize antigens. We have employed the soluble enzyme immune complex method which gives excellent results on paraffin-embedded tissues (BOENISCH 1989). This technique uses a preformed soluble enzyme–antienzyme immune complex which consists of an enzyme (the antigen) and the antibody directed against the enzyme.

The primary antibody and the antibody of the enzyme immune complex are both made in the same species so the secondary antibody can link the two together. The secondary antibody must be directed against immunoglobulins of the species which produced the primary antibody and the enzyme immune complex. The secondary antibody must be added in excess to ensure binding to the primary antibody and the enzyme immune complex. This will act as to link the primary antibody to the enzyme immune complex.

This soluble enzyme immune complex method is named for the particular enzyme immune complex used. The PAP method utilizes a peroxidase–antiperoxidase complex while the APAAP method uses an alkaline phosphatase–antialkaline phosphatase complex. The PAP complex consists of three molecules of peroxidase and two antibodies against peroxidase while the APAAP complex has two molecules of alkaline phosphatase and one antibody against the enzyme.

The deparaffinized tissue sections were stained using the universal Dako double-stain kit system 40 (Dako, Carpinteria, Calif.). The kit is designed to simultaneously detect two different tissue antigens using double-immunoenzymatic staining with peroxidase–antiperoxidase (PAP) and alkaline phosphatase-antialkaline phosphatase (APAAP) techniques (Shapiro et al. 1992a, c). The smooth muscle and epithelium were labeled with rabbit anti-desmin and a mouse anti-human prostatic acid phosphatase (PSAP), respectively. The optimal dilutions for anti-desmin and PSAP were 1:500 and 1:200, respectively. The staining procedure included incubations with hydrogen peroxide and blocking serum to quench endogenous peroxidase activity and reduce nonspecific staining. The tissue sections were sequentially incubated with the following reagents: PSAP, rabbit anti-desmin, and the provided mouse APAAP immune complex and rabbit PAP immune complex. A rabbit PAP complex was linked to the rabbit anti-desmin by a secondary antibody to rabbit antibody. The PAP complex was labeled brown using the chromogen DAB. A mouse APAAP complex was linked to the mouse anti-PSAP by a secondary antibody to mouse antibody. The APAAP complex was labeled red using the chromogen fast red. The epithelium, glandular lumen, smooth muscle, and connective tissue stained red, colorless, dark brown, and light brown, respectively, using the double immunoenzymatic staining technique.

The stained tissue sections were viewed under the Wild-Leitz Microscope using the 6.3 × plan fluotar objective and a Variolum adapter. A high-resolution JVC color video camera head (TK870U) captures the image of the histologic section which is displayed on a Sony RGB 12-inch color monitor. The image is simultaneously digitized using the AT Vista inside the Dell System 220 personal computer. The automated analysis is performed by the Bioquant Image Analysis System (BQ MEG IV-Vista: R & M Biometrics, Nashville, Tenn). The BQ MEG IV-Vista is a color system image analysis which discriminates color differences of stained tissue sections. The BQ MEG IV-Vista was utilized to discriminate smooth muscle (dark brown), glandular epithelium (red), fibrous tissue (pale brown), and glanular lumina (colorless). The thresholds were set to identify each of these components of the prostate. The area densities corresponding to each of these tissue components were calculated per full screen of the Sony RGB color monitor. At least 30 different fields were examined from each tissue section. The mean percentage of smooth muscle, fibrous tissue, glandular epithelium, and glandular lumina were determined from the tissue sections obtained from eight males with symptomatic BPH.

5.7 Results of Immunoenzymatic Studies

The percent area densities of smooth muscle, connective tissue, epithelium, and epithelial lumen were 22% ± 4%, 54% ± 4%, 16% ± 6%, and 9% ± 1%, respectively. The stroma–epithelial ratio was 4.8:1. This study demonstrated that a significant component of the prostate adenoma was smooth muscle (SHAPIRO et al. 1992a).

(SHAPIRO et al. 1992c). recently reported that mouse anti-actin is a more sensitive label for prostate smooth muscle than rabbit anti-desmin. Double immunoenzymatic staining was performed on 19 transrectal biopsy specimens obtained from males with clinical BPH using mouse anti-actin/rabbit anti-human PSAP and rabbit anti-desmin/mouse anti-human PSAP. The area densities of smooth muscle, connective tissue, epithelium, and epithelial lumen in the anti-actin/anti-human PSAP stained tissues were 39% ± 3%, 38% ± 3%, 12% ± 1%, and 11% ± 1%, respectively. The area densities of smooth muscle, connective tissue, epithelium, and glandular lumen in the anti-desmin/anti-human PSAP were 19% ± 2%, 59% ± 2%, 12% ± 1%, and 11% ± 1%, respectively. These data show that the area density of anti-actin stained smooth muscle was twofold greater than anti-desmin. A direct relationship has been observed between the area density of anti-actin and anti-desmin labeled smooth muscle. Anti-actin and anti-desmin labeling was performed on different tissue sections obtained from the same prostate specimens. The apparent variability between these different smooth muscle labeling techniques reflects the inherent heterogeneity of the prostate.

5.8 Summary

The application of computer-assisted color image analysis and double immunoenzymatic staining provides an accurate and efficient methodology for determining the cellular composition of the prostate. The application of this technique to the prostate has provided important insights related to the pathophysiology of BPH.

References

Barry MJ (1990) Epidemiology and natural history of benign prostatic hyperplasia. Urol Clin North Am 17:495

Bartsch G (1977) Stereology, a new quantitative morphological approach to study prostatic function and disease. Eur Urol 3:85–95

Bartsch G, Muller HR, Boerholzer M, Rohr HP (1979) Light microscopic stereologic analysis of the normal human prostate and benign prostatic hyperplasia. J Urol 122:487–491

Boenisch T (1989) Staining methods. In: Naish SJ (ed) Handbook of immunochemical staining methods. DAKO Corporation, Carpinteria, Calif., p 13

DeKlerk DP, Coffey DS (1978) Quantitative determination of prostatic epithelial and stromal hyperplasia by a new technique: biomorphometrics. Invest Urol 16:240–245

Franks LM (1975) Benign prostatic hyperplasia: gross and microscopic anatomy. In: Grayhack JT, Wilson JD, Scherbenske MJ (eds) Benign prostatic hyperplasia. National Institutes of Health, Bethesda, Md., p 63

Shapiro E, Hartanto V, Lepor H (1992a) Quantifying the smooth muscle content of the prostate using double-immunoenzymatic staining and color assisted image analysis. J Urol 147: 1167–1170

Shapiro E, Becich MJ, Hartanto V, Lepor H (1992b) The relative proportion of stromal and epithelial hyperplasia is related to the development of symptomatic BPH. J Urol 147:1293–1297

Shapiro E, Hartanto V, Lepor H (1992c) Anti-desmin vs. anti-actin for quantifying the area density of prostate smooth muscle. Prostate 20:259–267

Siegel YI, Zaidel L, Hanmel I (1990) Morphometric evaluation of benign prostatic hyperplasia. Eur Urol 18:71–73

Weibel ER, Bolender RP (1973) Stereological techniques for electron microscopic morphometry. In: Hayat MA (ed) Principles and techniques of electron microscopy, vol 3. Van Nostrand Reinhold, New York, pp 237–296

Weibel ER, Kistler GS, Scherle WF (1966) Practical stereological methods for morphometric cytology. J Cell Biol 30:23

6 Evaluation of End Points in the Treatment of Benign Prostatic Hyperplasia

REGINALD C. BRUSKEWITZ and MORTEN RIEHMANN

CONTENTS

6.1 Introduction

Benign prostatic hyperplasia (BPH) is variously described as a histologic entity with the characteristic stromal epithelial prostatic changes, as a symptom complex referred to as prostatism which includes both irritative and obstructive-type symptoms, as nearly synonymous with prostatic enlargement, and as a urodynamic event which is heralded by progressive outflow obstruction. The obstructive sequelae are related to a decrease in urinary flow and a concomitant increase in detrusor pressure which may eventually progress to decompensation of the lower urinary tract. This may be associated with bladder changes such as trabeculation and with upper urinary tract deterioration including hydronephrosis and renal compromise.

In a given individual the symptom complex prostatism varies considerably and may be predominated by obstructive-type symptoms including a decrease in the force of the urinary stream, intermittency, hesitancy, and terminal dribbling. In addition, the so-called irritative symptoms of frequency, urgency, nocturia and, when severe, urge incontinence may be noted. This mix of symptoms

REGINALD C. BRUSKEWITZ, MD, Professor of Surgery, and MORTEN RIEHMANN, MD, Research Fellow, Department of Surgery, Division of Urology, University of Wisconsin, Clinical Sciences Center, 600 Highland Avenue, Madison, WI 53792, USA

Petrovich/Baert (Eds.)
Benign Prostatic Hyperplasia

is quite variable as well. As will be described, prostatic enlargement is also quite variable with some men with the BPH complex having substantial prostatic enlargement whereas in others the degree of change in prostate size is minimal or nonexistent.

As new treatments emerge for the treatment of BPH, a variety of different measures are available with which to assess their efficacy. So-called objective measures including urodynamic studies of detrusor pressure and urinary flow rate are readily available, and a number of measures of deterioration of the urinary tract, including postvoid urinary residual, bladder trabeculation, and upper tract hydronephrosis measured radiographically are also commonly utilized. A very frustrating aspect of BPH assessment is the fact that these parameters vary considerably within a given patient, with some suggesting the BPH complex and others not. These same variables may change over either a short or a longer period of time in a given individual. Certainly within a group of patients undergoing assessment for BPH there is wide variability in these measurements. This presentation will summarize some of these variabilities and highlight some of the controversies regarding the assessment of BPH and the clinical efficacy of various treatments and trials in BPH.

6.2 Acute Urinary Retention

There is no agreement on whether patients with acute total urinary retention should be considered in clinical trials of various alternative managements for BPH. As an example, prostatic stents are often championed as a treatment for men in retention who are otherwise unfit for prostatectomy. The same has been true for prostatic hyperthermia or thermal therapy. On the other hand, drug therapies are often avoided in patients in acute urinary retention, with authors often stating that these patients deserve standard most effective treatment, i.e., prostatectomy. For some drugs such as antiandrogens, which have a slow mechanism of action, this would seem to be appropriate, whereas for other short-acting drugs such as α-blockers the same may not be true.

Acute urinary retention is often viewed as a final event in the progression of the BPH process. In fact, not all patients in acute urinary retention may require surgical treatment. Of 70 patients with acute retention and BPH who were initially treated by catheter drainage, 70% had recurrent retention within a week, and 90% required treatment (although did not necessarily develop retention) within 1 year (BREUM et al. 1982). Another study indicated that of patients presenting in acute urinary retention who did not undergo immediate prostatectomy, 58% required an operation within the first 3 months; requiring an operation is apparently not synonymous with recurrent retention in this report (CRAIGEN et al. 1969). These two studies highlight the importance of defining who, in fact, is relieved of obstruction and who progresses to additional treatment despite having had relief of obstruction. Unless this is clarified in a report, it is difficult to be certain how successful the intervention may have been.

6.3 Prostate Size

Recent reports on the efficacy of alternative treatments for BPH have often hinted that selection based on prostate size is important. It has become commonplace to exclude patients with a certain overall prostate size or configuration from entering into a clinical trial. In the case of balloon dilation, patients with smaller prostates and no median lobe enlargement are often selected, perhaps for technical reasons, because of the inability of the prostatic balloon to accommodate a particular configuration. On the other hand, transurethral resection of the prostate (TURP) appears to be less sensitive to size, and patients with small and large prostates fare approximately equally well from a urodynamic and symptomatic standpoint over the short run (Jensen et al. 1983b). However, patients with smaller prostates have an increased incidence of bladder neck contracture over the immediate or longer range (Bruskewitz et al. 1986).

Estimation of prostatic size by digital palpation alone is an unreliable guide to the determination of actual prostatic size. It appears that transrectal ultrasonography and more expensive approaches such as magnetic resonance imaging and computed tomography give more reliable estimations of overall size. It is clear that prostate size does not correlate well with symptomatology or postoperative outcome (Castro et al. 1969; Andersen et al. 1979).

It would seem reasonable to initially include patients with all size and configuration of prostate in the treatment scheme and to eliminate certain categories after the initial trial establishes that patients with that size or configuration clearly do not do well. This has been the case with transurethral incision of the prostate, which would serve as a good model for other emerging technologies. It would also be important to carefully analyze the data to conclude that a particular prostate size is not applicable for treatment rather than have an investigator make a rough estimate of this, and then have it become ingrained in future trials and treatments. In that prostate size does not correlate well with symptoms or outcome of surgical treatment, it is not likely that the patient should be excluded from an emerging treatment initially. This approach would prevent a reduction in generalizability occurring as new treatments emerge.

6.4 Postvoid Urinary Residual

Benign prostatic hyperplasia associated with chronic outflow obstruction is believed to be accompanied by slowly increasing volumes of postvoid urinary residual. As the volume increases the bladder decompensates, leading to retention or overflow incontinence and eventually hydronephrosis and renal compromise. While excretory urography used to be the predominant method of assessing the bladder volume following urination, it is now clear that this is a relatively inaccurate measurement. Catheterization is accurate to within 30 cc of actual postvoid residual measured by radionucleotide studies. However, in ongoing clinical trials where repeated catheterizations may be necessary, this invasion is not acceptable because of the slight chance of introducing urinary tract infection and a decrease in patient compliance. The current standard for studies is ultrasonic measurement, often with a hand-held portable unit.

Elevated postvoid residual of urine as a measure of obstruction or as an efficacy parameter is a controversial measurement in that residual urine might originate from conditions other than outflow obstruction (Abrams and Griffiths 1979; Bruskewitz et al. 1982). Furthermore, severely obstructed patients may present with no postvoid urinary residual, and the absence of residual urine is not proof that treatment can be postponed.

However, the biggest issue with postvoid urinary residual volumes and studies of efficacy of treatments for BPH is that in the same patient on repeated measurements over the short term, residual urine volumes may vary greatly. For this reason, the study is not reproducible. Nor does residual urine correlate with symptoms or urodynamic studies suggesting obstruction. Postvoid urinary residual should probably be relegated to a safety measure in BPH trials and not looked on as an efficacy measure.

6.5 Urodynamic Studies

6.5.1 Uroflowmetry

As indicated earlier, BPH may be viewed as a syndrome leading to bladder outflow obstruction. Uroflow studies generally using an electronically calibrated uroflow machine are widely used both in clinical practice and in the conduct of BPH clinical trials.

Uroflowmeters allow recording of voided volume, peak urine flow rate, mean urine flow rate, and flow as well as voiding time. Others will calculate the time to peak flow, but in general the voided volume and peak urinary flow rate are of the greatest utility and are the most widely utilized.

Authors have indicated that a maximum flow rate of 10 ml/s in older men with symptoms of prostatism is usually related to outflow obstruction; perhaps 90% of men would actually be found to be obstructed if additional urodynamic studies were performed (Abrams and Griffiths 1979). Patients with a maximum flow rate of 10–15 ml/s may or may not be obstructed, whereas those with flows in excess of 15 ml/s are considerably less likely to be obstructed and are far less likely to respond to surgical treatment. As a general rule of thumb, approximately 90% of patients with flow rates less than 15 ml/s will respond favorably to TURP in terms of symptom scores and patient global assessment whereas patients with flow rates of greater than 15 ml/s can be expected to have improvement in symptom scores and patient global assessment in about 60% of cases. This has led people advocating the use of flowmetry to suggest that TURP be restricted to patients with flow rates less than 15 ml/s or to those with flow rates greater than 15 ml/s but with documented outflow obstruction on pressure-flow studies (GERSTENBERG et al. 1982; IVERSEN et al. 1983). It is not clear that the less morbid alternate therapies should necessarily follow this directive. Nonetheless, studies have usually restricted patients in entry to flow rates less than 15 ml/s or perhaps less than 12 ml/s peak urine flow rate. While it is true that if you wish to be able to show statistical improvement in peak urinary flow rates you should pick patients with lower flows, it may not be appropriate to restrict these treatments to patients with these lower flows.

Other concerns regarding uroflowmetry include the observation that studies in asymptomatic elderly men have shown that a substantial portion of men in this age group have urinary flow rates which are well within the probably obstructed range. Despite the fact that they may be obstructed, they are asymptomatic and probably not likely candidates for treatment, be it surgical or alternative therapy (JØRGENSEN et al. 1986). These same investigators have shown that there is considerable intraindividual variation in peak flow rate when multiple testing is done over a very short period. The fact that asymptomatic males may be obstructed and that there is considerable intraindividual variability in peak flow rates decreases the utility of this measure as a parameter for BPH treatment.

Other concerns include the possible effect of voided volume on the peak urinary flow rate. Flow nomograms and corrected flow formulas have been constructed to correct for possible effects of voided volume on the peak urinary flow rate. It appears that over the range of 150–600 ml the effect of volume on peak flow in the male with presumed BPH and obstruction is negligible and can be ignored. However, there is a minimum voided volume, probably 150 ml, below which there can be considerable effects of volume on peak flow rate. Patients should probably be required to void a minimum of 150 ml before the flow curve is interpretable, and this should probably constitute an entry criteria for BPH clinical trials.

There also may be a learning curve for the individual with repetitive testing – with repeat uroflow testing the peak flow improves. Although investigators have been split as to the presence of this learning curve, it may be that up to two to three voids may result in progressive improvement despite no effect from voided volume. It may be reasonable to require three baseline studies upon entering a trial.

A final point about uroflow testing would be that following TURP, patients may have improvement in symptoms, but not improvement in flow or vice versa (although the latter is far less common). This association between peak urinary flow rate and symptomatology following surgical treatment has been observed for other alternative therapies for BPH as well. It would seem that this well-established finding would decrease the utility of peak urine flow testing in BPH trials. Nonetheless, uroflowmetry must be included in the clinical trials and computed as an efficacy measure.

6.5.2 Pressure–Flow Studies

There are two camps on the utility of pressure–flow studies; one believes that these studies are essential, while the other opts for minimal urodynamic studies such as uroflowmetry in conjunction with symptom analysis.

Pressure–flow studies are performed when bladder pressure is measured via a urethral or suprapubic catheter during voiding. Urine flow is measured simultaneously. The most frequent parameters studied are intravesical pressure, which implies the total pressure in the bladder, and detrusor pressure, which is the subtraction of intravesical pressure minus abdominal pressure measured with a rectal sensor. The bladder opening pressure, maximum intravesical and detrusor pressure, and pressure at maximum flow are often measured, but it is the pressure at maximum flow which appears to be most important. With obstruction the pressure within the bladder elevates during voiding, but other dysfunctions, including deficient relaxation of the external sphincter or bladder neck obstruction, would cause similar findings. A pressure–flow relationship is sometimes used to calculate a urethral resistance factor also. But there are many different formulas for this urethral resistance calculation, and this study is probably not as useful (BATES et al. 1979).

With surgical treatment of BPH such as TURP, the flow tends to improve and the detrusor pressure tends to decrease. However, this finding is quite variable, with some patients not showing any significant change in intravesical pressure. None of these intravesical measurements has been found to be predictive of successful outcome following TURP when studied prospectively (JENSEN et al. 1983a).

One of the primary issues in a large prospective clinical trial is the need to have a reproducible test which can be performed repeatedly over time in subjects under study. Although urodynamic studies are moderately reproducible, the need to repetitively catheterize patients for this study raises problems of patient compliance. Our own experience has been that patients do not submit to repeated catheterizations and this progressively reduces the number of patients available for follow-up study. The utility of pressure–flow study in clinical trials is very controversial, with some groups advocating such studies to clearly define outlet obstruction, whereas other groups find its utility or practicality less favorable.

Another issue is that as BPH becomes more narrowly defined as a syndrome of obstruction in patients with other manifestations of BPH, such as increased prostatism symptoms consistent with the disease, more patients are excluded from a trial who might in fact benefit from a particular treatment, including some of the less invasive approaches.

At this time, most large-scale studies are not employing pressure–flow studies, and it is certainly not mandatory that they be performed to document the efficacy of a treatment.

6.5.3 Cystometry

The cystometrogram is a bladder-filling study (as opposed to a pressure–flow voiding study) which allows documentation of bladder compliance capacity and checks for the presence of uninhibited detrusor contraction. The terms unstable, uninhibited, and bladder hyperreflexia have been applied when a patient cannot willfully suppress an increase in intravesical pressure secondary to a bladder contraction.

Uninhibited contractions can be associated with many neurologic disorders including Parkinson's disease and following cerebrovascular accidents, whereas uninhibited contractions also occur with advancing age, with BPH, and in the absence of outflow obstruction. The incidence of uninhibited bladder contractions in healthy asymptomatic elderly males range between 25% and 53% (Andersen et al. 1978; Jensen et al. 1984).

The etiology of unstable bladder contractions in BPH is not well understood. It is clear that uninhibited detrusor contractions contribute to the symptom complex of prostatism and may be associated with the irritative symptoms of urge incontinence, nocturia, and frequency, but the degree of correlation with these symptoms is generally poor (Frimodt-Møller et al. 1984). Postprostatectomy uninhibited contractions are found in 20%–30% of patients, having been found preoperatively in 50%–65% (Abrams et al. 1979; Andersen 1976; Chalfin and Bradley 1982; Andersen 1982). Some reports show that postoperative, uninhibited bladder contractions are associated with symptom treatment failure (Cote et al. 1981; Arams 1980). Generally there is a feeling that symptoms of prostatism associated with uninhibited contractions without obstruction should not be treated surgically. In addition, as pointed out, patients who have uninhibited contractions after transurethral resection for BPH are much more likely to have symptomatic treatment failure and failure by patient global assessment. In view of these problems that have been identified with standard surgical treatment of BPH in the presence of uninhibited detrusor contractions, there are many patients who fall into this category of significant irritative-type voiding symptoms who, according to one school of thought, should not be considered for surgery. It would be prudent to investigate these patients with less invasive alternative treatment and clinical trials by performing cystometrographic studies and documenting the presence of obstruction with uroflowmetry at least. This would then investigate the possible utility of these new treatments in this particular symptom complex which has not fared well with surgical treatment. A subset of patients should be investigated with cystometric studies before and after alternative treatment on a prospective basis.

6.6 Symptom Scores

In the beginning of this century surgeons were mainly concerned with and focused on resectability, operative techniques, and end points like operative mortality, morbidity, and complication rates. Gradually patients' subjective feelings played an increasing role in the choice of treatment, and patients' responses were more often monitored through follow-up studies and systematic questionnaires.

A number of BPH-related symptom scores have been developed and utilized in the last several decades (Castro et al. 1969; Abrams 1977; Boyarsky et al. 1977; Madsen and Iversen 1983; Peters and Walsh 1987; Fowler et al. 1988; Epstein et al. 1991; Barry et al. 1992). All of the questionnaires referenced are probably sensitive to clinical BPH.

Ideally symptom-scoring schemes for evaluation of BPH measure physical health in terms of urinary complaints, bother due to these symptoms, and the possible impact on perception of quality of life. The criteria listed in Table 6.1 should be met. Quality of life traditionally is a global measure and a much broader concept than health. Quality of life provides an aggregate for dimensions such as daily living and function, activity, health, and outlook.

The Fowler Index is validated though items such as quality of urinary stream and nocturia are not included in the questionnaire. Besides the Fowler Index, two other questionnaires, Epstein and Barry, have been validated. All of these three scores also measure bother due to urinary symptoms. Validity can be broadly defined as the ability of a score to measure what is claims to measure. Validity can further be subclassified in categories such as content, construction, and discriminative ability of the questionnaire. Validity is often determined by examining the relationship of the score or item to a variety of other items (Cronbach 1951).

The AUA Symptom Score has recently been introduced and has been extensively validated in more than 200 BPH patients and more than 100 control subjects. The validation process began with the construction of 15 questions covering BPH symptoms. Additional questions about the degree of bother from the urinary symptoms, sexual function, and the impact on quality of life were

Table 6.1. Criteria for BPH symptom scores

1. Questions should be exhaustive, mutually exclusive, and reflect areas of importance for the patient, and be relative to BPH and prostatism.
2. The questionnaire should be reliable and have a high test–retest reliability.
3. The questionnaire should be discriminative.
4. The questionnaire should be capable of being self-administered.
5. A validated bothersome score should be included.
6. Health-related quality of life questions should include validated questions about daily living and sexual and social function.

presented to the patients as well. Six questions that correlated best with each other and the global questions were statistically selected as a tentative symptom index. Hesitancy was not an item identified by these highly correlated questions, but was regarded a classic symptom of BPH and was added to the index. The symptom score was believed to be sensitive to clinical changes and met five of the six criteria listed in Table 6.1. Generally, patients with scores of 7 or less have mild symptoms, patients with scores of 8–19, moderate symptoms, and patients with scores of 20–35, severe symptoms.

A review of the symptom scores identifies considerable variability in the way in which questions are presented covering the same item. As an example, nocturia is rated by some score systems as the number of voidings each night (Abrams 1977; Madsen and Iversen 1983; Peters and Walsh 1987; Epstein 1988). Boyarsky adds that the patient has to awaken at night because of the need to void, while Barry adds how many times the patient typically got out of bed to void. While these different methods of asking questions about nocturia might present the same data, they as well may not.

The Madsen and Boyarsky questionnaires have been the most frequently utilized. Obstructive and irritative scores are substratified, but quality of life and a bothersome index are not included in these scores. The lack of validation and the absence of a bothersome index detract from these symptom score systems. As an example, a patient who gets up to void five or six times per night may be terribly bothered by this and insist on treatment, while the next patient feels this is totally acceptable and does not seek relief.

The validated symptom indices are designed to be self-administered whereas the others are not. A questionnaire which is not self-administered induces potential bias from the interviewer, particularly if the interviewer is not blinded as to the treatment given, such as in a randomized trial.

The need for outcome indicators is obvious in order to provide reliable data from clinical studies, from which can be derived guidelines for offering patients the optimal therapy. Many BPH symptom score questionnaires have been introduced; this has resulted in some confusion when interpreting and comparing results from different studies. Though reasonably well-validated questionnaires are now available, there are still some important questions to be addressed and some limitations for comparison of outcomes. For instance, may a nonuniform follow-up time be a potential source of bias? This can create difficulties in interpretation as one may look at outcomes of a selected group of patients who survived and whose symptoms and postoperative complications have resolved. Comparison across studies also may be difficult because of case mix, operative procedures, stage or degree of disease, and age. Older people generally seem to suffer more losses than younger people when exposed to similar stresses. Symptom indices for different age, sex, race, geographic, and socioeconomic groups of patients have to be assessed. Frequently no baseline preintervention measurements are made in clinical studies. Another important consideration is the ease of usage of a symptom score. An index may be too difficult to use because too many questions are asked or because of the possibility of misunderstanding, though the initial series of studies showed excellent validation. When assessing quality of life, the concept of good quality has a different meaning for different people in different places and at different times.

The ultimate applicability of the AUA questionnaire is an issue which only can be assessed when it has been extensively evaluated in a broad spectrum of different groups of patients.

6.7 Conclusions

Usually urodynamic tests are performed to confirm the clinical impression, but also to evaluate parameters that might alter diagnosis or treatment. The ultimate goal of urodynamic investigations in BPH patients is that these tests identify men with bladder outlet obstruction, and among those, the fraction who would benefit from intervention. However, there is controversy about the need for urodynamic procedures in the assessment of infravesical obstruction (GAMMELGAARD et al. 1983; HINMAN 1979).

Symptoms correlate poorly with more objective measurements of bladder outlet obstruction. This implies the need for an alternative form of objective data confirming infravesical obstruction or other factors, such as detrusor dysfunction unrelated to BPH. Though patients with maximum flow rates greater than 15 ml/s generally have poorer postoperative results, more than 50% of patients with the worst urodynamic combination – high peak flow rates combined with no elevation of detrusor pressure during flow, and uninhibited bladder contractions – still have a favorable outcome following TURP. This implies that the presently used schemes for using urodynamic investigations to select patients for treatment leave much to be desired.

In the design of a clinical trial it is important to be prospective and precise as the trial is designed. The preceding discussion about symptom score indices highlights the fact that careful attention to detail, validation, and reproducibility are important criteria when designing the study and subsequently determining efficacy in all parameters being investigated. Ideally, studies should be prospective, controlled, and blinded, and the data presented in a complete and statistically acceptable format to allow the reviewer to come to meaningful determinations about the specific alternative therapy for BPH.

References

Abrams PH (1977) Prostatism and prostatectomy: the value of urine flow rate measurement in the preoperative assessment for operation. J Urol 117: 70–71

Abrams PH (1980) Investigation of postprostatectomy problems. Urology 15: 209–212

Abrams PH, Griffiths DJ (1979) The assessment of prostatic obstruction from urodynamic measurements and from residual urine. Br J Urol 51: 129–134

Abrams PH, Farrar DJ, Turner-Warwick RT, Whiteside GC, Feneley RCL (1979) The results of prostatectomy: a symptomatic and urodynamic analysis of 152 patients. J Urol 121: 640–642

Andersen JT (1976) Detrusor hyperreflexia in benign infravesical obstruction. A cystometric study. J Urol 115: 532–534

Andersen JT (1982) Prostatism. III. Detrusor hyperreflexia and residual urine. Clinical and urodynamic aspects and the influence of surgery on the prostate. Scand J Urol Nephrol 16: 25–30

Andersen JT, Jacobsen O, Worm-Petersen J, Hald T (1978) Bladder function in healthy elderly males. Scand J Urol Nephrol 12: 123–127

Andersen JT, Nordling J, Walter S (1979) Prostatism. I. The correlation between symptoms, cystometric and urodynamic findings. Scand J Urol Nephrol 13: 229–236

Barry MJ, Fowler FJ Jr, O'Leary MP, Bruskewitz RC, Holtgrewe HL, Mebust WK, Cockett ATK, The Measurement Committee of the American Urological Association (1992) The American Urological Association's symptom index for benign prostatic hyperplasia. J Urol 148: 1549–1557

Bates P, Bradley WE, Glen E, et al. (1979) The standardization of terminology of the lower urinary tract function. J Urol. 124: 551–554

Boyarsky S, Jones G, Paulson DF, Prout GR Jr (1977) A new look at bladder neck obstruction by the Food and Drug Administration regulators: guidelines for investigation of benign prostatic hypertrophy. Trans Am Assoc Genitourin Surg 68: 29–32

Breum L, Klarskov P, Munck LK, Nielsen TH, Nordestgaard AG (1982) Significance of acute urinary retention due to infravesical obstruction. Scand J Urol Nephrol 16: 21–24

Bruskewitz RC, Iversen P, Madsen PO (1982) Value of postvoid residual urine determination in evaluation of prostatism. Urology 20: 602–604

Bruskewitz RC, Larsen EH, Madsen PO, Dørflinger T (1986) Three-Year follow-up of urinary symptoms after transurethral resection of the prostate. J Urol 136: 613–615

Castro JE, Griffiths HJL, Shackman R (1969) Significance of signs and symptoms in benign prostatic hypertrophy. Br Med J II: 598–601

Chalfin SA, Bradley WE (1982) The etiology of detrusor hyperreflexia in patients with infravesical obstruction. J Urol 127: 938–942

Cote RJ, Burke H, Schoenberg HW (1981) Prediction of unusual postoperative results by urodynamic testing in benign prostatic hyperplasia. J Urol 125: 690–692

Craigen AA, Hickling JB, Saunders CRG, Carpenter RG (1969) Natural history of prostatic obstruction. A prospective survey. J R Coll Gen Pract 18: 226–232

Cronbach LJ (1951) Coefficient alpha and the internal structure of tests. Psychometrika 16: 297–334

Epstein RS, Deverka PA, Chute CG, et al. (1991) Urinary symptom and quality of life questions indicative of obstructive benign prostatic hyperplasia. Suppl Urol 38: 20–26

Fowler FJ, Wennberg JE, Timothy RP, Barry MJ, Mulley AG, Hanley D (1988) Symptom status and quality of life following prostatectomy. JAMA 259: 3018–3022

Frimodt-Møller PC, Jensen KM-E, Iversen P, Madsen PO, Bruskewitz RC (1984) Analysis of presenting symptoms in prostatism. J Urol 132: 272–276

Gammelgaard PA, Andersen JT, Meyhoff HH (1983) Clinical significance of urodynamic measurements. In: Hinman F Jr (ed) Benign prostatic hypertrophy. Springer, New York Berlin Heidelberg, pp 502–506

Gerstenberg TC, Andersen JT, Klarskov P, Ramirez D, Hald T (1982) High-flow infravesical obstruction in men: symptomatology, urodynamics and results of surgery. J Urol 127: 943–945

Hinman F Jr (1979) Urodynamic testing: alternatives to electronics. J Urol 121: 643–645

Iversen P, Bruskewitz RC, Jensen KM-E, Madsen PO (1983) Transurethral prostatic resection in the treatment of prostatism with high urinary flow. J Urol 129:995–997

Jensen KM-E, Bruskewitz RC, Iversen P, Madsen PO (1983a) Predictive value of voiding pressures in benign prostatic hyperplasia. Neurourol Urodyn 2:117–125

Jensen KM-E, Bruskewitz RC, Iversen P, Madsen PO (1983b) Significance of prostatic weight and prostatism. Urol Int 38:173–178

Jensen KM-E, Bruskewitz RC, Madsen PO (1984) Urodynamic findings in elderly males without prostatic complaints. Urology 24:211–213

Jørgensen JB, Jensen KM-E, Bille-Brahe NE, Mogensen P (1986) Uroflowmetry in asymptomatic elderly males. Br J Urol 58:390–395

Madsen PO, Iversen P (1983) A point system for selecting operative candidates. In: Hinman F Jr (ed) Benign prostatic hypertrophy. Springer, New York Berlin Heidelberg, pp 763–765

Peters CA, Walsh PC (1987) The effect of nafarelin acetate, a luteinizing hormone-releasing hormone agonist on benign prostatic hyperplasia. N Engl J Med 317:599–604

7 Contemporary Imaging of the Prostate

RAYMOND H. OYEN

CONTENTS

7.1 Introduction

Relatively recent changes and improvements in equipment have vastly increased the image resolution of transrectal ultrasonography (TRUS) of the prostate.

RAYMOND H. OYEN, MD, Adjunct Clinic Head, Department of Radiology, Catholic University of Leuven, Herestraat 49, 3000 Leuven, Belgium

Petrovich/Baert (Eds.)
Benign Prostatic Hyperplasia

TRUS is now routinely used for diagnosis, staging, and monitoring of prostatic cancer, as well as for guided biopsy, implantation of local radiotherapy, and urodynamic studies. New areas of technical development such as color Doppler studies, image reconstruction, and computer analysis should further increase the scope of applications for TRUS. Similar considerations account for magnetic resonance imaging (MRI) of the prostate. The development of endorectal surface coils has improved visualization of the internal structure of the prostate. MRI has thus become a valuable tool for the local staging of prostatic cancer. The value of other imaging techniques such as intravenous urography and computed tomography (CT) is of decreasing interest in patients with prostatic diseases.

This chapter focuses mainly on the normal anatomy of the prostate and on the imaging of prostatitis, benign prostatic hyperplasia, and prostatic cancer.

7.2 Normal Anatomy

A clear understanding of the normal anatomy of the prostate in several spatial planes is an important prerequisite for the interpretation of radiologic images of the prostate. Therefore, a brief review of the anatomy is necessary as it relates to the commonly used imaging techniques, i.e., TRUS and MRI.

7.2.1 Development, Gross Anatomy, and Histology (Table 7.1)

7.2.1.1 Development

The prostate develops from the pelvic portion of the urogenital sinus in the 11th week of gestation (WILSON 1970). Multiple endodermal buds arise from the primitive urethra in the region of the entrance of the mesonephric ducts. The endodermal buds invade the surrounding mesenchyma of the urogenital sinus, which is responsible for the development of the connective tissue and muscular components of the prostate (GRAYHACK and KOZLOWSKI 1987). The central zone, however, is believed to be of wolffian duct origin (MCNEAL 1983). The gland is well differentiated by the 4th month of gestation and reaches its normal structural morphology at puberty.

7.2.1.2 The Fibromuscular Tissues

The adult prostate is a chestnut-shaped conical gland enveloped in a fibrous capsule positioned between the base of the bladder and the urogenital diaphragm. The "prostatic capsule" is in fact a laminated structure of dense connective tissue located between the glandular structures of the prostate and

Table 7.1 Details of development and histology of the prostate

	Peripheral zone (PZ)	Central zone (CZ)	Transition zone (TZ)	Peri-urethral glands (PUG)
Origin	Urogenital sinus	Intrusion of wolffian duct	Urogenital sinus	Urogenital sinus
% glandular tissue	70	20–25	5–10	< 1
Duct origin	Double row Posterolateral recesses of distal prostatic urethra	Convexity of verumontanum	Posterolateral recesses just proximal to the verumontanum	Laterally, anteriorly, and posteriorly along the proximal prostatic urethra
Extension	Base of verumontanum to apex	Verumontanum to base	Lower border of proximal sphincter	Within periurethral smooth muscle stroma
Acini	Small, round smooth walls 0.15–0.3 mm ∅	Large, irregularly contoured $\geq$ 0.6 mm ∅	0.15–0.3 mm ∅	
Stroma	Abundant loose stroma with randomly arranged muscle bundles	Compact smooth muscle fibers	Compact interlacing smooth muscles blending with anterior fibromuscular stroma and preprostatic sphincter	
Stroma/epithelium ratio	High	Intermediate	High	
Secretory cells	Pale cells	Darker granular cytoplasm	= PZ	= PZ
	Small nuclei in a uniform basal location	Moderately large nuclei in different levels		
	PSA and PAP	PSA and PAP	PSA and PAP	PSA and PAP
	Substrate for pepsinogen II and tissue plasminogen?	Pepsinogen II and tissue plasminogen		
Basal cells	Flattened layer parallel to basement membrane Slender filiform dark nuclei Little or no discernible cytoplasm forming a complete envelope Proliferative compartment?			
Endocrine–paracrine cells	Paracrine function? Serotonin-containing granules Neuron-specific enolase Somatostatin, calcitonin, bombesin			
Transitional epithelium	Urethra and main prostatic ducts Cells with scant cytoplasm No maturation to umbrella cells Luminal surface consists of a single layer of secretory cells = PZ, positive for PSA and PAP stainings			

the loose periprostatic tissue. It is not a true capsule since it cannot be separated from the prostate and is incomplete (AYALA et al. 1989). The prostatic capsule is fixed to the pubic symphysis by the puboprostatic ligaments, and the endopelvic fascia or investing fascia of the levator ani muscles is attached to the lateral aspects of the prostate. The two layers of Denonvillier's fascia separate the posterior surface of the prostate from the anterior surface of the rectum. The posterior aspect of the prostatic apex and proximal urethra is attached to the anterior aspect of the rectum by the recto-urethral muscle.

The fibromuscular tissues of the prostate also include the anterior fibromuscular stroma and the preprostatic sphincter and account for approximately one-third of the prostatic mass in adults.

The anterior fibromuscular stroma is composed mainly of smooth muscle fibers that extend from the bladder neck inferolaterally around the anterior aspect of the prostatic urethra. The thickness of this apron of tissue increases distally to about the level of the verumontanum; distal to the verumontanum it becomes narrower and thinner as it approaches the apex of the prostate. Its lateral margins blend with the prostatic capsule.

The preprostatic sphincter surrounds the proximal urethral segment from the level of the bladder neck to the verumontanum and is composed of tightly packed smooth muscle fibers that are continuous with the superficial layer of the trigone. The fibers of the anterior fibromuscular stroma and the preprostatic sphincter extend across the distal urethral segment and intermingle with the striated muscle fibers that surround the distal urethral segment to form the postprostatic sphincter.

7.2.1.3 The Glandular Tissues

The urethra serves as the key anatomic reference point dividing the gland into the anterior fibromuscular portion and the posterior glandular portion (Fig. 7.1). The urethra angles approximately 35° anteriorly midway between the apex and the base of the prostate, dividing the prostatic urethra into a proximal and a distal segment. The ejaculatory ducts pass through the prostate to end in the distal urethral segment at the verumontanum or within the slit-like orifice of the prostatic utricle. Its course is nearly a direct extension of the long axis of the distal urethral segment, though usually offset a few millimeters posteriorly.

Surrounding the prostatic urethra and the prostatic sphincters, two major and two minor glandular zones are described (MCNEAL 1981). The major glandular region consists of the central zone (CZ) and the peripheral zone (PZ), while the minor zones consist of the paired transition zone (TZ) and the tiny periurethral zone (PUZ). There is more glandular tissue posterior than anterior to the urethra at the base level, while this ratio tends to equalize at the apex. Differences in acinar architecture, in cellular structure, and in stromal composition among the zones are reflected in differences in echogenicity and intensity on ultrasonography and MRI respectively.

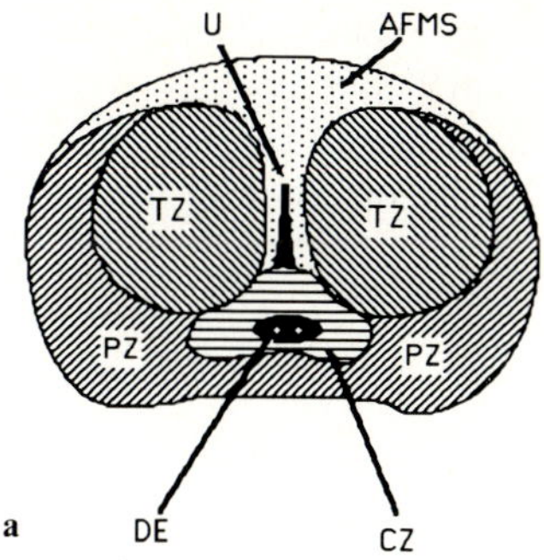

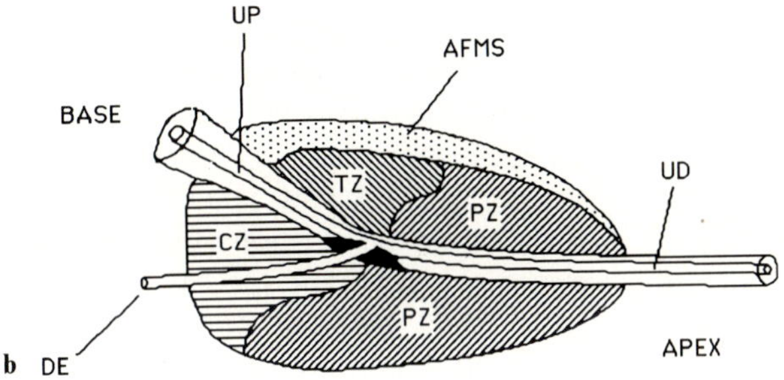

Fig. 7.1a, b. Normal anatomy. Schematic drawing of the prostate: **a** transverse section through the midportion and **b** sagittal section. The urethra (*U*) is divided into the proximal prostatic (*UP*) and distal prostatic segment (*UD*) and is surrounded by sphincters. The central zone (*CZ*) has a pyramidal configuration immediately surrounding the ejaculatory ducts (*DE*) at the base. The paired transition zone (*TZ*) is located anterolaterally to the proximal prostatic urethra. The peripheral zone (*PZ*) surrounds both the TZ and the CZ from the base to the apex. The anterior surface of the prostate is covered by an apron of fibromuscular tissue: the anterior fibromuscular stroma (*AFMS*)

The PZ accounts for approximately 75% of the glandular tissue of the normal prostate. It surrounds the urethra from the verumontanum distally to the apex of the gland. The ducts of the PZ drain into the distal urethral segment between the verumontanum and the apex on a double lateral line. The PZ and TZ and the periurethral glands have fairly similar histologic appearances and are derived embryologically from the urogenital sinus. The histology of the PZ is characterized by small, smooth-walled, round acini with a stroma of loosely interwoven, randomly oriented muscle bundles.

The CZ accounts for approximately 25% of the glandular tissue of the normal prostate. Its ducts arise in a small focus on the convexity of the verumontanum and immediately surrounding the ejaculatory ducts throughout their course through the prostate. The CZ has a distinctly different histology and, as mentioned above, is derived from the wolffian ducts. Histologically, the CZ is characterized by large, irregular acini partially subdivided by intraluminal ridges and a stroma of long, tightly arranged muscle fibers.

The TZ accounts for approximately 5%–10% of the glandular tissue only. It comprises two small lobules on either side of the proximal urethral segment immediately lateral to the preprostatic sphincter. The ducts of the TZ empty into the posterolateral recesses of the proximal urethral segment at the level of the verumontanum. The histology of the TZ is identical to that of the PZ except for the stroma, which appears more compact.

The periurethral glands constitute less than 1% of the glandular tissue of the prostate and are embedded in the smooth muscle wall of the urethra entirely within the preprostatic sphincter. The ducts of these tiny glands drain into the posterolateral recesses of the proximal urethral segment.

The glands of the PUZ and the adjacent prostatic glands in the TZ are the site of benign prostatic hyperplasia and the PZ is the site of origin of the vast majority of carcinomas and of inflammation.

7.2.1.4 Areas of Anatomic Weakness

Several areas of anatomic weakness in the prostate have been recognized. These particular areas should be assessed when staging for prostatic cancer. The sites of anatomic weakness are different for the PZ and CZ, and the TZ. For the PZ and CZ they include the prostatic capsule, the entrance of branches of the neurovascular bundle at the posterolateral aspect of the gland, the trapezoid area in the apical portion of the gland, the seminal vesicle beak, the invaginated extraprostatic space accompanying the ejaculatory ducts, and the bladder neck at its junction with the CZ and TZ. The sites of weakness of the TZ include the junction of the surgical capsule and the anterior fibromuscular stroma, the apex, and the base.

There is no capsule at the bladder neck or where the ejaculatory ducts enter the prostate. The bladder neck margin of resection consists predominantly of prostatic stroma, which merges imperceptibly with the bladder musculature and the stroma of the seminal vesicles.

The ejaculatory ducts and the intraglandular part of the seminal vesicles produce a site of anatomic weakness due to the absence of an encompassing capsule. The seminal vesicles and ejaculatory ducts are separated from the glandular elements of the CZ by only loose connective tissue, an inward extension of the extraprostatic space, which is called the "invaginated extraprostatic space." Thus a path exists in the center of the gland connecting the extraprostatic space at the base with the apical portion of the gland at the verumontanum.

Another area of anatomic weakness is to be found at the apex of the prostate, where the prostatic capsule is thin or even absent. Consequently there is a more intimate admixture of glandular tissue with extraprostatic sphincteric striated muscle. A distinct area can be described bounded by the PZ proximally, the membranous urethra anteriorly, the rectourethral muscle distally, and the serosal surface of the rectum posteriorly. Because of its shape it is known as the "trapezoid area."

The entrance of branches of the neurovascular bundle at the dorsolateral aspect of the gland in fact creates other "invaginated extraprostatic spaces" along which tumor spread likely occurs. It has indeed been shown that extracapsular extension can occur exclusively in the perineural spaces at the level of a cranial and caudal (apical) nervous plexus emerging from the neurovascular bundle (STAMEY et al. 1988; VILLERS et al. 1989).

Finally another architectural particularity is the presence or the absence of an anterior commissure (MYERS et al. 1987), i.e., the development of glandular tissue anterior to the urethra. When the anterior commissure is absent the ventral aspect of the distal prostatic urethra is located more cranially (the anterior notch). This has consequences during radical prostatectomy since transection of the urethra at this level can result in a portion of the posterior apical prostate (and tumor) being left behind. In prostates with a well-developed anterior commissure this problem does not exist.

7.2.1.5 Blood Supply

A branch of the prostatovesical trunk, the prostatic artery, serves as the main blood supply to the prostate. The prostatovesical trunk is a variable branch from the internal pudendal, inferior vesical, and superior or middle rectal arteries. The prostatic artery courses along the lateral surface of the prostate, giving off several branches that further divide into the external capsular branches, which in turn further divide into the external capsular branches and internal urethral branches (MULDOON and RESNICK 1990). The venous drainage of the prostate occurs via the lateral capsular veins, the venous channels along the anterior inferior aspect of the prostate, and the veins of the vasa deferentia. The capsular veins drain to Santorini's plexus and ultimately to the vesical and internal iliac veins.

Lymphatic channels surrounding the prostatic acini drain into the periprostatic lymphatic plexus, which in turn drains into the hypogastric, sacral, vesical, and external iliac nodes.

7.2.1.6 Innervation

The pelvic plexus of nerves supplies the parasympathetic innervation via the hypogastric nerve. The prostatic nerves course along the posterior and lateral aspect of the prostate as part of the neurovascular bundle and merge into the substance of the prostate in two distinct areas (VILLERS et al. 1989). The superior pedicle arises at the level of the base of the prostate, subdivides, then spreads along and penetrates through the prostatic capsule before arborizing into the parenchyma of approximately 80% of the gland. The inferior pedicle arises at the level of the apex, subdivides, and then spreads along and penetrates the apical surface of the prostate.

7.2.2 Normal Anatomy on Ultrasonography

The expanded use of TRUS has greatly furthered knowledge of the zonal anatomy of the prostate and permitted clinical evaluation of internal prostatic architecture (HARDT et al. 1988; JONES et al. 1989; LEE et al. 1989c). Unfortunately,

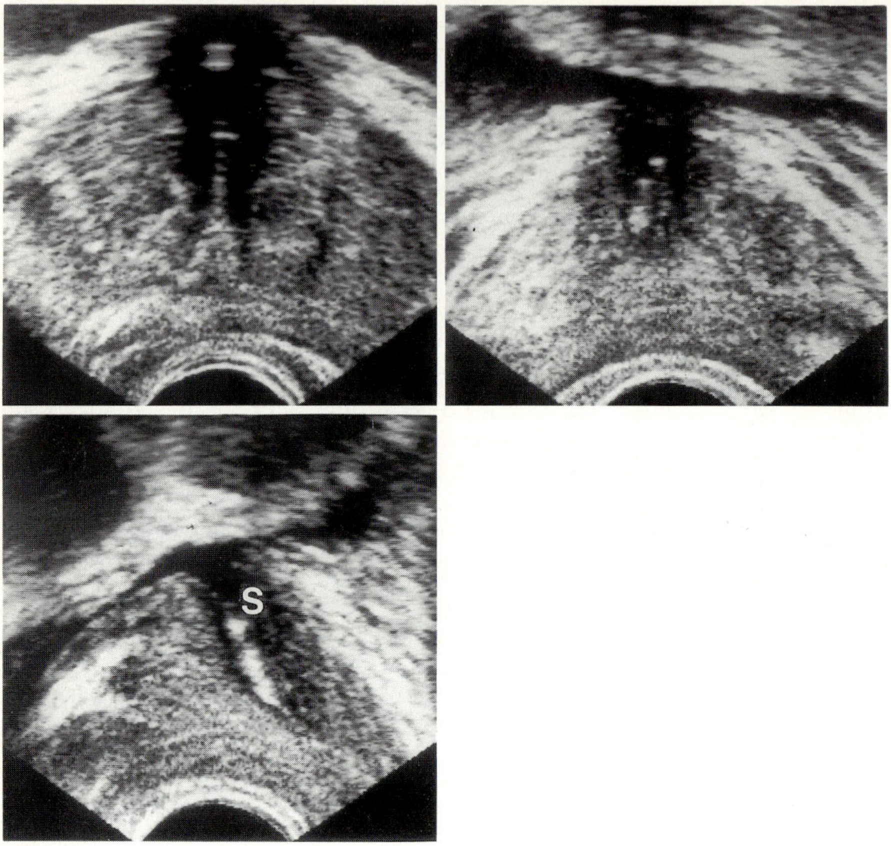

Fig. 7.2a–c. Normal anatomy. **a, b** At an oblique transverse scan through the midportion of the prostate, the verumontanum has an "Eiffel tower" appearance. The reflections are due to incrustations of the tiny periurethral glands. **c** Sagittal scan of the proximal prostatic urethra showing hyperechoic areas within the confines of the preprostatic sphincter (*S*) due to calcifications of these tiny glands

the technique is operator dependent, and the quality of the results is related directly to that person's knowledge and experience.

A variety of transrectal transducers are now available for imaging the prostate in the axial and/or the sagittal plane. Scanning techniques will vary depending upon the probe design. A very convenient probe design is an end-firing and therefore end-viewing transducer which allows multiplanar imaging in oblique coronal and sagittal projections. Some manufacturers have produced separate probes for transverse and sagittal scanning.

Most clinicians prefer the patient to be in a left lateral decubitus position for transrectal scanning. Others feel more comfortable with a lithotomy position.

In ideal circumstances, in men under the age of 30 years the zonal anatomy can be fully illustrated. The urethra and its surrounding sphincters are seen as an

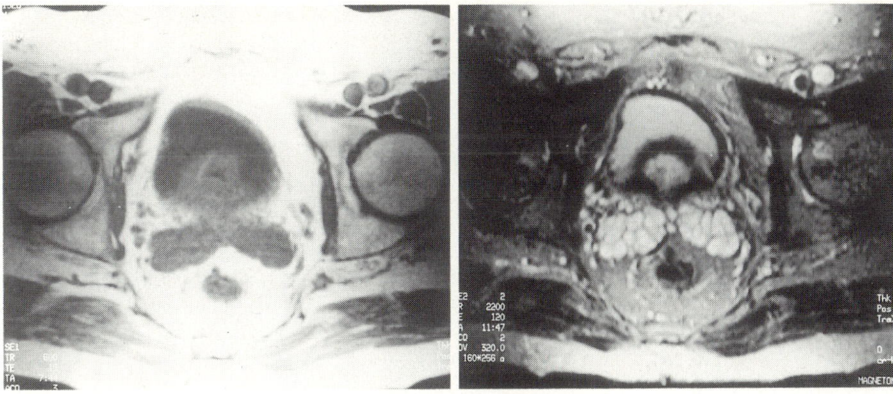

a b

Fig. 7.8a, b. Normal anatomy. T1-weighted image (TR 600, TE 15) and **b** T2-weighted image (TR 2000, TE 120) displaying the symmetric seminal vesicles as hypointense and hyperintense respectively. The prostate is enlarged and protrudes into the bladder. The veins of the periprostatic plexus are hypointense on T1- and hyperintense on T2-weighted images

The reference plane of MRI is the transverse plane. Depending upon the pathology involved, complementary coronal and/or sagittal imaging planes can be applied.

Several parameters have been reported to optimize MRI of the prostate (Poon et al. 1991). Spin-echo techniques are now used routinely. On T1-weighted images (TR 500–600 ms, TE 15–20 ms), the prostate and the seminal vesicles are of a uniform medium signal intensity (Fig. 7.8a) regardless of the magnetic field strength, and the internal zonal anatomy cannot be appreciated. T1-weighted images offer the best contrast between the prostate, seminal vesicles, periprostatic fat, blood vessels, and surrounding muscle.

On T2-weighted images (TR 2000 ms, TE 20–120 ms), the internal anatomy of the prostate becomes obvious. The intensity of the smooth muscle of the preprostatic sphincter is isointense with that of the bladder wall. Although the lumen of the proximal prostatic urethra is normally collapsed during voiding, the urethral mucosa and periurethral stroma are visible as a single hyperintense region that can be distinguished from the surrounding CZ and sphincteric muscle. This is most likely due to the high vascularity of the urethral mucosa, which in turn explains the increase in the signal intensity after injection of gadolinium. The distal prostatic urethra can never be seen. Because of its higher water content and lesser amount of stroma, the PZ displays the highest signal intensity (Fig. 7.9). The hypointense CZ can be recognized using the hyperintense ejaculatory ducts as the key reference. Distinction between the PZ and CZ is possible in 90% of males under the age of 35 years but in only 25% above that age. The intensity of the TZ increases after the injection of gadolinium, whilst the PZ does not increase in intensity.

The low-intensity large crescentic anterior region seen in the normal prostate on T2-weighted images corresponds well to the anterior fibromuscular stroma, consisting of muscle components.

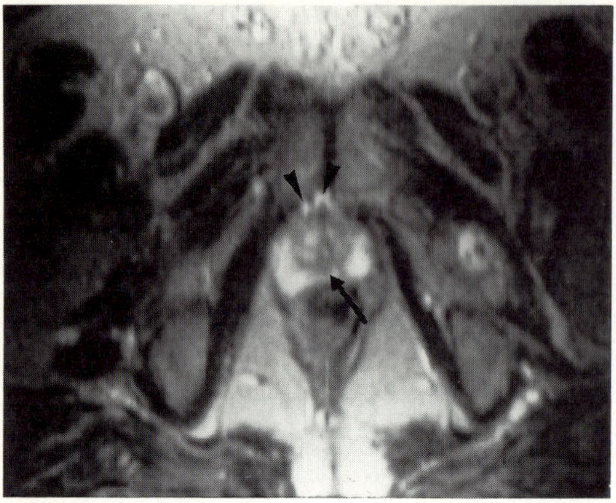

Fig. 7.9. Normal anatomy. T2-weighted image (TR 2200, TE 120). The PZ, due to its highest water content, has the highest intensity. The TZ is hyperplastic and therefore heterogeneous, the intensities depending upon the ratio of stromal to glandular hyperplasia. The CZ lies between the hyperplastic TZ and the posterior prostatic surface at the midline (*arrow*) Venous structures are seen as hyperintensities retropubically (*arrowheads*)

The prostatic capsule is discernible as a hypointense line in parts of the gland, but can be seen in no more than 50% of the cases. However, it is still not known whether the thin prostatic capsule, consisting of a few layers of tissue only, is visible with the present techniques.

The fluid in seminal vesicles has high signal intensities on T2-weighted images, whereas their walls have a lower signal (Fig. 7.8b). The internal anatomy of the seminal vesicles is well judged after injection of gadolinium because of the vascularity of the muscular wall.

The periprostatic venous plexus appears as a hyperintense structure surrounding the prostate, particularly laterally and posterolaterally (Figs. 7.8, 7.9). The plexus becomes less visible with aging, especially when the prostate is large and compresses the surrounding veins.

In older age groups, the zonal anatomy of the prostate is more clearly defined than in young patients, both because of morphologic changes in the structure of the prostate and because of physiologic changes resulting in differing zonal MR signal intensities (ALLEN et al. 1989; GEVENOIS et al. 1990). Because in older men the TZ is hyperplastic to some degree, the TZ has heterogeneous intensities on T2-weighted images, depending upon the ratio of glandular and stromal fibrosis and cystic alterations.

A technique combining ultralong TE (120–160) and a narrow bandwidth, which suppresses fat has been reported to increase the detection of prostatic carcinoma. Fat suppression can also be carried out by the inversion recovery technique using inversion times of 160–180 ms to suppress the periprostatic and intraprostatic fat signals. This allows better visualization of the boundaries of the gland. Longer TEs of up to 300 ms create an edging effect around the prostate, rectum, seminal vesicles, and other periprostatic tissues, which may be extremely useful in local staging of disease.

7.3 Inflammatory Conditions

7.3.1 Definitions

Although inflammatory conditions are common and account for a significant portion of urologic practice, they remain an ill-defined and poorly understood group of diseases. Based on clinical features together with microscopic examination of expressed prostatic fluid (EPS), four clinical types are identified: acute and chronic bacterial prostatitis, nonbacterial prostatitis, and prostatodynia (DRACH et al. 1978).

1. *Acute bacterial prostatitis* is diagnosed when positive bacterial cultures are obtained from purulent EPS in a patient with systemic signs of infectious disease. Gram-negative enteric bacteria and *Escherichia coli* account for 80% of the cases (ORLAND et al. 1985). Other common causative agents are staphylococcus and gonococcus.
2. A patient with *chronic bacterial prostatitis* has no symptoms or systemic signs of infection. Frequently there is no history of acute prostatitis at all. The diagnosis is established when the prostatic fluid is purulent by microscopic examination and bacterial cultures are positive. The diagnosis is frequently made on the basis of EPS obtained by prostatic massage.
3. *Nonbacterial prostatitis* is diagnosed when the prostatic fluid is found to be purulent by microscopic examination but bacterial cultures remain negative. Prostatitis caused by *Mycoplasma*, *Trichomonas*, and *Chlamydia* is included in this category.
4. *Prostatodynia* is in fact a diagnosis of exclusion. The patient has symptoms of prostatitis, including pelvic pain and obstructive urinary symptoms, but the prostatic fluid is not purulent on microscopic examination and bacterial cultures are negative. Prostatodynia thus is not to be considered as a real inflammatory condition but probably as an acquired functional disorder.

Granulomatous prostatitis is a histologic diagnosis characterized by infiltrates composed of histiocytes, lymphocytes, and giant cells. It accounts for approximately 1% of benign inflammatory diseases of the prostate. According to EPSTEIN and HUTCHINS (1984), three different groups can be distinguished:

1. *Specific* granulomatous prostatitis is caused by *Mycobacterium tuberculosis*, fungi, *Brucella abortus*, and *Treponema pallidum*. Tuberculosis of the prostate is seldom diagnosed clinically; it is usually an unexpected finding in biopsies, in surgical specimens, or at autopsy. It has been described after BCG instillations in the bladder, too.
2. *Nonspecific* granulomatous prostatitis is characterized by prostatic granulomas without demonstrable infectious agents. They account for at least 70% of granulomatous prostatitis. The patient presents with symptoms of acute prostatitis or is recovering from acute prostatitis. The etiology of nonspecific

granulomatous prostatitis is not clear; however, it is now believed to be the result of resolving acute bacterial prostatitis (Orland et al. 1985). In 25% of the cases this inflammatory disease is related to a transurethral resection as a consequence of glandular duct obstruction.

3. Patients with *eosinophilic* granulomatous prostatitis usually have peripheral eosinophilia and a history of asthma and mucocutaneous allergies (Towfighi et al. 1972).

Prostatic abscesses are uncommon. Most of them are seen in males with a history of urinary tract infection, *E. coli* being the most common infectious agent. Patients usually have fever and pain, but may be asymptomatic. The gland is typically enlarged and tender on digital rectal examination (DRE). Fluctuation, when present, is a diagnostic clue (Papanicolaou et al. 1987).

Prostatic calculi are common at all ages. They are located within the ducts and acini, and are thought to be the result of calcification of corpora amylacea and precipitated prostatic secretions (Klimas et al. 1985). Prostatic calcifications seem to be directly related to age, are clinically silent in most cases, and are considered to be an insignificant finding. There are no specific symptoms clearly related to calcifications even though inflammatory disease is often associated with calcifications (Bock et al. 1989). Only rarely, in younger males, is there an obvious association with acute or chronic inflammation (De la Rosette et al. 1992).

7.3.2 Ultrasonography

Seven TRUS features having a significant correlation with a diagnosis of prostatitis have been identified previously: high-density and mid-range echoes, echolucent zones, capsular irregularity and thickening, ejaculatory duct echoes, and periurethral zone irregularity (Doble and Carter 1989). It is felt, however, that several of these features are not typical for acute prostatitis and not helpful in the individual patient. Increase in prostatic volume, be it diffuse (Fig. 7.10) or focal (Fig. 7.11), scattered hypogenicity of the PZ (Fig. 7.12), and loss of the zonal differential echogenicity (Fig. 7.10) are more consistent findings in acute prostatitis, especially in younger patients. The volume of the gland, however, is not a reliable feature either, since the initial volume of the gland is mostly unknown. Sometimes TRUS is normal even in an obvious clinical setting of acute prostatitis; therefore the value of TRUS in such a setting remains doubtful. Color Doppler might be helpful in these circumstances as the inflammatory area is hypervascular compared to the normal PZ. TRUS is very useful in the diagnosis or exclusion of abscess formation, a complication of acute prostatitis. Typically a thick-walled hypoechoic area with internal scattered echoes or a fluid level may be found, usually in the PZ (Figs. 7.13, 7.15). Occasionally a previously existing (utricular or müllerian) midline cyst undergoes abscess transformation (Fig. 7.14). Transperineal TRUS-guided biopsy with an 18 g

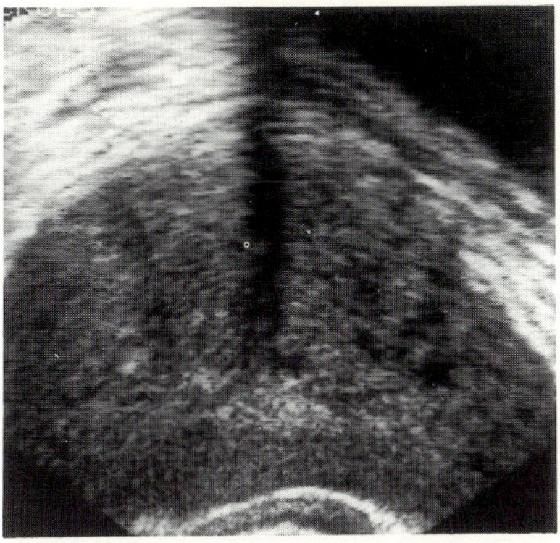

Fig. 7.10. Acute prostatitis in a 24-year-old male with a large (28 g) hypoechoic prostate without zonal differentiation. The top of the CZ is recognizable as a triangular area with normal echogenicity behind the verumontanum

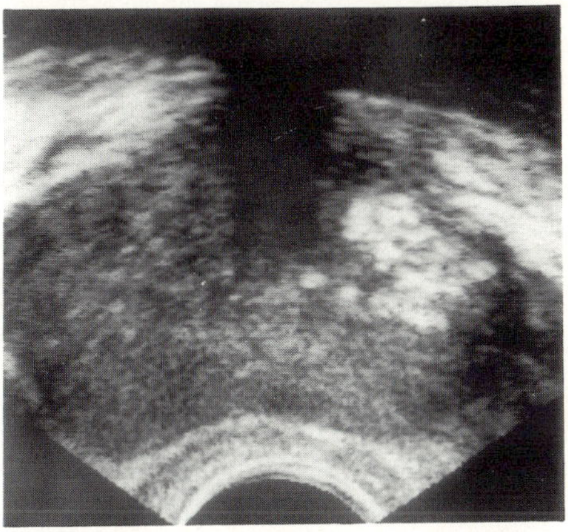

Fig. 7.11. Acute prostatitis. Asymmetric enlargement and decreased echogenicity of the right PZ in a young male with acute prostatitis

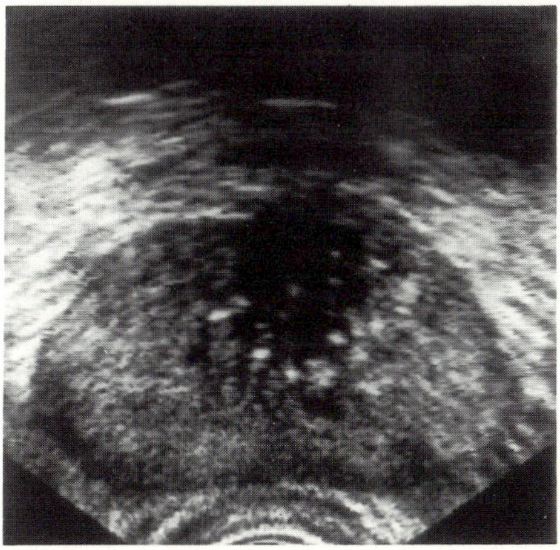

Fig. 7.12. Acute prostatitis. Transverse scan of the prostate showing scattered hypogenicity throughout the PZ. The volume of the prostate is normal. There are no areas of abscess formation

a 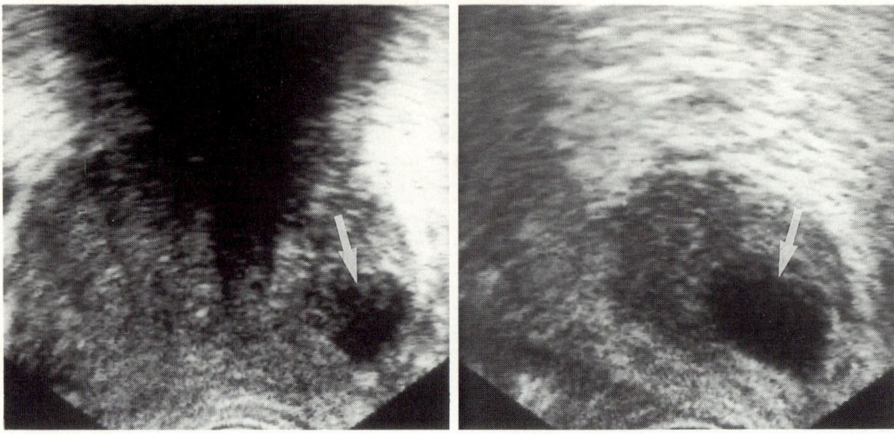 b

Fig. 7.13a, b. Prostate abscess. **a** Transverse and **b** sagittal views of a prostatic abscess (*arrow*) in the PZ on the left side. The abscess disappeared without drainage after appropriate antibiotic therapy and never recurred

needle or temporary drainage – with or without local injection of antibiotics – is effective and has become the treatment of choice compared to transurethral resection, which may cause retrograde ejaculation (Fig. 7.15) (Cytron et al. 1988; Oyen et al. 1991c).

Sonographic findings in patients with chronic prostatitis syndrome have been reported to consist in heterogeneity of the prostate, constant dilatation of the periprostatic venous plexus ($> 150\ mm^2$), dilated and elongated seminal vesicles with thickening of the inner septa, and bladder neck hypertrophy (Di Trapani et al. 1988). In contrast, in another study constant dilatation of the periprostatic venous plexus and elongation of the seminal vesicles were more commonly seen in a control group of normal men.

We rely on the heterogeneity of the PZ. This heterogeneity consists in scattered hypoechoic foci which unfortunately are indiscernible from cancer without biopsy. On the other hand, hyperechoic lesions without acoustic shadowing can be expected, too (Fig. 7.16). It should be stressed that there is no correlation between the severity of the symptoms in chronic abacterial prostatovesiculitis and the extent of changes visualized by TRUS (Christiansen and Purvis 1991). Moreover, the TRUS changes are irreversible even if the patient has been cured.

A diffusely heterogeneous hyperechoic gland, i.e., PZ, may indicate a functional organic stricture and warrant further investigations (retrograde urethrocystography or micturition urethrography) (Fig. 7.17). This especially accounts for heterogeneity of the residual peripheral gland after transurethral prostatectomy.

Cystic cavities in the PZ have been described in patients with chronic prostatitis, too. They seem to be related to fibrosis and compression of the

a b c

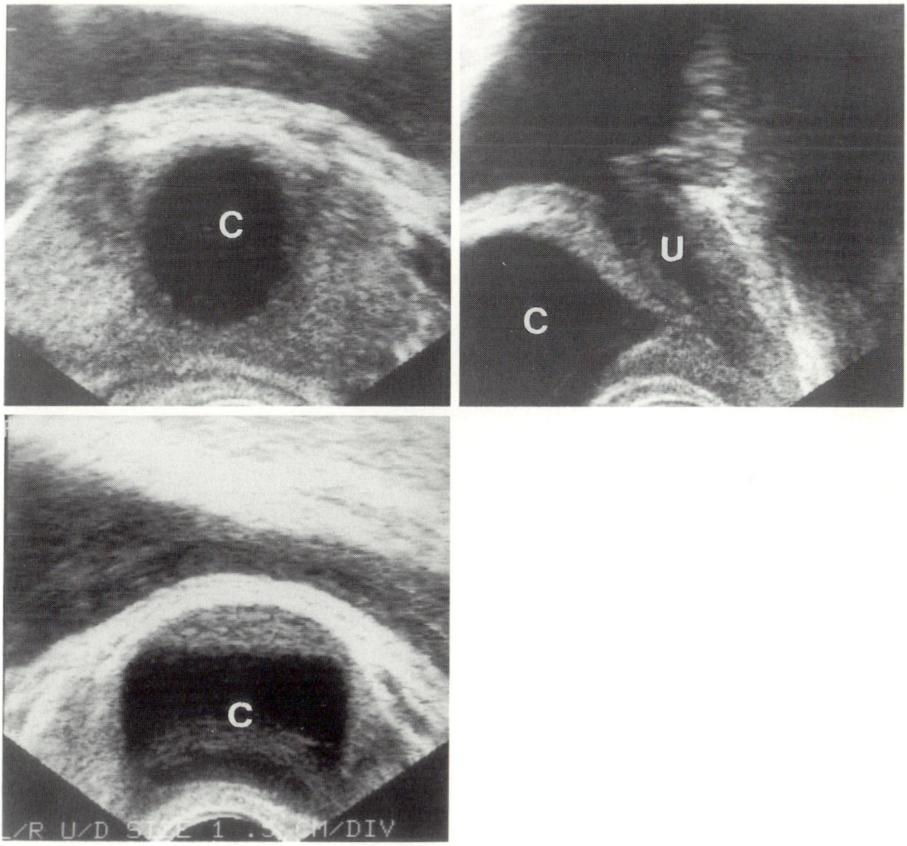

Fig. 7.14a–c. Infected midline cyst. A large midline cyst (*C*) (transverse scan, **a**) is present posterior to the urethra (*U*) and extends beyond the confines of the gland (sagittal scan, **b**). Note the rather thick wall and the fluid level in the lower part of the lesion (**c**). This was proven at transperineal biopsy to be a cyst that had undergone abscess transformation

glandular ducts (Nghiem et al. 1990). Others have reported that cystic lesions in the prostate are most frequently related to a growth phenomenon related to the presence of BPH, inflammatory conditions, or anatomic variants (Hamper et al. 1990).

In chronic vesiculitis one of the seminal vesicles appears small and hyperechoic, sometimes with calcifications (Fig. 7.18).

TRUS-guided transperineal biopsies of abnormal areas of the prostate to ascertain the role of *Chlamydia trachomatis* revealed that there is no evidence that chlamydiae are directly implicated in chronic abacterial prostatitis (Doble et al. 1989).

Chronic prostatitis can be treated with intraprostatic antibiotic injections under sonographic control in individual cases (Jimenez-Cruz et al. 1988). The

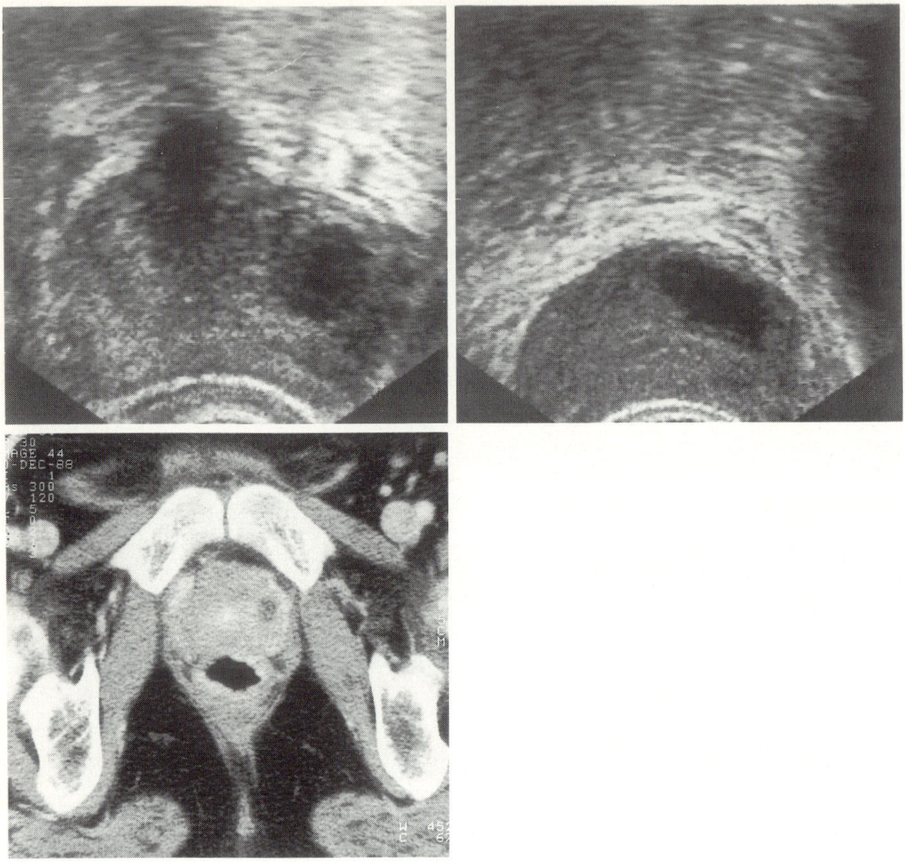

a b c

Fig. 7.15a–c. Prostatic abscess. Thick-walled hypoechoic lesion in the PZ on the left side (**a** transverse and **b** sagittal sections) in a patient with symptoms of acute prostatitis not resolving under therapy. The abscess is seen as a hypodense lesion on CT (**c**). It was successfully treated by transperineal TRUS-guided drainage and injection of antibiotics

most specific sign is the presence of hypoechoic foci in the PZ (specificity of 94%); the other criteria have a specificity of less than 50% (DOBLE et al. 1989).

Calcifications along the course of the ED in a normal-appearing gland, are more commonly seen in patients with prostatodynia (DOBLE and CARTER 1989). If there are calcifications in the TZ and the PZ is entirely normal, these calcifications are not likely to be due to prostatitis. If, however, calcifications are located in the PZ, they are probably due to prostatitis.

On DRE as well as on TRUS, nonspecific granulomatous prostatitis may be confused with carcinoma because the prostate is usually enlarged, nodular, hard, and fixed, with hypoechoic areas diffusely spread throughout the PZ (Figs. 7.19, 7.20). This distribution pattern might be the key for the differential diagnosis from a carcinoma. Focal hypoechoic lesions due to granulomatous

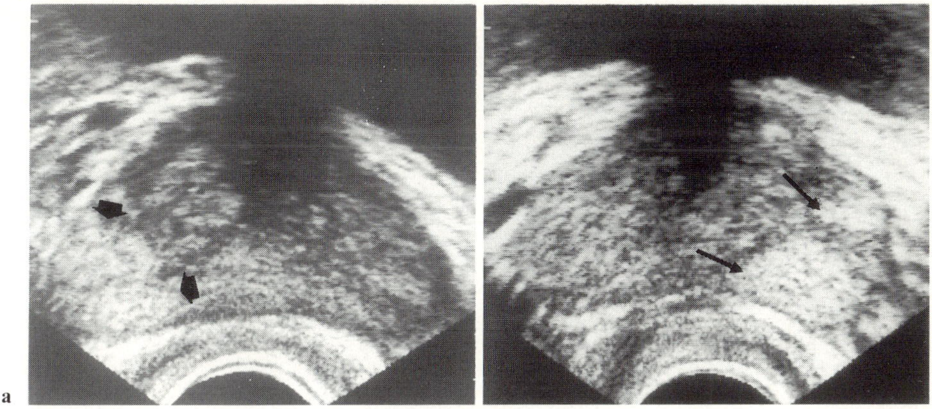

Fig. 7.16a, b. Chronic prostatitis. Hyperechoic area in the PZ on the right and left sides (*arrows*) in two different patients with chronic prostatitis

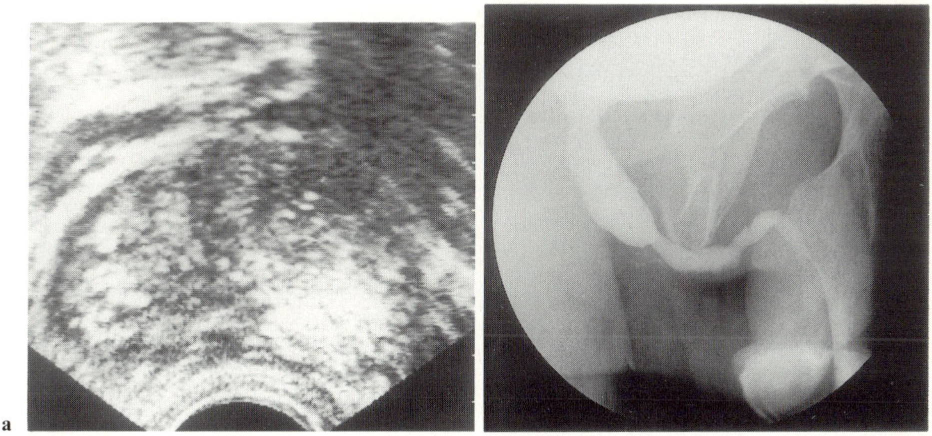

Fig. 7.17a, b. Chronic prostatitis. **a** Transverse scan of the prostate in a young male showing scattered hyperechogenicity throughout the gland, including the TZ, the CZ, and the PZ. Because of the extent of the calcifications it was thought to be due to a urethral stricture. **b** This was confirmed by micturition urethrocystography

prostatitis are indiscernible from a carcinoma without biopsy. Granulomatous prostatitis normally appears to be hypovascular on color Doppler. Hypervascularity, in contrast, may indicate the presence of a prostatic carcinoma and is an indication for TRUS-guided biopsies for further differential diagnosis (Figs. 7.21, 7.22).

The dramatically but temporarily elevated serum prostate specific antigen (PSA) levels in bacterial prostatitis can cause confusion in the diagnosis of prostatic carcinoma. Persistent elevation of the PSA levels after appropriate

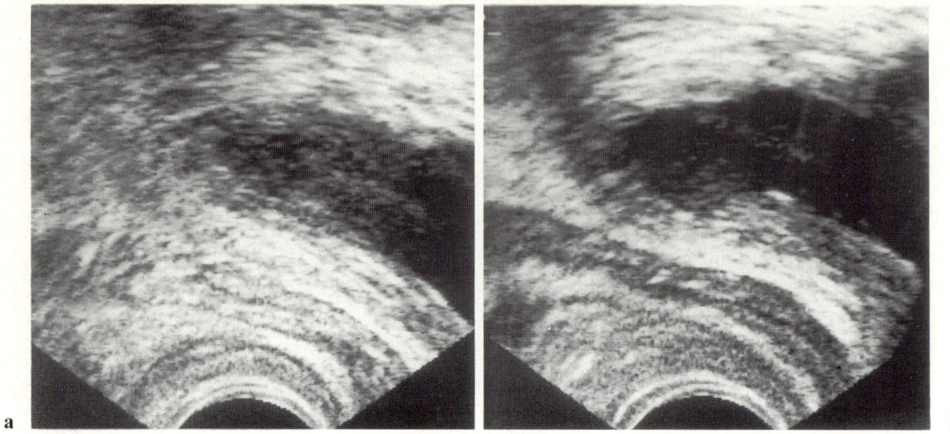

Fig. 7.18a, b. Chronic vesiculitis. Longitudinal TRUS of the seminal vesicles. Note the increased echogenicity of the left seminal vesicle (**a**) and the focally increased echogenicity of the right seminal vesicle (**b**) due to chronic vesiculitis

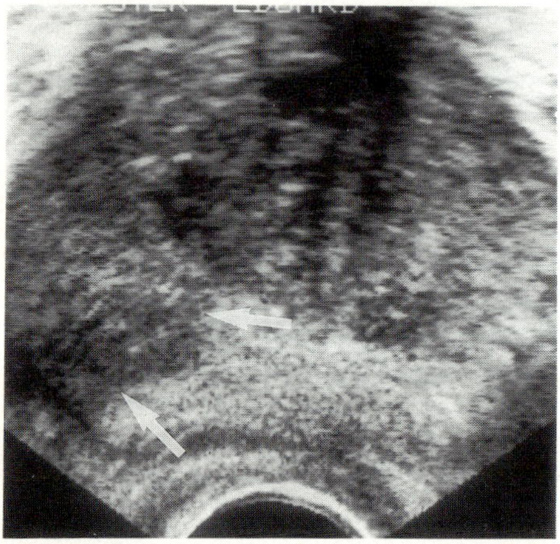

Fig. 7.19. Nonspecific granulomatous prostatitis. Transverse section of the prostate. The prostate was firm on DRE and the PZ was heterogeneous on TRUS; biopsy proved the disease to be benign. The hypogenicity in the right PZ (*arrows*) cannot be differentiated from a carcinoma in the PZ

therapy may indicate concomitant carcinoma (Neal et al. 1992) and therefore is an indication for TRUS-guided biopsies, especially in the presence of hypoechoic lesions in the PZ.

7.3.3 Computed Tomography

Computed tomography is only rarely indicated in the evaluation of patients with acute prostatitis or abscess formation. A prostatic abscess, confined to the prostate or extending into the surrounding tissues, can be seen as a hypodense mass lesion with an enhancing periphery after intravenous injection of iodinated

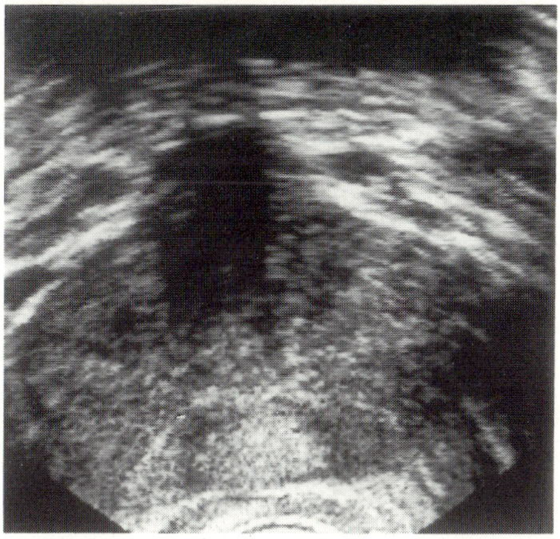

Fig. 7.20. Granulomatous prostatitis. Evolution of acute prostatitis (4 weeks): a hyperechoic area bordered by a hypoechoic halo in the PZ was proven at biopsy to be nonspecific granulomatous prostatitis. It was felt as a firm nodule on DRE

a 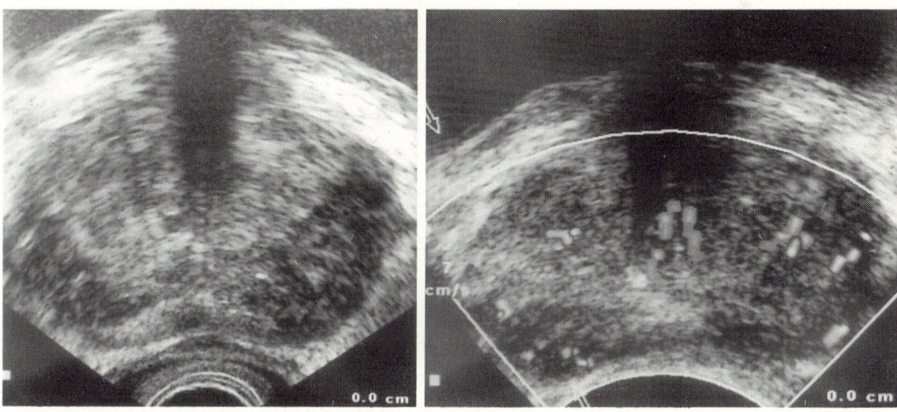 b

Fig. 7.21a, b. Granulomatous prostatitis. **a** Transverse TRUS showing scattered hypogenicity in the PZ. **b** On color Doppler ultrasonography the hypoechoic area is hypervascular (*gray blocks*). Note the normal vascularity of the periurethral area at the verumontanum. Although the distribution of the lesions in the PZ might suggest prostatitis rather than carcinoma, the two diseases are indistinguishable. Moreover both pathologies may occur simultaneously in one patient

contrast medium (Fig. 7.15) (Thornhill et al. 1987). The CT appearance of tuberculous prostatitis has occasionally been reported (Wang and Chang 1991).

Computed tomography can be used as an alternative to TRUS to guide percutaneous drainage of larger prostatic and periprostatic abscesses.

7.3.4 Magnetic Resonance Imaging

On MRI prostatic or periprostatic abscesses are seen as a hyperintense lesion on T2-weighted images. There are reports that chronic prostatitis can cause heterogeneity indistinguishable from carcinoma (Buonocore et al. 1984).

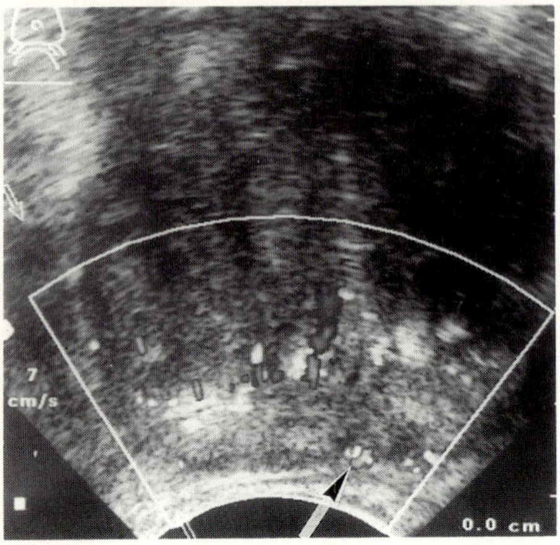

Fig. 7.22. Focal granulomatous prostatitis. Small hypoechoic, hypervascular focus in the PZ near the midline (*arrow head*), proven at biopsy to be nonspecific granulomatous prostatitis

7.4 Benign Prostatic Hyperplasia

7.4.1 Definitions

The incidence of nodular hyperplasia of the prostate varies in different parts of the world. It is high in whites and U.S. blacks, and relatively low in Asians and African blacks. This difference in incidence, as well as the higher rates among Chinese-Americans, suggests an environmental influence, in addition to genetic factors, in the origin of prostatic hyperplasia (Lytton 1983).

The etiology and pathogenesis of this tissue growth remain poorly and only partially understood. There is some evidence that disturbance of the testosterone and estrogen metabolism within the prostate is involved in the pathogenesis. Tissue concentrations of dihydrotestosterone and the enzymes that regulate its level, such as 5α-reductase, appear to play a major role in the pathogenesis of benign prostatic hyperplasia (BPH) (Geller 1989) (See Chaps 1, 2). BPH produces a steady enlargement in prostatic size throughout life. The total prostatic volume increases statistically significantly with aging and the growth rate is calculated to be 0.81%/year ($\pm$ 0.25%), corresponding to 0.2 ml/year. The growth rate of the periurethral area (TZ and PUZ) is 1.5%/year ($\pm$ 0.5%) (Jakobsen et al. 1988).

Microscopically, the nodular hyperplasia has a stromal (smooth muscle and fibroblast) and an epithelial component. The resultant nodules thus demonstrate a spectrum of cellular composition varying from exclusively stromal at one extreme to virtually exclusively acinar (adenomatous) at the other (Franks 1954). Most commonly the nodules are composed of a mixture of stroma and proliferating glandular epithelium (fibromyoadenomatous nodules). The size of the nodules depends upon the degree of hyperplasia. In moderate hyperplasia (< 50 g), the nodules tend to be small and predominantly localized adjacent to

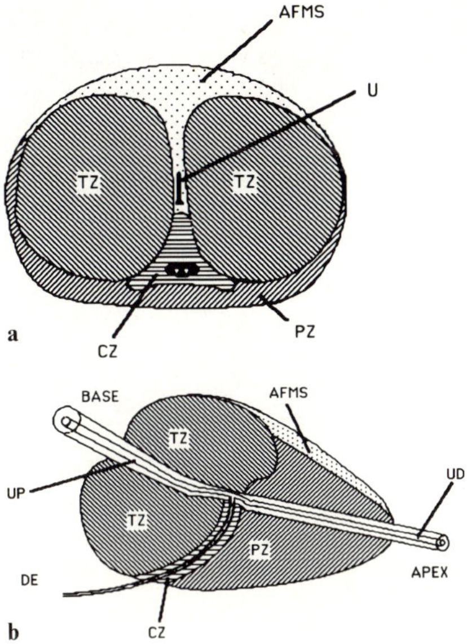

Fig. 7.23a, b. BPH. Schematic drawing (**a** transverse, **b** sagittal). In BPH the volume of the transition zone (*TZ*) increases and flattens and elongates the proximal prostatic urethra (*UP*). Depending upon the degree of hyperplasia, the central zone (*CZ*), the peripheral zone (*PZ*), and the anterior fibromuscular stroma (*AFMS*) become compressed. The ejaculatory ducts (*DE*) are displaced as well. UD (distal prostatic urethra)

the urethra and seem to be stromal, at least in the early stages. In pronounced hyperplasia, the nodules are larger, measuring more than 8 mm in diameter in 50% of the cases. The fact that stromal nodules are more vascular than glandular nodules explains why, on color Doppler and on gadolinium-enhanced MRI, these nodules display the highest vascularity. The hyperplastic epithelium is commonly found in papillary configurations with variable dilatation of the hyperplastic ducts. Intraglandular corpora amylacea are commonly associated with these cystically dilated hyperplastic ducts. Prostatic infarcts of varying age are found in approximately 20% of surgical specimens. Approximately 10% of prostatic specimens removed with a clinical diagnosis of prostatism harbor a focus of adenocarcinoma.

Hyperplasia of the TZ develops lateral to the proximal prostatic urethra (Fig. 7.23). Hyperplasia of the TZ is frequently asymmetric, explaining lateral deviation of the proximal prostatic urethra.

Hyperplasia of the glands of the tiny PUZ is clinically irrelevant and seldom attains a significant mass, except as an occasional midline dorsal nodule at the bladder neck protruding into the bladder, the so-called median lobe. Hyperplasia of the lateral and median lobes may occur either separately or simultaneously, i.e., trilobar hyperplasia (McNeal 1988).

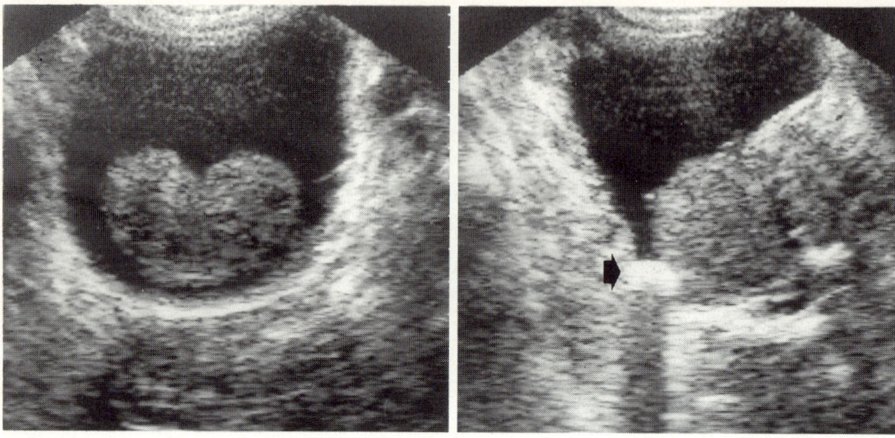

a b

Fig. 7.24a, b. Suprapubic sonography. **a** Transverse section of the intravesical portion of the hyperplastic prostate. Note the bladder calculus (*arrow*) on the sagittal section (**b**)

Stamey et al. (Stamey 1987) concluded that benign hyperplastic tissue elevates the serum PSA level at a rate of 0.3 nl/ml/gr BPH tissue.

Others however did not observe any correlation between the quantity of hyperplastic tissue and the serum PSA concentration (Weber 1989, Partin 1990).

Based on these findings it appears unlikely that a series of normal ranges for given prostate sizes could be established.

7.4.2 Ultrasonography

Transabdominal ultrasonography is useful for measuring the size of the prostate and for depicting intraglandular calcifications and cysts. The intravesical extension of the prostate can be estimated (Fig. 7.24). The glandular architecture of the PZ, however, cannot be evaluated routinely. Postvoid residual bladder volume measurement and a survey of the kidneys can be readily performed at the same time. Some sonographers feel that patients with prostatism can be screened completely by ultrasonography of the kidneys and of the prostate (Hendrikx et al. 1988).

Transrectal ultrasonography is the more effective method for imaging BPH, differentiating lateral from median lobes (Figs. 7.25, 7.26), and evaluating the PZ. The different tissue elements present in the hyperplastic nodules are reflected by the variable appearance ranging from hypoechoic stromal nodules to hyperechoic glandular nodules (Fig. 7.27) (Burks et al. 1986; Dahnert et al. 1986; Lee et al. 1986). Sometimes the nodules are surrounded by a hypoechoic halo or pseudocapsule (Burks et al. 1986). This, however, is not related to the presence or absence of a carcinoma. The echo texture of BPH is so variable that

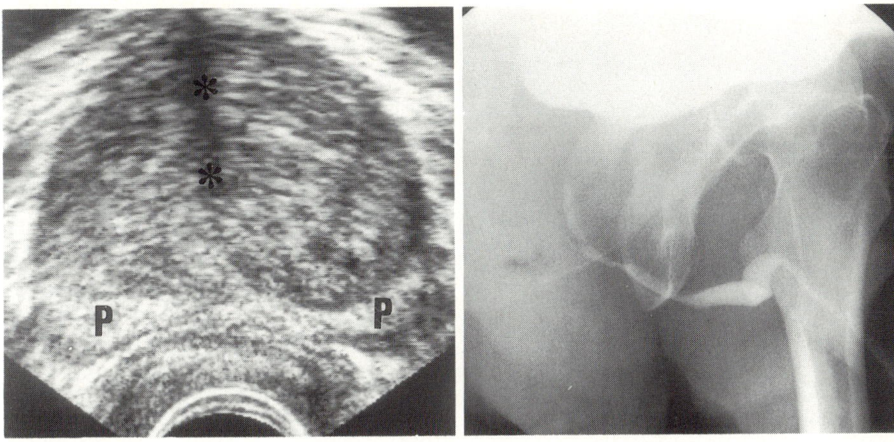

a b

Fig. 7.25a, b. BPH. TRUS showing diffuse hyperplasia of the TZ compressing the urethra and its surrounding sphincters, now recognizable as a thin hypoechoic line only (*). The PZ (*P*) is compressed. In pronounced hyperplasia it may become difficult to evaluate the compressed PZ conclusively. **b** Voiding urethrocystography showing normal expansion of the bladder neck. The proximal prostatic urethra, however, is elongated and flattened due to hyperplasia of the TZ

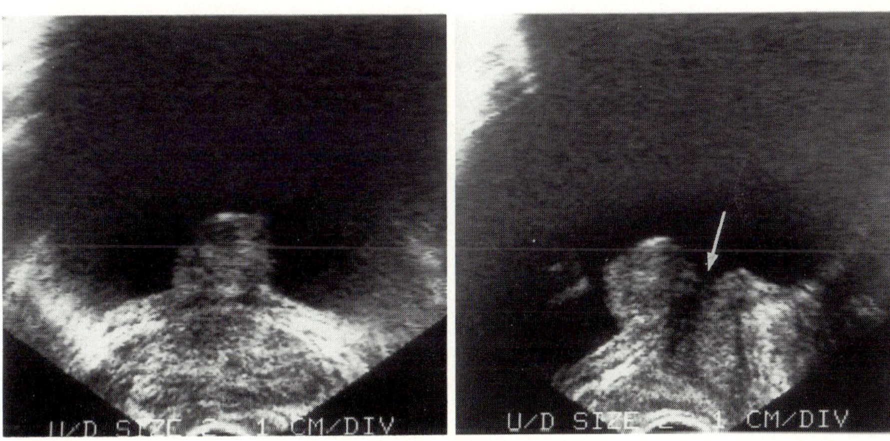

a b

Fig. 7.26a, b. Typical median lobe on **a** transverse and **b** sagittal ultrasonography. The hyperplastic periurethral glands are protruding into the bladder behind the bladder neck (*arrow*). During micturition it will further narrow the bladder neck. Although the prostate is small (12 g), this man had severe symptoms of bladder outlet obstruction

it is impossible to detect tumoral foci. An exclusively stromal hyperplastic nodule is represented as a hypoechoic lesion (Fig. 7.28). A hypoechoic nodule in the hyperplastic TZ is not suggestive of a carcinoma as it would be located in the PZ. A hypoechoic rim is commonly seen between the hyperplastic TZ and the CZ and PZ: the surgical pseudocapsule. Echogenic foci, with or without

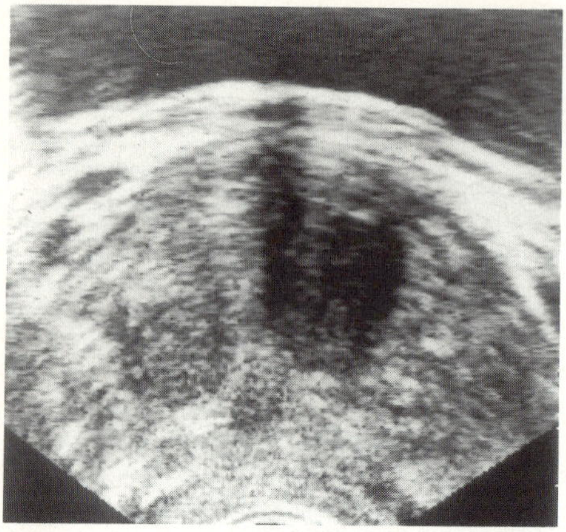

Fig. 7.27. BPH. Transverse scan showing several nodules in the TZ. The echogenicity depends upon the ratio of stromal and glandular hyperplasia, the stromal nodules being hypoechoic, the purely glandular nodules hyperechoic. Because of the nodular appearance of the hyperplastic TZ, it is referred as benign nodular hyperplasia (BNH), too

a 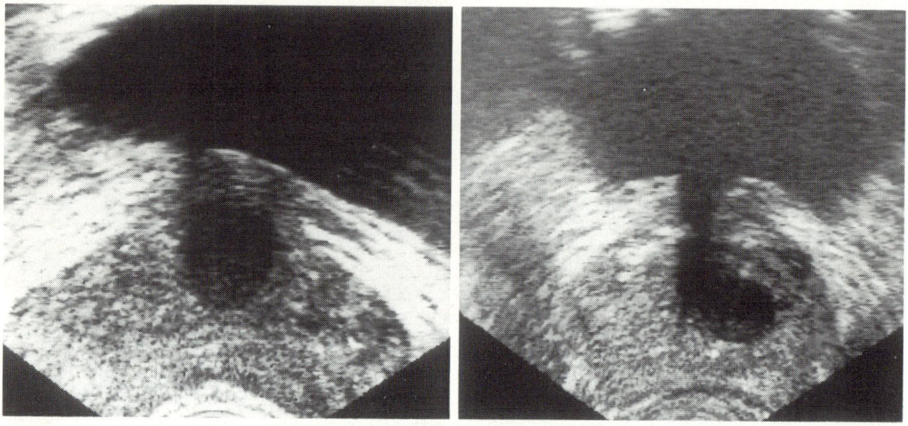 b

Fig. 7.28a, b. BPH. Transverse scans. **a** A hypoechoic, stromal nodule is present in the TZ on the left side (8 mm) although the volume of the prostate is normal. **b** A similar stromal nodule is present in another patient, who has diffuse hyperplasia of the contralateral TZ. Hypoechoic nodules in the TZ do not have the same significance as those in the PZ

shadowing, are often seen against the surgical capsule (Fig. 7.29). Cystic lesions are frequently present in glandular nodules but can be seen in diffuse (glandular) hyperplasia, too (Fig. 7.30). Prostatic cysts have the typical sonographic features of a cyst: a sharp back wall, enhanced through transmission, and lack of internal echoes. These prostatic cysts are clinically rare masses seldom large enough to be palpable on DRE. Prostatic cysts are retention cysts and thus are lined by a flattened acinar epithelium. They contain clear viscous fluid, are roughly spherical, and are usually laterally located within the prostate.

From the moment the TZ becomes hyperplastic, it becomes hypervascular on color Doppler as well. The vascularity is prominent in hypoechoic stromal nodules, and poor as in the PZ in hyperechoic glandular nodules. Sometimes,

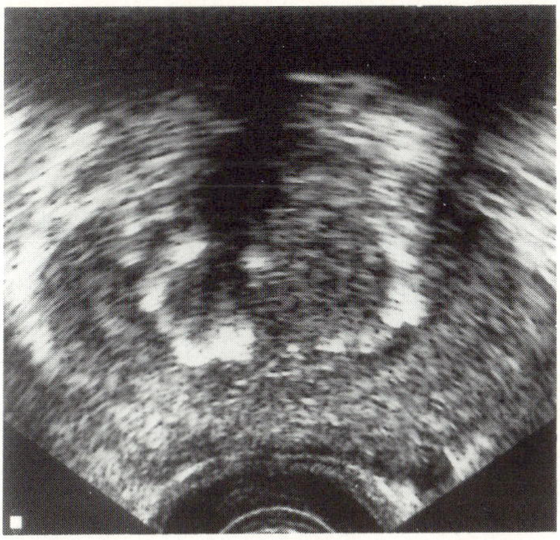

Fig. 7.29. BPH. Transverse scan. Calcifications surrounding the asymmetric hyperplastic TZ at the junction between the TZ and the PZ and CZ: the surgical capsule

a 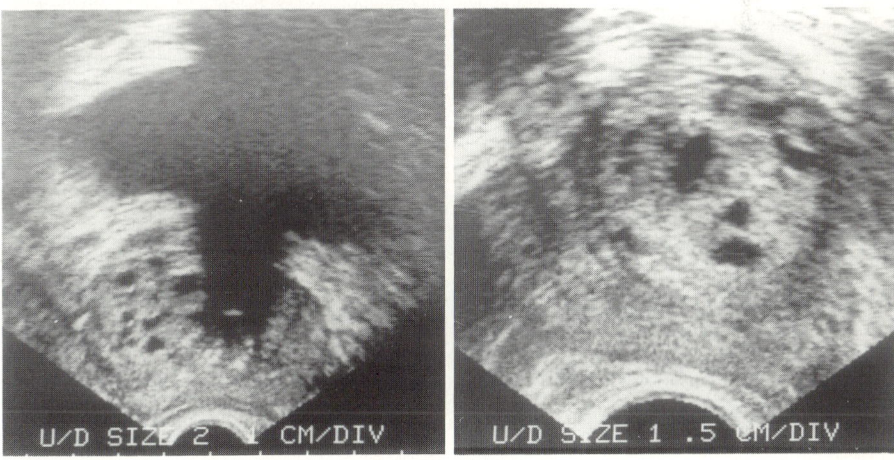 b

Fig. 7.30a, b. BPH. **a** Transverse and **b** sagittal scans of the prostate, showing asymmetric hyperplasia of the TZ. The hyperplasia is pronounced on the right side. Several anechoic areas are produced by cystic dilation of acinar and ductular structures

however, the nodules display no vascularity, which might be a partial explanation for the areas of infarction frequently encountered on resection specimens.

Volume measurement of the prostate or the hyperplastic TZ can be performed according to the techniques described in Sect. 7.2.2.

Insertion of an intraprostatic spiral using sonographic guidance is a valuable alternative to an indwelling catheter in patients awaiting prostatic surgery and in those who are either unfit or unwilling to undergo prostatectomy (Nielsen et al. 1990; Van Poppel et al. 1991). The better results are obtained with TRUS guidance, since correct positioning of the spiral relative to the bladder neck and to the external sphincter is extremely important to ensure sufficient voiding

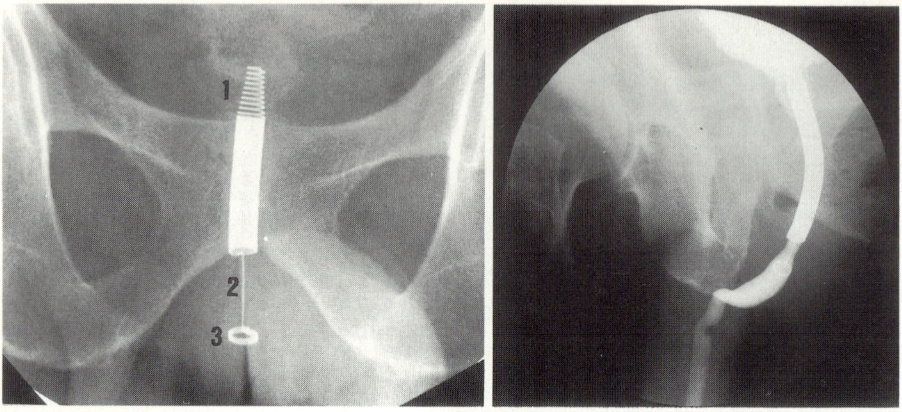

a b

Fig. 7.31a, b. Intraprostatic spiral. **a** Anteroposterior film of the pelvis. Note the position of the spiral. The thinner portion of the spiral (*2*) should be located within the external sphincter (at the urogenital diaphragm); the ring has to be located in the membranous urethra (*3*), while the cone (*1*) protrudes into the bladder. Knowledge of the normal anatomy of the prostate is an important prerequisite for correct insertion of the spiral. **b** Micturition cystogram illustrating the position of the spiral relative to the prostatic urethra, the membranous urethra, and the bulbous urethra

ability and continence respectively (Fig. 7.31). In a similar way, prostate balloon dilatation can be monitored by TRUS (SLOAN 1991).

After transurethral resection, or open enucleation, the hyperplastic TZ is removed, thus producing typical images on TRUS or cystourethrograms (Fig. 7.32) or any other imaging modality.

7.4.3 Computed Tomography

The prostate is enlarged, sometimes with undulating contours, and it may protrude into the bladder or behind it. A median lobe expands into the bladder and is seen as a "filling defect" originating at the bladder base on the midline. The latter may be confused with a bladder carcinoma by the inexperienced radiologist.

Computed tomography cannot distinguish nodular hyperplasia from carcinoma since both processes produce enlargement of the gland with a rather homogeneous internal density.

7.4.4 Magnetic Resonance Imaging

With a 1.5-T or 1-T imager, diffuse BPH has the same signal characteristics as the normal prostate, whereas nodular BPH is isointense on T1-weighted images

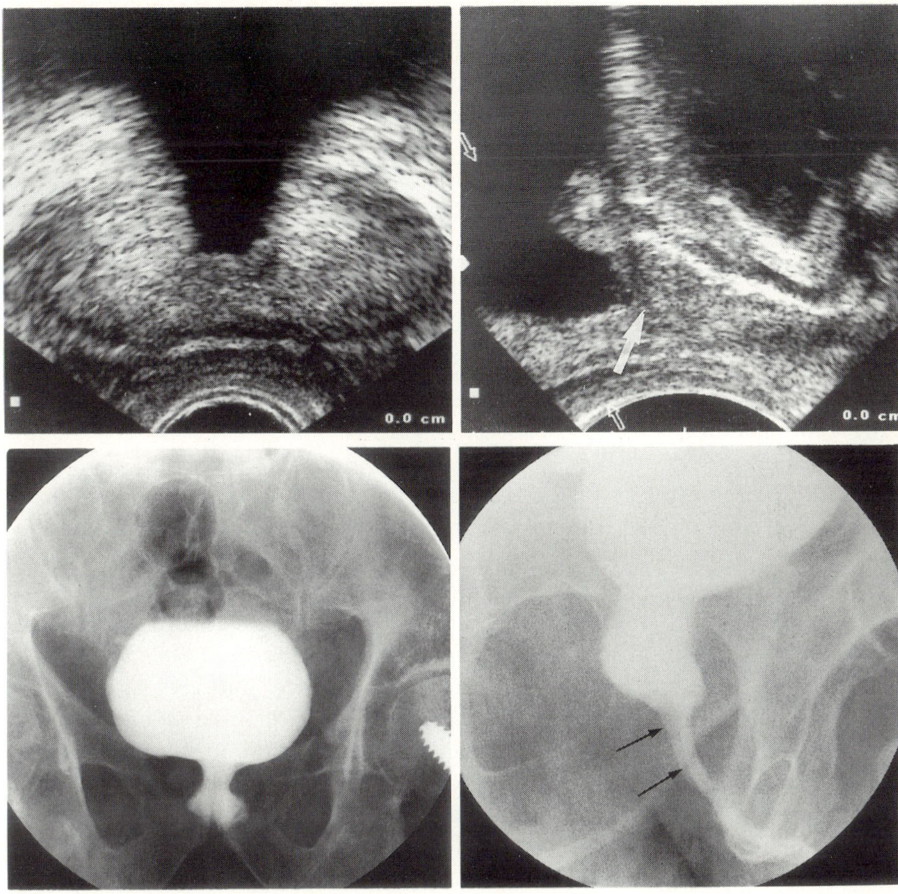

a b c d

Fig. 7.32a–d. Appearance after transurethral resection. **a** Transverse and **b** sagittal scans showing the residual prostate predominantly consisting of PZ after transurethral resection of the hyperplastic transition zone. Note that the resection cavity extends up to the level of the verumontanum only (*arrow*). **c** Cystogram and **d** voiding urethrogram after transurethral resection. Widening of the bladder neck and the proximal prostatic urethra. The verumontanum (*arrows*) is preserved as the hyperplastic transition zone develops anterolaterally and proximally to it

and demonstrates a mixture of hyperintense, isointense, or hypointense foci on T2-weighted images. The MRI characteristics are relatively predictable, depending upon the distribution and size of the glandular elements as well as the composition of the surrounding stroma (Schiebler et al. 1989; Lovett et al. 1992). Given the variety of tissues constituting the BPH process, it is inevitable that the MRI appearance will vary, and it is unlikely that a specific diagnosis of BPH will be achieved on the basis of MRI. This also explains why different authors have variously characterized BPH as hyperintense nodules (purely glandular hyperplasia) or hypointense nodules on T2-weighted images (predominantly stromal hyperplasia), or as indistinguishable from normal tissue (Bryan et al. 1986; Carrol et al. 1987; Dooms and Hricak 1986; Larkin et al. 1986; Ling et al. 1986; Poon et al. 1985). A low signal halo (pseudocapsule) is sometimes seen surrounding the nodules on T2-weighted images, especially when endorectal surface coils are used (Carrol et al. 1987; Kahn et al. 1989). After the injection of gadolinium, the glandular nodules remain hypointense, while the stromal nodules become hyperintense.

Accurate determination of prostate volume can be achieved with MRI, but this is not a cost-effective method compared with ultrasonography.

7.5 Malignant Tumors of the Prostate

7.5.1 Introduction

Adenocarcinoma of the prostate is a very common malignancy of older males and ranks second only to lung cancer in frequency: it accounts for 10% of male cancer deaths in the United States. The incidence increases with age, rising to 50% in patients over age 75 and to 80% in patients over age 80 (Von Eschenback and Johnson 1978). However, only about one-sixth to one-third of the cases found at autopsy are manifest clinically (Catalona and Scott 1978).

There is a wide variation in incidence between races and geographic areas. American blacks have the highest rate of prostatic carcinoma, while Orientals have the lowest rates. The rate in African blacks is low and in sharp contrast to the rate in American blacks. A similar rise in the incidence of prostatic carcinoma is seen in Japanese and Polish immigrants to the United States, compared to the ethnic groups in their native land, suggesting an etiologic role of environmental factors (Kovi 1983). In contrast, the prevalence of latent prostatic carcinoma appears to be uniformly high among all of these racial, ethnic, and geographic groups. This suggests that through aging males in all population groups are prone to develop carcinoma, but they are subject to different cancer-promoting factors (Dhom 1983; Kovi 1983). The majority of carcinomas (70%) originate in the PZ; 20% originate in the TZ and 10% in the CZ. Carcinomas of the TZ are most frequently found incidentally during transurethral resection, operative enucleation, or random biopsies. Adenocarcinomas of acinar origin account for 95% of all prostatic carcinomas and predominantly arise in the PZ.

Malignant mesenchymal tumors of the prostate are extremely rare, accounting for only about 0.1% of primary prostatic neoplasms (Tannenbaum 1975). Most of them occur before the age of 50, and a third of them are seen in children. Rhabdomyosarcoma is the most common prostatic malignancy of childhood.

Leiomyosarcoma is a malignant tumor of smooth muscle and occurs in older age groups. This neoplasm has a typical prolonged course, with multiple recurrences (Smith and Dehner 1972).

Other soft tissue sarcomas, including malignant schwannoma and malignant fibrous histiocytoma, have also been described in the prostate (Bain et al. 1985).

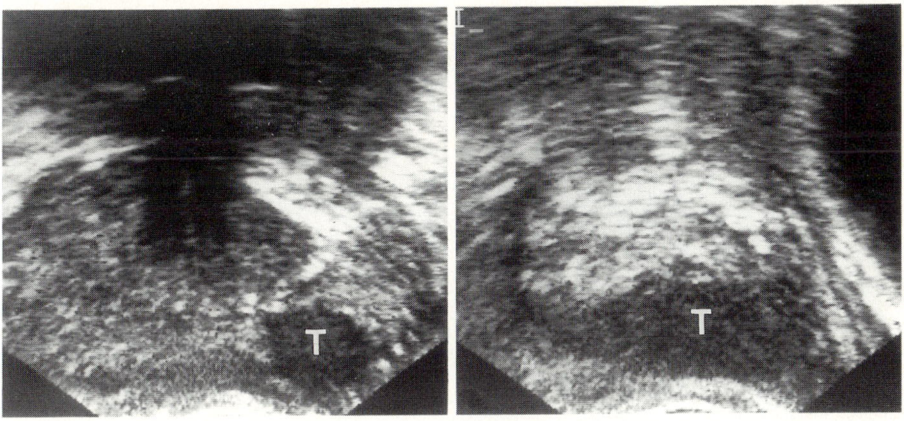

a b

Fig. 7.33a, b. Adenocarcinoma. Typically hypoechoic tumor (*T*) of the PZ on the left side on both **a** axial and **b** sagittal sonograms

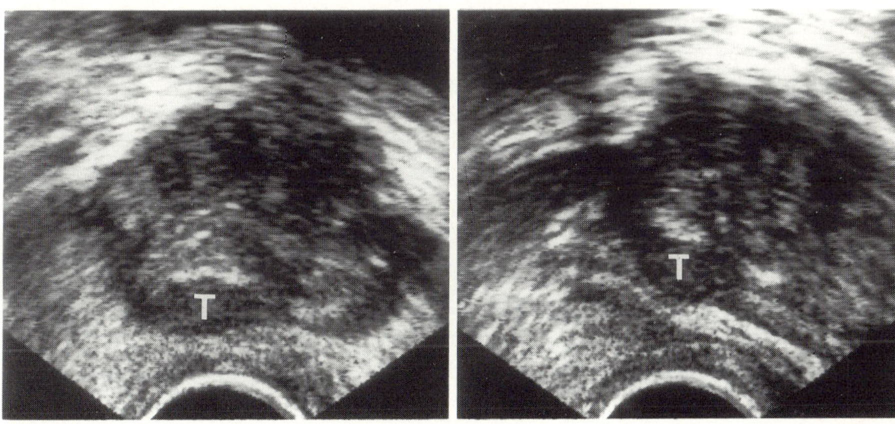

a b

Fig. 7.34a, b. Adenocarcinoma of the prostate (T2a). **a** Transverse and **b** sagittal scans showing a well-circumscribed hypoechoic nodular lesion (*T*) in the PZ at the base of the gland, bulging the surface of the prostate. Note that the PZ is heterogeneous, and it thus might become impossible to detect smaller tumors sonographically

7.5.2 Diagnosis of Prostatic Carcinoma

7.5.2.1 Ultrasonography

The majority of carcinomas are believed to arise in the PZ, whereas BPH arises in the TZ or PUZ (McNeal 1969, 1983, 1988). Lesions in the PZ that have a hypoechoic appearance are highly suspicious for malignancy (Figs. 7.33, 7.34) (Burks et al. 1986; Dahnert et al. 1986; Lee et al. 1985, 1986). This is effective for

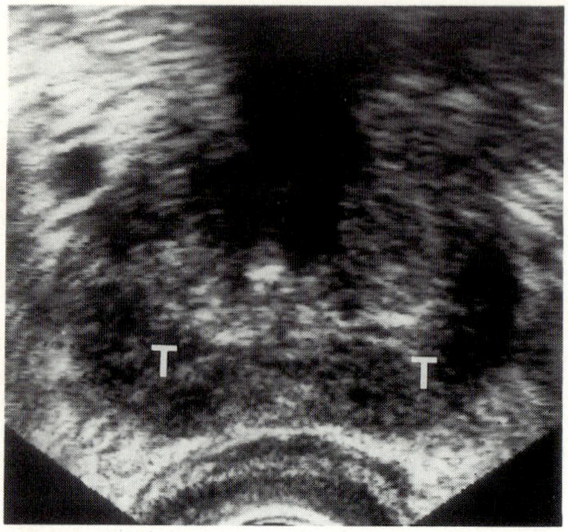

Fig. 7.35. Adenocarcinoma of the PZ (T). Diffusely hypoechoic PZ is infiltrating the TZ. Although the prostatic capsule seems to be intact, microscopic infiltration or transgression cannot be excluded

the vast majority of cancers originating in the PZ. Small carcinomas begin as echopenic foci subcapsularly in the PZ. As the tumors grow, they extend to the CZ, to the – hyperplastic – TZ, and to the capsule. This behavior explains why more advanced tumors have a heterogeneous appearance, i.e. they envelop preexisting brighter echoes from corpora amylacea or calculi. This is probably the explanation for the positive biopsies of echogenic regions in advanced carcinomas in earlier series (GLEASON and Veterans Administration Cooperative Research Group 1977). It should, however, be stressed that at least 25% of carcinomas are only slightly hypoechoic or even completely isoechoic (DAHNERT et al. 1986; LEE et al. 1985, 1989a; RIFKIN and CHOI 1988; RIFKIN et al. 1993; SHINOHARA et al. 1989).

The differences in appearance on TRUS are also correlated with histologic grade and the degree of stromal fibrosis. The more hypoechoic cancers are, in general, the better differentiated cancers with less fibrosis. There seems to be a tendency for the isoechoic cancers and those with subtle hyperechoic areas to display poor cellular differentiation more frequently and to have a greater degree of stromal fibrosis, but considerable overlap among histologic types is seen (RIFKIN et al. 1989). Hyperechoic tumors can be unusual ductal adenocarcinomas with central necrosis and dystrophic calcifications (EGAWA et al. 1992). In bilateral carcinoma, there may be no normal tissue for comparison: the disappearance of the normal internal zonal architecture thus may be the only sonographic indication of a diffuse carcinoma involving the prostate (Fig. 7.35) (HERNANDEZ and SMITH 1990). Rarely cystic (endometroid) carcinomas may be seen (Fig. 7.36).

Normal glandular tissue and several benign processes such as chronic and acute prostatitis, postinflammatory atrophy, infarction, and cysts may have similar hypoechoic TRUS findings. Prostatic intraepithelial neoplasia (PIN), a presumed premalignant lesion, may occasionally produce similar lesions on TRUS. These patients merit careful monitoring since the incidence of prostatic carcinoma increases with the presence of PIN lesions (BRAWER et al. 1989;

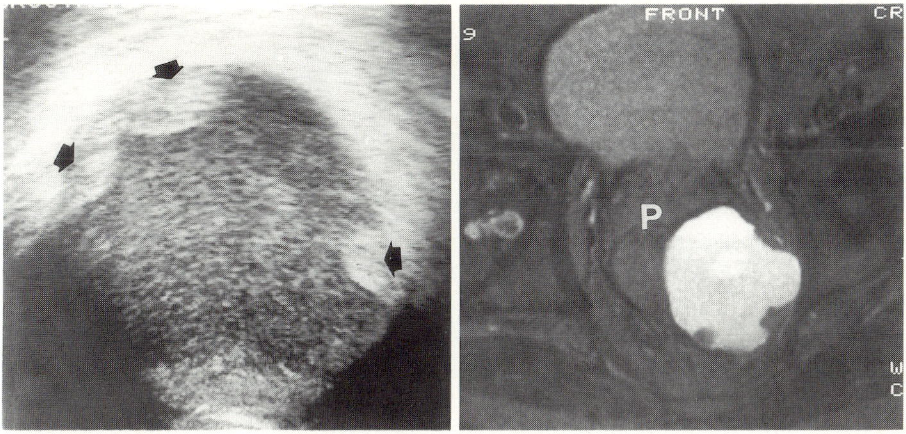

a b

Fig. 7.36a, b. Cystic (endometroid) adenocarcinoma of the prostate. **a** TRUS reveals a large cystic lesion with wall proliferations (*arrows*) and internal echoes due to hemorrhage. **b** Transverse T2-weighted MR image of the pelvis. The tumor is hyperintense on T2-weighted images. The masses at the internal wall of the tumor are visible as hypointense protrusions. *P*, prostate

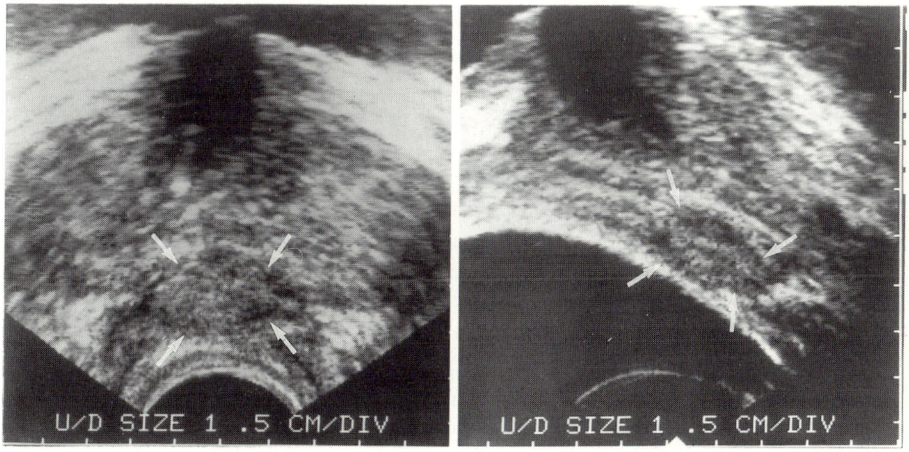

a b

Fig. 7.37a, b Benign hyperplastic nodule in the PZ. **a** Transverse and **b** sagittal scans of the prostate. A midline nodule (*arrows*) is present at the apex, bulging the prostatic surface and bounded by a hypoechoic halo. On DRE these nodules are felt either as a firm nodule or a soft lesion

Devonec et al. 1989, 1990). We recently described a benign lesion in the PZ of the prostate mimicking prostatic carcinoma of the PZ: hyperplastic nodules (Fig. 7.37) (Oyen et al. 1993). These are ovoid, slightly hypoechoic lesions surrounded by a hypoechoic halo and bulging the prostatic capsule. Although the diagnosis is likely on TRUS, TRUS-guided biopsies seem to be necessary to exclude malignancy.

TRUS-guided transrectal biopsy is a safe and valuable diagnostic tool that can be performed on an out-patient basis and with only minor complications (TORP-PEDERSEN et al. 1989).

Hematuria and/or hemospermia occurred in two-thirds of the patients and in all cases ceased spontaneously. Since in this study 6.2% of the patients had an *E. coli* infection of the urinary tract after the procedure, and half of them required hospital cure with parenteral antibiotics for 1-8 days, prophylactic antibiotics are proposed when core biopsy of the prostate is performed transrectally (GUSTAFSSON et al. 1990). Prostatitis has been described as a complication in some cases, too (2%) (BILLEBAUD et al. 1990).

Transient elevations of PSA are seen after biopsies, but DRE and TRUS without biopsy had no such effects (AUS and SKUDE 1992).

In one case a large hematoma in the rectal wall with nearly total occlusion of the rectal lumen was reported following a TRUS-guided biopsy of the prostate (SEYMOUR and OESTERLING 1992). Three cases of tumor seedling in the tract following a transperineal biopsy of prostatic cancer with a Tru-cut needle have been reported (RYAN and PEELING 1990).

Preliminary reports on the value of color Doppler in the diagnosis of malignant prostatic neoplasia emphasize the value of this technique in the discrimination of prostatic neoplasms in the PZ, the cancers being hypervascular and either hypoechoic or isoechoic (GUERCINI et al. 1991). In prostatic cancer there is an increased flow within (Figs. 7.38, 7.39) or surrounding (Fig. 7.40) the lesion. Diffuse prostatitis exhibits a diffusely abnormal flow; in focal prostatitis the flow is not significantly different from that in cancer. In BPH a significant abnormal flow was seen, usually in the central gland or in the area of the surgical capsule. This is consistent with our earliest findings with color-encoded Doppler (OYEN et al. 1991a). Biopsies are still necessary to obtain histologic diagnosis since focal granulomatous prostatitis may have similar characteristics (Figs. 7.21, 7.22). According to more recent results, color Doppler can provide additional information and may increase the specificity and sensitivity in the evaluation of potential prostatic malignancy (RIFKIN et al. 1991, 1993). All of the prostatic cancers studied by RIFKIN et al. had an abnormal blood flow on color Doppler. Of the 132 cancers, 123 (93%) had corresponding gray-scale abnormalities and 114 (86%) demonstrated abnormal blood flow on color Doppler imaging. Nine of the 132 cancers (7%) had no obviously identifiable abnormalities on gray-scale scanning but had distinctly abnormal flow on color Doppler scanning. Abnormal findings on color scanning without abnormal findings on gray-scale scanning occurred in 8 of the 33 cases of inflammatory foci (24%) and in 24 of the 469 (5%) benign lesions.

Some sonologists routinely perform random biopsies of the contralateral lobe in patients with a prostatic nodule. The incidence of contralateral cancer in patients with a tumor digitally localized to one prostatic lobe ranges between 14% and 50% (CARTER S.S. et al. 1989; DANIELS et al. 1992; DYKE et al. 1990; HODGE et al. 1989a, b; LEE F. Jr et al. 1991). These patients have higher serum PSA levels and a larger tumor volume than those with negative contralateral a 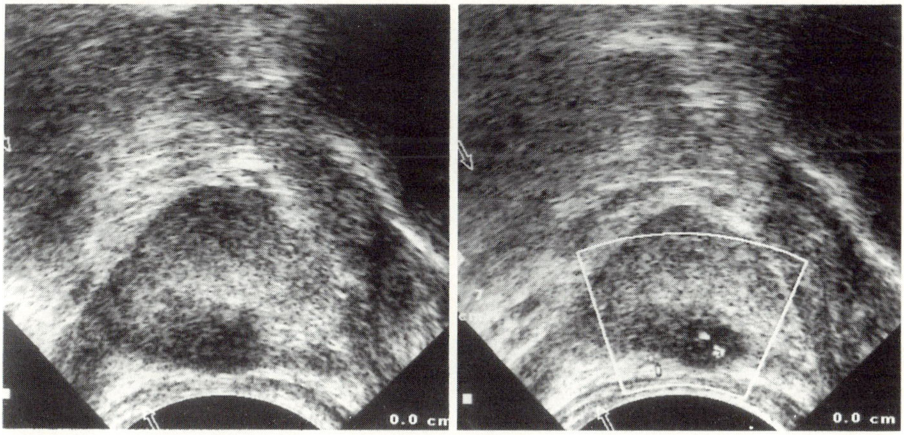 b

Fig. 7.38a, b. Adenocarcinoma. Hypoechoic nodule in the PZ (**a**) with only focal hypervascularity (*white area* within the tumor) on color Doppler ultrasonography (**b**)

a 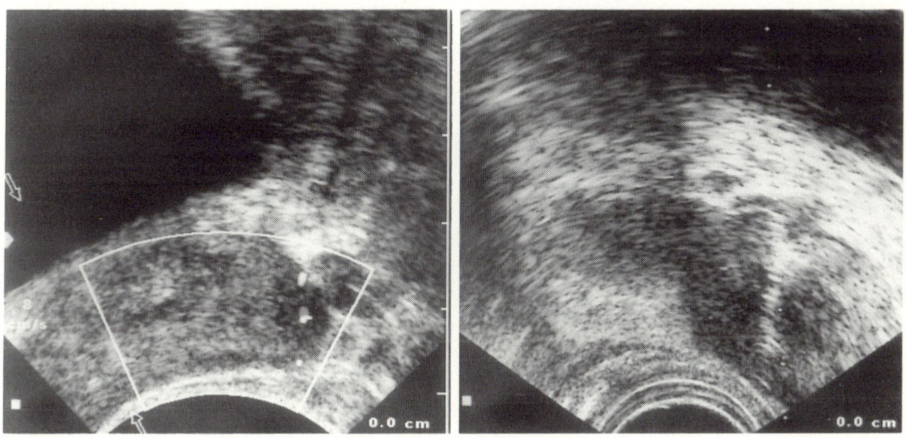 b

Fig. 7.39a, b. Adenocarcinoma of the prostate. **a** Transverse section of the left PZ showing focal hypervascularity of the hypoechoic area of the PZ. **b** Sagittal section: after the biopsy the course of the needle is recognizable as a hyperechoic line throughout the suspicious lesion

biopsies. The findings demonstrate that contralateral negative biopsies in patients with unilaterally palpable disease predict low-volume, localized tumor and a negligible likelihood of surgical margin compromise when using a contralateral nerve-sparing approach. Bilaterally positive biopsies suggest larger tumor volume with a greater likelihood of adverse pathologic findings and recurrence (Daniels et al. 1992). It has been confirmed by others that random biopsy does not result in significant alteration of clinical staging. Although the additional yield from random prostatic biopsy is small but distinct, except for the series of Hodge and Carter (Carter H.B. et al. 1989; Hodge et al. 1989a), this

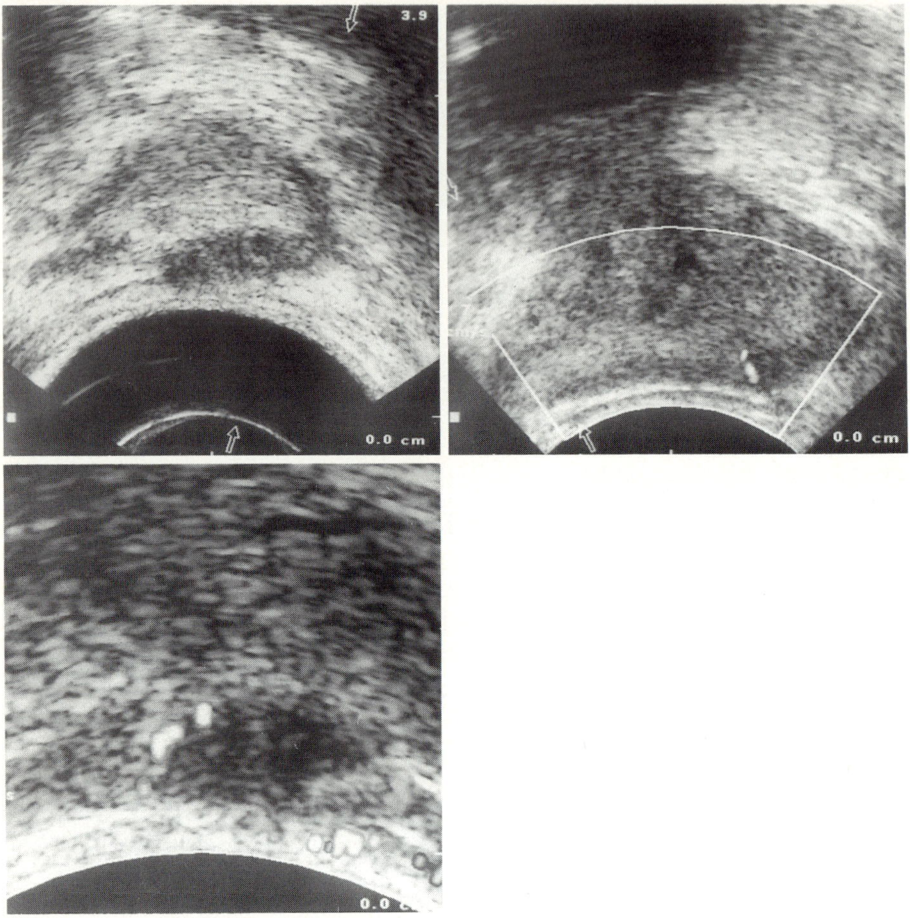

Fig. 7.40a–c. Adenocarcinoma of the PZ. There is only hypervascularity at the periphery of the hypoechoic tumor (**a**) on both the transverse section (**b**) and sagittal color Doppler (**c**)

policy may have clinical relevance (DYKE et al. 1990). In the latter series, while the palpable nodule was benign in 7% of cases (five patients), an impalpable isoechoic tumor of significant volume was detected in the contralateral lobe in three patients. HODGE et al. (1989a) even proved that if one neglects the presence of a nodule on TRUS, the diagnosis of a palpable tumor is possible with six systematic random biopsies of both lobes in the majority of cases. Nevertheless, they admit that 5% of the cancers are missed if no directed biopsy of the nodule is performed.

The value of TRUS guided multiple systematic biopsies in the early diagnosis of cancer of the prostate is well established (BILLEBAUD et al. 1990). These authors reported that systematic prostatic biopsies (Fig. 7.41) detected 14 cancers in men without suspicion of cancer on DRE. This method detects 41% of all prostatic cancers in men with normal rectal examination when the PSA

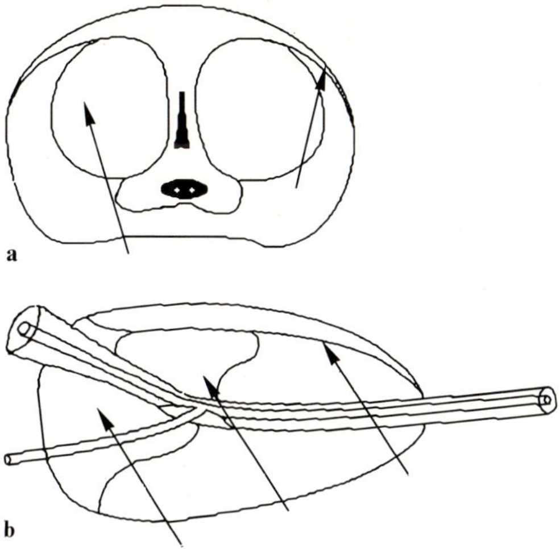

a

b

Fig. 7.41a, b. Systematic random biopsies. Biopsies are taken halfway between the urethra and the prostatic capsule (**a**) at the base, in the midportion, and at the apex of the gland and on both sides. Thus the different zones are sampled. However, it may be useful to take more anteriorly oriented biopsies to **a** in order to sample the anterior extension of the PZ, too

level is 10 ng/ml or more. The real question is whether this early diagnosis is useful for the patient, since presently there is no certainty of any therapeutic benefit in terms of quantity and quality of life (Terris et al. 1992a; Vallancien et al. 1991b).

In a study of the value of ultrasonography in the detection of prostatic cancer, post-mortem specimens were correlated with histologic whole-mount step-sectioned specimens. The sensitivity (32%) and the specificity (64%) of TRUS appear too low to justify its use in clinical screening for prostatic adenocarcinoma. PSA and TRUS together appear more effective than ultrasonography alone in the detection of prostatic adenocarcinoma (Coffield et al. 1992). When DRE, TRUS, and PSA are summated, the detection rate for prostatic cancer is twice as high as when a single parameter is used (Perrin et al. 1991). TRUS is not more sensitive than DRE for the detection of prostatic cancer stage T1a-b (Grups et al. 1990).

Several ratios between PSA and prostate volume (V) have been proposed. In patients with prostatic carcinoma, the ratio PSA/V was 1.73; in normal subjects and in those with BPH, the mean PSA/V ratio was 0.090 and 0.099, respectively (Veneziano et al. 1990). TRUS-guided biopsies are (a) necessary when there is a suspicious area and the PSA/V ratio exceeds 0.15, and especially when it exceeds 0.30, (b) not indicated when sonographic abnormalities are associated with a PSA/V of less than 0.15, because they are most frequently due to benign lesions (Veneziano et al. 1990; Wasserman et al. 1991).

There seems to be no correlation between the PSA level and the Gleason grade in prostatic cancer in patients with a negative bone scintigram (Amiel et al. 1989).

The overall predictive value of a hypoechoic lesion in the PZ has been reported to be 41%, increasing to 61% when combined with the finding of a positive DRE and to 52% if the PSA level is elevated (LEE F. et al. 1989b). Biopsy of small suspicious hypoechoic lesions ($\leq$ 1.0 cm) may not be indicated if the results of both DRE and PSA are normal (LEE et al. 1989b). In our series, 58% of all focal hypoechoic lesions in the PZ were proven to be carcinoma, regardless of the findings at DRE (OYEN et al. 1991d). The sensitivity and specificity of DRE are 69% and 79%, while the values were 88% and 77% for TRUS (NAITO et al. 1988). The incidence of impalpable hypoechoic nodules ranges from 18% to 44%, the majority of the nodules being localized in the PZ. Biopsies of these hypoechoic nodules are positive in 5%–41% of cases.

7.5.2.2 Computed Tomography

With CT, carcinoma usually cannot be distinguished from normal tissue or nodular hyperplasia. In early stages the tumor is thus imperceptible. Evaluation of invasion or breakthrough of the capsule is very difficult unless it is gross. In these advanced stages, tumor extension can be reasonably appreciated with DRE, TRUS, or MRI, too.

7.5.2.3 Magnetic Resonance Imaging

PHILLIPS et al. (1987) retrospectively reviewed 31 patients with benign and malignant prostatic lesions who had MRI at 1.5 T and concluded that the prostate had no specific signal intensity that enabled differentiation between benign and malignant changes. However, CARROL et al. (1987), working at 1.5 T, reported that prostatic carcinoma has a low signal intensity, whereas JAEGER et al. (1987), working at 0.15 T, reported that prostatic cancer is hyperintense. Since 1988, dramatic improvements in MRI technology (particularly endorectal coil design), coupled with better appreciation of tumor biology, have markedly increased the potential of MRI in the detection and staging of prostatic carcinoma. During this period, a number of reports have emerged explaining the varying appearance and rate of detection of prostatic carcinoma, and these reports have documented that MRI is much more useful than previously thought.

At least two factors affect the ability to detect carcinoma nodules on MRI: tumor grade and tumor size. The signal intensity of prostatic cancer is a function of its cellularity and differentiation (grade), as shown by SCHIEBLER et al. (1989) in their in vitro work at 1.39 T. These investigators noted that well to moderately well differentiated carcinomas grow in nodules of densely packed glandular elements with little central space for mucin storage. Therefore, the high cellularity and reduced fluid content of this grade of cancer generate a low signal intensity. On the other hand, poorly differentiated carcinomas tend to grow in

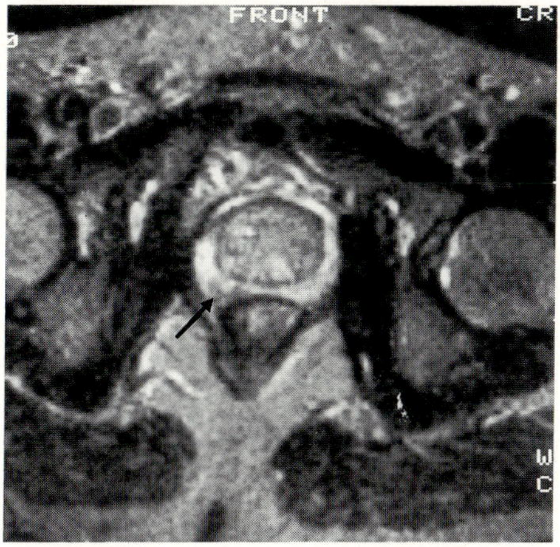

Fig. 7.42. Prostatic cancer. T2-weighted image (TR 2200, TE 120) showing a hypointense lesion in the PZ on the right side (*arrow*). The TZ is hyperplastic and displays heterogeneous signal intensities

an infiltrative pattern, causing little distortion of the normal architecture of the gland and thereby averaging their intensity with adjacent normal cells, making them poorly visible on MRI. Although direct extrapolation of these in vitro results to in vivo studies at lower fields is not straightforward, current in vivo studies strongly suggest that different grades of carcinoma have different signal intensities at 1.5 T. It appears that a typical cancer nodule on MRI is a hypointense lesion in the PZ of the prostate (Fig. 7.42); conversely, any hypointense lesion in the PZ should be regarded with great suspicion. High-intensity lesions should be interpreted with great care, especially if they appear in the hyperplastic TZ, because the majority of BPH nodules in this region are also hyperintense. There is also a rare mucin-secreting prostatic carcinoma that appears as a hyperintense lesion regardless of its location in the prostate.

The size of the tumor is the less important of the two factors mentioned as influencing the ability to detect the cancer. As the well-differentiated tumor grows in size, it loses differentiation in the periphery, making margin identification and volume estimation on MRI inaccurate (QUINT et al. 1991). THICKMAN et al. (1990) showed that 37% of tumors over 5 mm in greatest diameter were underestimated in volume and that 22% were overestimated; KAHN et al. (1989) reported that there was a 25%–70% (mean, 40%) underestimation of tumor volume by MRI in 43% of their patients. No tumors in that series were overestimated in volume. Furthermore, there was no correlation between tumor size and detection, i.e., a small tumor could be identified, whereas a larger tumor could be missed. In KAHN et al.'s study (1989), tumor grades were not taken into account, but from the discussions above it is evident that a small well to moderately well differentiated carcinoma can be readily detected by MRI whereas a large, poorly differentiated one may be missed or underestimated in volume. Therefore, discrepancies in the reported figures for the sensitivity and specificity of MRI of the prostate arise from differences in tumor grade and volume in those series. For example, 67% of carcinomas in the series of CARROL et al. (1987) and 71% of carcinomas in the series of KAHN et al. (1989) were detected by MRI on long TR/TE images, whereas in another study only 36% of all cancers and 82% of the cancers greater than 5 mm in diameter were identified. It should be noted that all studies mentioned above used body coils for image generation.

With increasing popularity of the nerve-sparing radical prostatectomy procedure, it is necessary to identify the neurovascular bundle before surgery. Extension of tumor to this structure is generally accepted as a sign of unresectability. Only high-resolution surface-coil images can identify the neurovascular bundle. Any lateral displacement of this structure or change in its signal intensity may be regarded as a sign of tumor spread. Invasion of the capsule typically takes place at the 5 and 7 o'clock positions on transverse images where the neurovascular bundle penetrates the gland. Once outside the gland, the tumor can spread to the periprostatic fat, seminal vesicles, and obturator internus, and even circumscribe the rectum. Any discontinuity in the prostatic capsule or irregularity of the margin of the gland on long TR/TE images may be a sign of capsular infiltration. In addition, any abnormality of the periprostatic venous plexus and abnormal signal intensity in periprostatic fat may be considered further evidence of capsular infiltration. The contour of the gland is best depicted on endorectal coil images. KAHN et al. (1989) demonstrated that MRI at 0.35 T is 37.5% sensitive, 100% specific, and 82% accurate in predicting extraglandular disease on long TR/TE images. The corresponding figures of BEZZI et al. (1988) at 1.5 T were 44% sensitivity, 81% specificity, and 65% accuracy. This must not be interpreted to mean that low-field MRI is more accurate than high-field MRI, but rather reflects the more stringent criteria used by BEZZI et al. (1988) in defining capsular infiltration.

There are three ways a tumor can spread to seminal vesicles, and this has been elegantly described by WHEELER (1989) in a study of 30 patients. Forty percent of the patients had a tumor in the seminal vesicles due to direct extension up the two ejaculatory ducts; 30% had direct invasion of the seminal vesicles, either from the base of the prostate or from the periprostatic area; and the remaining 30% showed isolated areas of cancer within the seminal vesicles without any evidence of extracapsular disease, presumably due to hematogenous spread. MRI appearance of seminal vesicle involvement is that of a low-signal-intensity lesion within the hyperintense seminal vesicle on long T2-weighted images. Replacement of normally fluid-filled tubules of seminal vesicles by highly cellular tumor produces the reduction in signal intensity. Depending on the path of spread, the low-signal lesion could be either centrally (through the ejaculatory ducts) or peripherally located. If the central portion of the prostate is large, centrally located seminal vesicle tumors may be difficult to see on axial images. In this case, it is necessary to obtain long TR/TE sagittal images.

The inflatable surface coil for transrectal MRI of the prostate now offers high spatial resolution and excellent contrast and substantially improves studies of the prostate (SCHNALL et al. 1991; MARTIN et al. 1988). With this technical improvement, MRI is now considered the most reliable method for staging prostatic carcinoma (POLLACK 1991).

7.5.3 Staging of Prostatic Carcinoma

Although the clinical-based staging system according to Jewett-Whitmore is still widely used, we feel that it should be replaced by the latest and well-balanced TNM system (SCHRÖDER et al. 1992). This staging system takes into account the latest developments such as random biopsies. Moreover tumor staging with TRUS and MRI can be accurately described according to the TNM classification.

7.5.3.1 Ultrasonography

T Staging Transabdominal ultrasonography only assesses prostate and seminal vesicle size. TRUS permits T staging of prostatic carcinoma by measuring the volume of the tumor and by demonstrating gross extension outside the capsule into periprostatic fat (Fig. 7.43), bladder, seminal vesicles, rectum (Fig. 7.44), and occasionally juxtarectal lymph nodes.

Although the internal anatomy of the prostate and its surroundings can be evaluated in detail, the superiority of TRUS to DRE for the purpose of staging has not been demonstrated unequivocally.

It is suggested that the tumor volume strongly correlates with the probability of capsular penetration and the presence or absence of extraglandular tumor spread. The metastatic potential of a prostatic tumor is indeed related to its volume and its histologic grade. The majority of tumors of less than 0.5 cm^3 (a sphere of 1 cm diameter) are latent and asymptomatic and are considered to be insignificant. Between 0.5 and 4 cm^3 (spherical lesion of 2 cm in diameter) extraprostatic spread and metastases are rare. Tumors larger than 4 cm^3 are

a 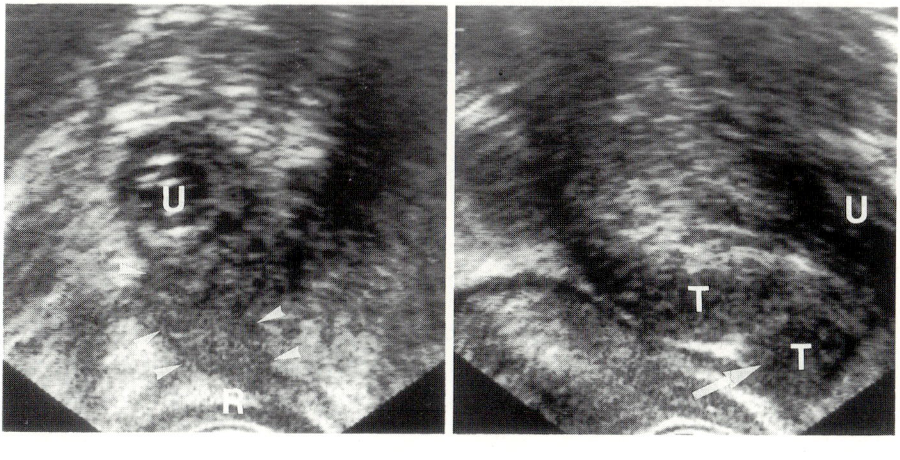 b

Fig. 7.43a, b. Adenocarcinoma of the prostate. **a** Transverse scan through the apex and **b** apical sagittal section. A hypoechoic tumor in the PZ is extending in the trapezoid area (*arrow*) and to the rectal wall (*arrowheads*). *T*, Tumor; *U*, urethra with a Foley catheter; *R*, rectum

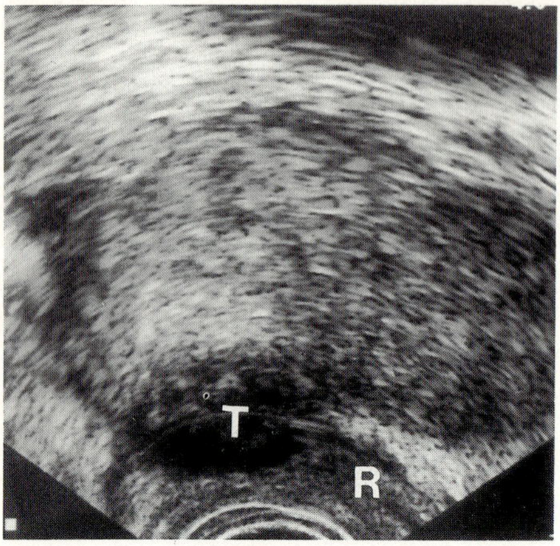

Fig. 7.44. Adenocarcinoma of the prostate (T4a). Hypoechoic tumor (*T*) in the PZ on the right side, invading the rectum (*R*)

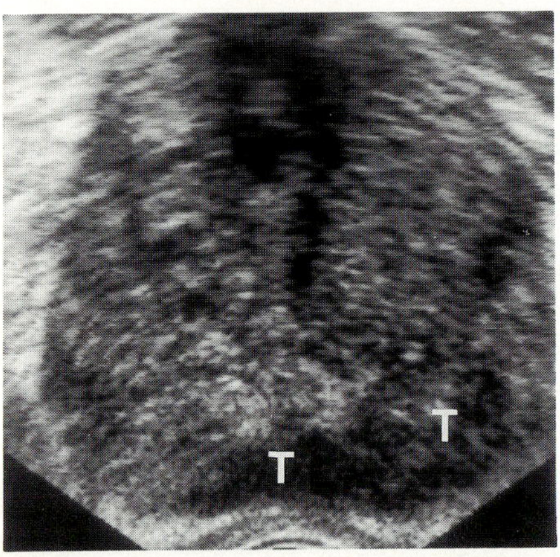

Fig. 7.45. Large tumor (*T*) in the PZ on the left side, extending over the midline. The prostatic capsule is irregular but this is not a reliable criterion for evaluating invasion or transgression

aggressive and there is a clear relation between the volume and the histologic grade: tumors between 4 and 12 cm^3 in volume are of histologic grade 4 or 5 in 50% of the cases, while tumors larger than 12 cm^3 are of grade 4 or 5 in at least 70% of the cases. Moreover invasion of the seminal vesicles, capsular transgression, lymph node metastases, and bone metastases become frequent with the latter volume. In conclusion, the critical tumor volume is 4 cm%. It takes about 4 years for a tumor to grow from 0.5 cm^3 to 4 cm^3 (SHINOHARA et al. 1989).

Tumor sizing, however, is fairly inaccurate and tumor volume is underestimated in 40%–60% of cases (LEE et al. 1989b; SHINOHARA et al. 1989). With the current technology, TRUS imaging alone does not appear to be a useful means of predicting cancer volume. Preoperative determinations of tumor volume by any modality do not correlate with pathologic tumor volume (SPIGELMAN et al. 1986; MCSHERRY et al. 1991). The infiltrative portion of the tumor cannot be estimated by any imaging modality at present.

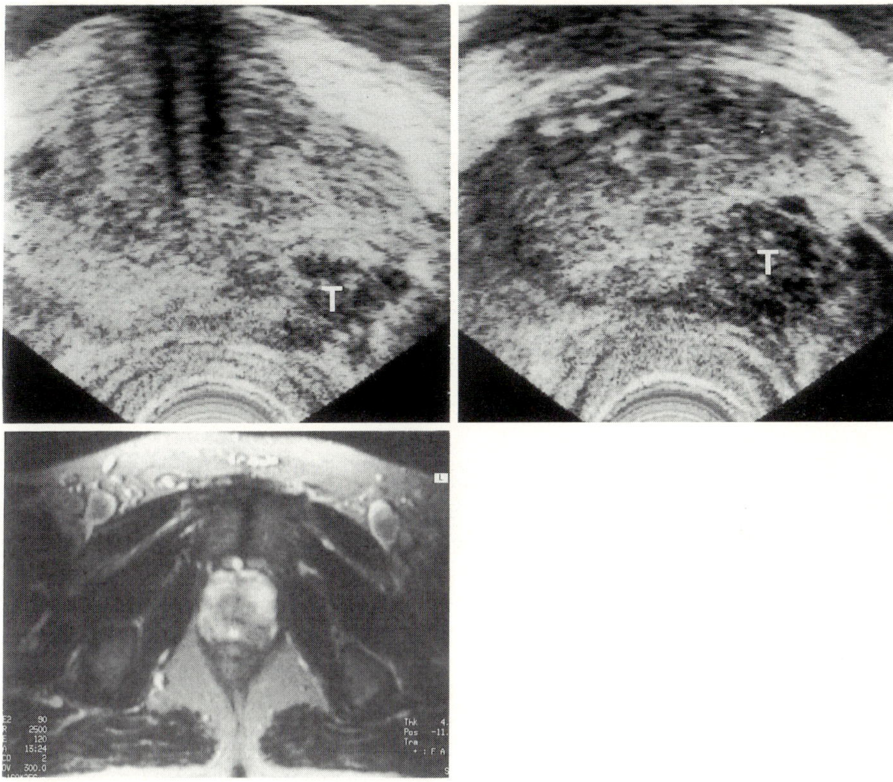

a b c

Fig. 7.46a–c. Adenocarcinoma of the prostate (T3a). Tumor (*T*) in the left PZ with capsular transgression (**a** transverse and **b** sagittal images). Note that the tumor displays scattered hyperechogenicity due to infiltration of the relatively echoic PZ. **c** The tumor is hypointense on a T2-weighted MR image (TR 2500, TE 120) and is indistinguishable from the TZ. It cannot be appreciated whether there is capsular invasion or transgression

With TRUS extension beyond the confines of the prostatic capsule is suggested by interruption or irregular thinning or irregularity (Figs. 7.45, 7.46) (Lee et al. 1986). Other investigators have determined that the value of TRUS in staging prostatic cancer is limited by its inability to detect microscopic invasion of the capsule or seminal vesicles (Fig. 7.47). A positive TRUS diagnosis of pericapsular tumor spread correlates only moderately well with the depth of penetration demonstrated at pathologic examination. Pericapsular tumor spread is incorrectly overdiagnosed in 9.1% of cases and missed in 31.3% (Hamper et al. 1991).

Seminal vesicle enlargement and changes in echogenicity are well shown but are not specific. Biopsy of the seminal vesicles improves the preoperative staging of prostatic cancer before radical prostatectomy: negative biopsies are good predictors of the absence of lymph node invasion (Vallancien et al. 1991a). It is

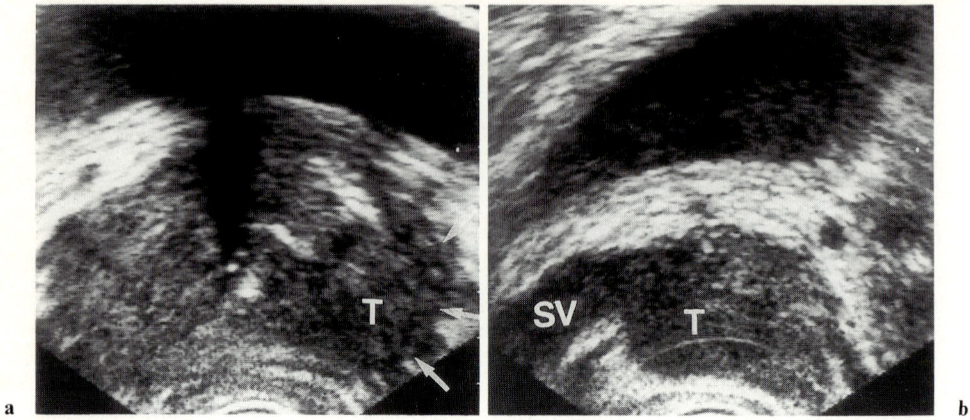

Fig. 7.47a, b. Adenocarcinoma of the PZ (T3b–c). **a** Transverse and **b** sagittal scans showing a hypoechoic tumor (*T*) in the PZ on the left side, with capsular transgression (*arrows*). Because the tumor is isoechoic to the seminal vesicle (*SV*), tumoral invasion of the SV cannot be evaluated. Targeted biopsies of the SV can be useful to stage this tumor correctly

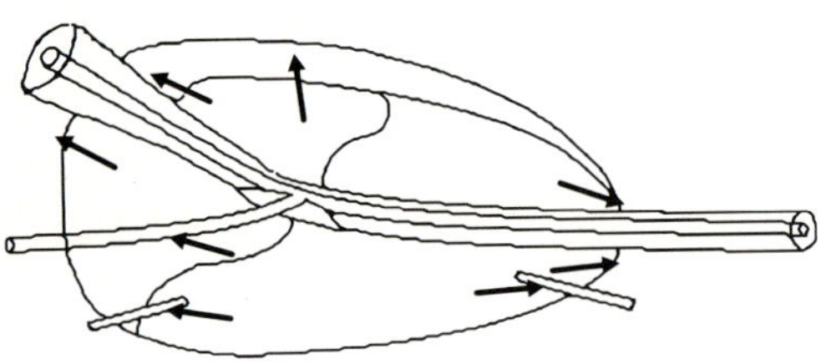

Fig. 7.48. Areas where tumor spread is likely to occur. These areas comprise the anterior fibromuscular stroma, the bladder neck, the apex, the invaginated extraprostatic space, and the neurovascular bundles

now believed that MRI is superior for evaluating tumor extension into the seminal vesicles (FRIEDMAN et al. 1988).

Following the completion of a recent multi-institutional cooperative trial it was concluded that TRUS was not highly accurate in staging early prostatic cancer, mainly because the examination did not have the ability to identify microscopic spread of disease (RIFKIN et al. 1990). A total of 230 patients were evaluated with TRUS and MRI prior to radical prostatectomy. Correlation of radiologic and pathologic findings revealed that TRUS correctly staged 66% of patients with advanced disease and only 46% with localized disease. In patients with advanced disease correctly staged by TRUS, there was an exact match between the site of periprostatic invasion detected by TRUS and that identified by pathologic examination only 71% of the time. The sensitivity of TRUS in detecting seminal vesicle invasion was determined to be 22% while the specificity was 88%.

The comprehensive description of the zonal anatomy has identified the likely sites of cancer within the gland and provides further understanding of the way in which prostatic tumors spread (Fig. 7.48). The primary sites of tumor escape

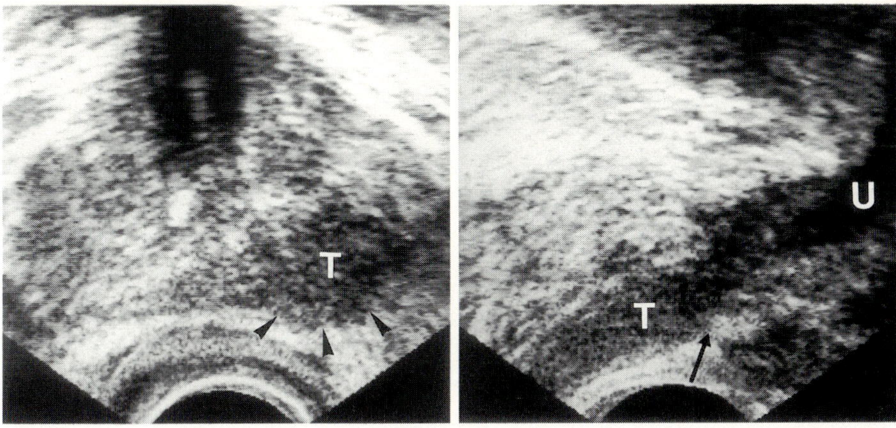

Fig. 7.49. Peripheral zone tumor (*T*) on the left side, with **a** capsular transgression and **b** extension to the apical urethra. There is tumoral invasion of the trapezoid area (*arrow*), too. *U*, Urethra. Microscopic invasion of the apical urethra and trapezoid area cannot be excluded by any method. Targeted biopsies are indicated if this information would be useful for further therapy planning

have been described. They are different for inner (TZ) and outer gland (CZ and PZ) cancers: PZ cancers escape through the prostatic capsule (38%), anterior fibromuscular stroma (5%), seminal vesicles (18%), the base of the gland at the neurovascular bundle (21%), and the apex (31%). TZ cancers escape through the anterior fibromuscular stroma (6%) and the apex (11%). Histologic differences have been noticed as well: Gleason scores are significantly different for TZ and PZ cancers. PZ carcinomas thus show increased aggressive behavior of both histologic and biologic nature. Strategic TRUS-guided biopsy affords accurate tumor mapping and staging when modes of internal spread and escape of cancer from the different zones are known (Fig. 7.49) (LEE F. et al. 1991). This might be important for future therapy planning. TRUS does allow directed biopsies of the seminal vesicles or other suspect areas such as the invaginated extraprostatic space, the trapezoid area, or penetrating fascicles of the neurovascular bundle, and thus may be helpful in accurate staging of the disease. Color Doppler may be helpful in targeting these particular areas. The latter technique has proven to be helpful intraoperatively as well (DREW et al. 1989).

7.5.3.2 Computed Tomography

T Staging The reported sensitivity of CT in detecting extracapsular extension is between 30% and 50%, with a specificity of about 90% and an accuracy of 60%–75% (DAHNERT et al. 1986; BIONDETTI et al. 1987). Invasion of the seminal vesicles must be significant before it is detectable (Fig. 7.50). Obliteration of the periprostatic fat or the angle between the seminal vesicles and the prostate and

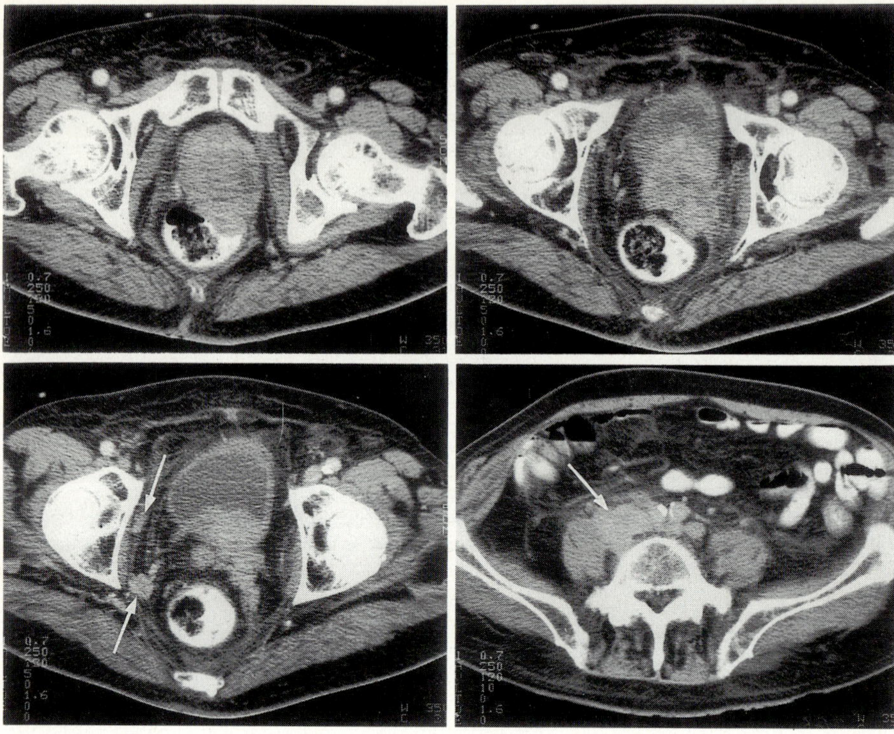

a b c d

Fig. 7.50a–d. A large prostatic tumor is extending beyond the confines of the prostate, infiltrating the rectum (**a**), the rectal fascia (**a, b**), and the pelvic wall (**b**). There are metastatically involved lymph nodes (*arrows*) in the right obturator area (**c**) and the right iliac communis chain (*arrow* in **d**)

asymmetry in the volume of the seminal vesicles are not reliable signs of extraglandular tumor spread.

N Staging There is growing controversy over whether CT is still the imaging modality of choice for detecting lymphadenopathy in patients with known prostatic cancer. Some authors consider CT to be ill-suited for the detection of lymph node metastases since the only criterion is lymph node enlargement. Yet, the overall accuracy of CT for detecting pelvic adenopathy is approximately 80%, with a high specificity (MORGAN et al. 1981). Size criteria of the lymph nodes are invaluable in the individual patient. Percutaneous CT-guided fine-needle aspiration biopsy can be used to confirm metastatic involvement of lymph nodes, thus increasing the sensitivity and specificity of CT as an N-staging modality (Figs. 7.51–7.53). Fine-needle aspiration biopsy of all suspicious lymph nodes is recommended to obtain a histologic diagnosis, especially in those cases where a diagnosis of metastases would alter further therapy (OYEN et al. 1991b; VAN POPPEL et al. 1992).

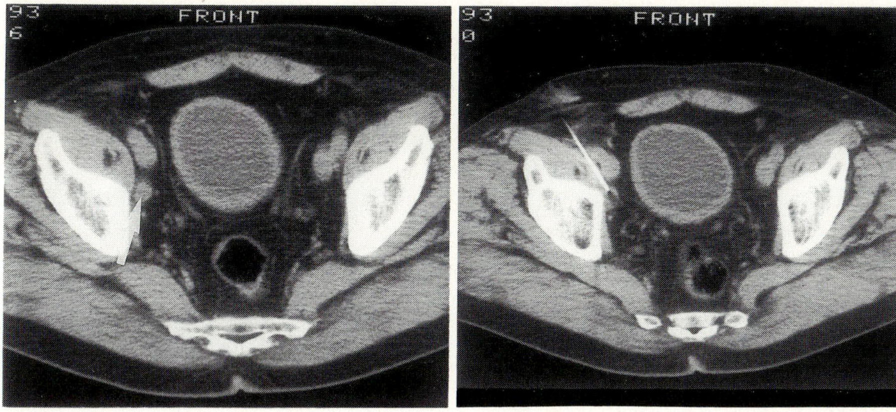

a b

Fig. 51a, b. Lymph node metastases. Solitary enlarged lymph node in the right external iliac chain (*arrow*); microscopically proven metastases from the known locally confined prostatic tumor. Needle biopsy by an anterior approach

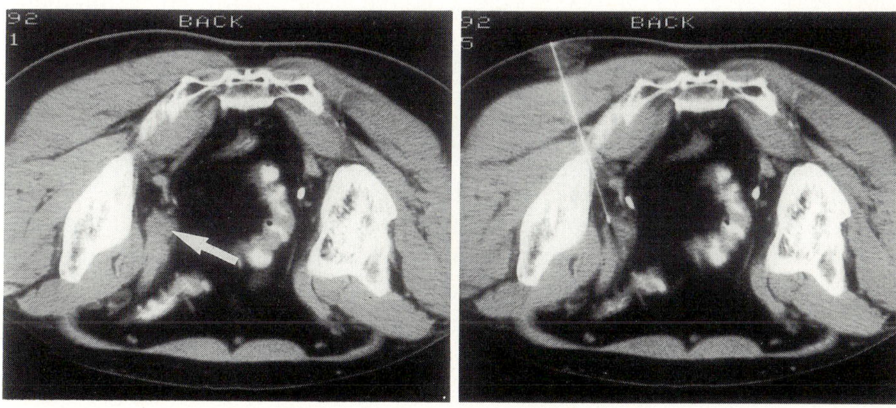

a b

Fig. 52a, b. Lymph node metastases in a patient with a prostatic adenocarcinoma (T2b). Nodule in the external iliac chain on the right side (*arrow*), proven to be metastatically involved by percutaneous fine-needle aspiration biopsy via a dorsal approach

Newer surgical developments, such as endoscopic lymphadenectomy, are gaining interest in the N staging for pelvic malignancies.

Bone windows should always be obtained in the clinical setting of prostatic carcinoma.

7.5.3.3 Magnetic Resonance Imaging

T Staging A carcinoma of the prostate which penetrates through the capsule into the periprostatic tissues interrupts or obliterates this rim, whereas an intact

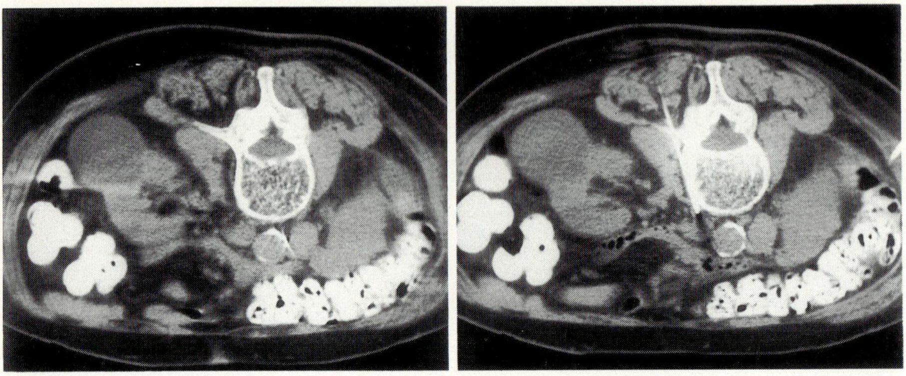

Fig. 7.53a, b. Para-aortic lymph node. Biopsy-proven lymph node metastases from a prostatic carcinoma (T2b) (dorsal approach)

rim indicates that the tumor is confined within the prostatic capsule. Agreement with clinical methods has been reported in 76% of the patients (BIONDETTI et al. 1987; POON et al. 1985, 1988). Tumor in the periprostatic fat is optimally demonstrated on T1-weighted images as hypointensities. Multiplanar images are often required to obtain optimal accuracy.

Involvement of the seminal vesicles, the bladder neck, and adjacent muscle or fasciae is best seen on T2-weighted images (FRIEDMAN et al. 1988; LEE and ROLLS 1986). Tumor extension to the bladder neck or muscles is hyperintense compared with normal muscle, while tumor spread in the seminal vesicles is hypointense. The specificity of the latter seems to be high, although it has been reported that atrophy, fibrosis, or hemorrhage may mimic tumor spread (BIONDETTI et al. 1987; LEE and RHOLL 1986).

Obliteration of the high tubular intensity venous plexus anterolateral to the prostate is a reliable sign of extracapsular tumor spread. The periprostatic venous plexus can be observed as a bright rim on coronal MR images obtained by the spin-echo technique.

The sensitivity of MRI in detecting invasion of the neurovascular bundle was 68%, the specificity 59%, and the overall accuracy 64% in a study where the whole body coil was used (CHADWICK et al. 1991). TRUS is more sensitive in the detection of tumor and extracapsular tumor spread. MRI is more sensitive in the detection of tumor involvement of the seminal vesicles and the bladder base, and allows the detection of lymphadenopathy and bone metastases in the lumbosacral spine and pelvis (CHADWICK et al. 1991).

Magnetic resonance imaging appears to have an overall accuracy of 80%–90% in differentiating stage B from stage C and D disease, with a sensitivity and specificity of 75%–90% (BEZZI et al. 1988; BIONDETTI et al. 1987; KAHN et al. 1989).

Endorectal surface coil MRI has an accuracy of 82% in the differentiation of stage T2 from stage T3 cancer. However, microscopic capsular invasion and minimal seminal vesicle invasion are still underestimated (RIFKIN et al. 1990; SCHNALL et al. 1991). Addition of inversion-recovery sequences with the endorectal coil may improve the usefulness of this technique (PARIVAR et al. 1991).

Recent findings suggest that gadopentetate dimeglumine is not warranted for routine use in endorectal MRI of the prostate but may be useful for evaluation of the seminal vesicles in selected patients (MIROWITZ et al. 1993).

Transrectal ultrasonography and MRI are considered complementary investigations and for the accurate staging of prostatic malignancy both investigations should be used.

N Staging Evaluation of pelvic lymph nodes is an integral part of the staging of the patient with prostatic cancer. Metastatic and inflammatory lymph nodes cannot be reliably differentiated on the basis of their signal intensities. For practical purposes, clusters of nodes larger than 1 cm in diameter are considered pathologic. Because of the necessity of a large field of view, pelvic nodes can only be screened by body coil MRI, and short TR/TE images provide the best contrast and resolution for this purpose. An accuracy of 69% and a specificity of 95% have been reported (LEE et al. 1984; HRICAK et al. 1987).

Lymph nodes can be demonstrated on T1-weighted images as hypointensities. Lymph node metastases are hyperintense compared with normal muscle on T2-weighted images.

The sensitivity of MRI in the detection of lymph node metastases is 69%, with a specificity of 95% and an accuracy of 88% (BEZZI et al. 1988; FRIEDMAN et al. 1988). MRI also allows the detection of bone metastases in the pelvis and lumbosacral spine.

7.5.4 Follow-up After Therapy

Suspicious appearing hypoechoic lesions suggestive of cancer, whether in the PZ or the TZ, should be biopsied after transurethral resection (TUR) before expectant management of stage T1 prostatic cancer is considered (EGAWA et al. 1991b). The sensitivity of tumor detection for cancers originating in the PZ was 81% after TUR or open enucleation. The sensitivity, however, was 0% for tumors confined to the TZ. Tumor staging is not compromised by previous prostatic enucleation or TUR (CARROLL et al. 1992; TERRIS et al. 1992b). TRUS-guided systematic biopsies in clinically stage T1 cancers revealed cancer in only 28%; with more anteriorly directed biopsies, cancer was detected in 47% of the patients (TERRIS et al. 1992b). Anteriorly directed biopsies are warranted to evaluate the anterior extension of the PZ rather than the anterior parts of the residual PZ (Fig. 7.41).

Transrectal ultrasonography is useful in the follow-up of patients with prostatic carcinoma who are receiving hormone therapy. The volume of the prostate decreases after 12 months and the echo pattern changes significantly in two-thirds of the patients (BROSETA et al. 1989). The mean volume reduction of the

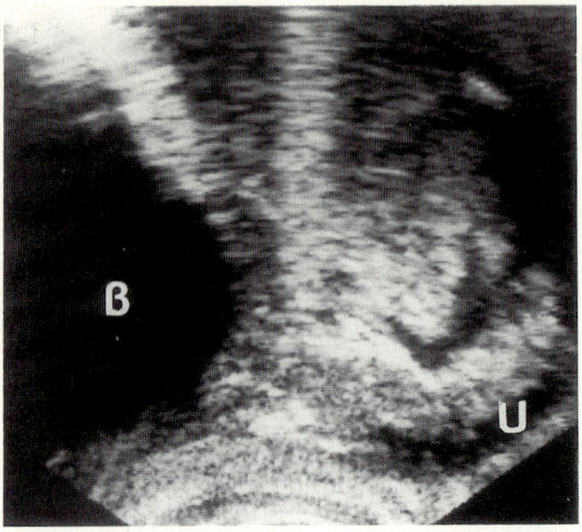

Fig. 7.54. Radical prostatectomy. Sagittal scan after radical prostatectomy at the junction between the bladder (*B*) and the membranous urethra (*U*)

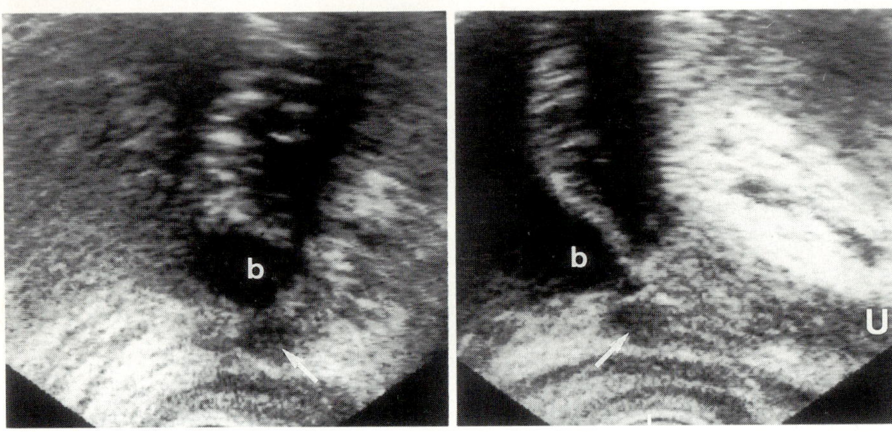

a b

Fig. 7.55a, b. Recurrent tumor after radical prostatectomy. **a** Transverse and **b** sagittal scans of the vesicourethral junction after radical prostatectomy. A small hypoechoic lesion (*arrow*) was proven on biopsy to be local recurrence 1 year after radical prostatectomy. There was a gradual increase in PSA, too. *b*, Bladder; *U*, membranous urethra

prostate at 3 months after the start of treatment was 37.1%. Patients in whom the volume of the prostate had regressed by 50% or more at 3 months had a better prognosis than those with a smaller volume reduction (SNELLER et al. 1992).

Knowledge of the baseline anatomic structures depicted on TRUS obtained after radical prostatectomy may be useful in the selection of tissue for TRUS-guided needle biopsy in patients with elevated levels of PSA (Fig. 7.54). The main value of TRUS-guided biopsies in patients after radical prostatectomy compared to digitally guided biopsy may be in accurate positioning of the biopsy needle about the vesicourethral anastomosis (WASSERMAN et al. 1992a, b). Since histologically the recurrent or residual tumor has the same appearance, it will present as hypoechoic foci around the anastomosis (Figs. 7.55, 7.56).

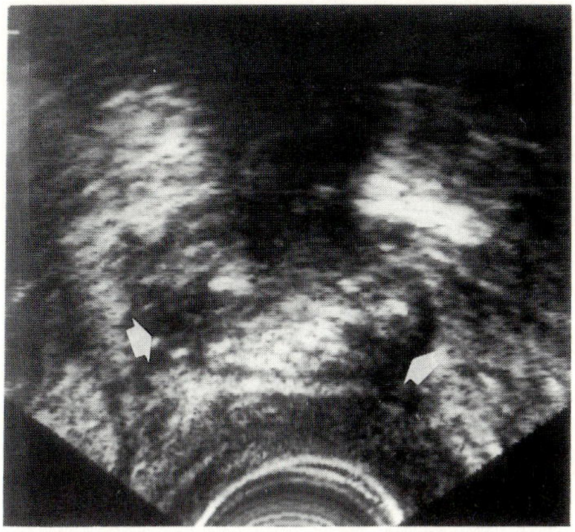

Fig. 7.56. Residual prostate following radical prostatectomy shows a heterogeneous pattern. Biopsy of the hypoechoic area on either side of the prostate (*arrows*) revealed PIN II lesions

The essence of nonsurgical treatment for prostatic cancer is the use of effective imaging. Experience has shown that TRUS is the ideal imaging system for targeting treatments because of its ease of use and the absence of adverse effects. Percutaneous transperineal TRUS-guided interstitial radiotherapy is an attractive and elegant technique for the administration of high-dose local radiotherapy to the prostate. The complications of seed implantation are those associated with the radiation rather than with the technique of implantation. However, radiotherapy has not provided impressive local control of the disease or prolonged survival. This seems to be due more to the inadequacy of iodine-125 in controlling the cancer than to poor seed placement (CARTER S.S. et al. 1989).

Transrectal ultrasonography is particularly valuable for monitoring the response of prostatic cancer to radiotherapy. Changes in the echo structure of the gland may be observed following treatment, but these may be difficult to interpret. The capsule may be restored, the tumor may appear smaller, and sometimes, the identification of the tumor may become impossible. The volume of the gland generally decreases, but this has not been established as a reliable indicator of the subsequent prognosis (CLEMENTS et al. 1989). In the irradiated patient, the prostate and seminal vesicles can develop several patterns of intensity abnormalities. In particular, diffuse low signal intensities in the prostate and seminal vesicles should establish radiation fibrosis as an important differential diagnosis (CHAN and KRESSEL 1991; EGAWA et al. 1991b). The use of TRUS for early detection and staging of recurrent disease after definitive radiation is crucial for patient selection for definitive salvage therapy. Persistent cancer retains its hypoechoic appearance after definitive radiotherapy. Hypoechoic lesions larger than 5 mm in diameter found more than 12 months after radiotherapy should be suspected of representing persistent local disease. TRUS-guided biopsy or serial measurement of hypoechoic lesions should be considered in such circumstances (EGAWA et al. 1989; KABALIN et al. 1989). TRUS-guided biopsy of a hypoechoic lesion showed 71.2% to have persistent carcinoma (SIDERS and LEE 1992). The TRUS criteria for the presence of cancer are the same for both the postirradiated prostate and the untreated prostate, and TRUS is the most sensitive test for the diagnosis of persistent local cancer following iodine-125 seed implantation (LEE et al. 1988).

7.6 Congenital Anomalies

7.6.1 Introduction and Definitions

Hypoplasia of the prostate is a consistent feature of prune-belly syndrome. Both the stromal smooth muscle and the glandular tissue are markedly reduced or completely absent. The prostatic urethra is dilated and sacculated (MOERMAN et al. 1984).

Heterotopia of the prostate has been described at the region of the verumontanum and may present as a pedunculated mass protruding into the bladder (BUTTERIC et al. 1971).

The prostatic utricle, a müllerian derivative, is enlarged or replaced by a vagina (vagina masculinus) in patients with intersex (DEVINE et al. 1980). Hypospadias without underlying intersex is also frequently associated with enlarged utricle. Some utricular cysts may be acquired due to inflammatory stricture of the utricular orifice. These cysts may cause urinary obstruction or obstruction of the ejaculatory ducts, or provide a site for recurrent infection and stone formation (POLSE and EDELBROCK 1968). The utricle cyst is lined with columnar or low cuboidal epithelium and filled with serous, mucoid, or purulent fluid.

7.6.2 Ultrasonography

Utricular and müllerian duct cysts are midline cysts and the content is either anechoic or echogenic with sometimes gravity-dependent fluid levels (GREGG and STY 1989; HOLM and FORSBERG 1984; VILLERS et al. 1990) (Figs. 7.57, 7.58). Because of their volume they may cause obstruction of the ejaculatory ducts. It may be impossible to distinguish a utriclar cyst from a müllerian duct cyst. Utricular cysts, however, are usually confined to the prostate, while müllerian duct cyst may develop well outside the confines of the prostate, sometimes offset from the midline: in fact they may develop at any place along the course of the müllerian duct.

Ejaculatory duct cysts are rare. Many small cysts are not associated with symptoms. Large cysts are associated with perineal pain, hematospermia, and ejaculatory pain. These cysts typically contain spermatozoa. Ejaculatory cysts are due to an obstruction of the duct that may be either congenital or secondary

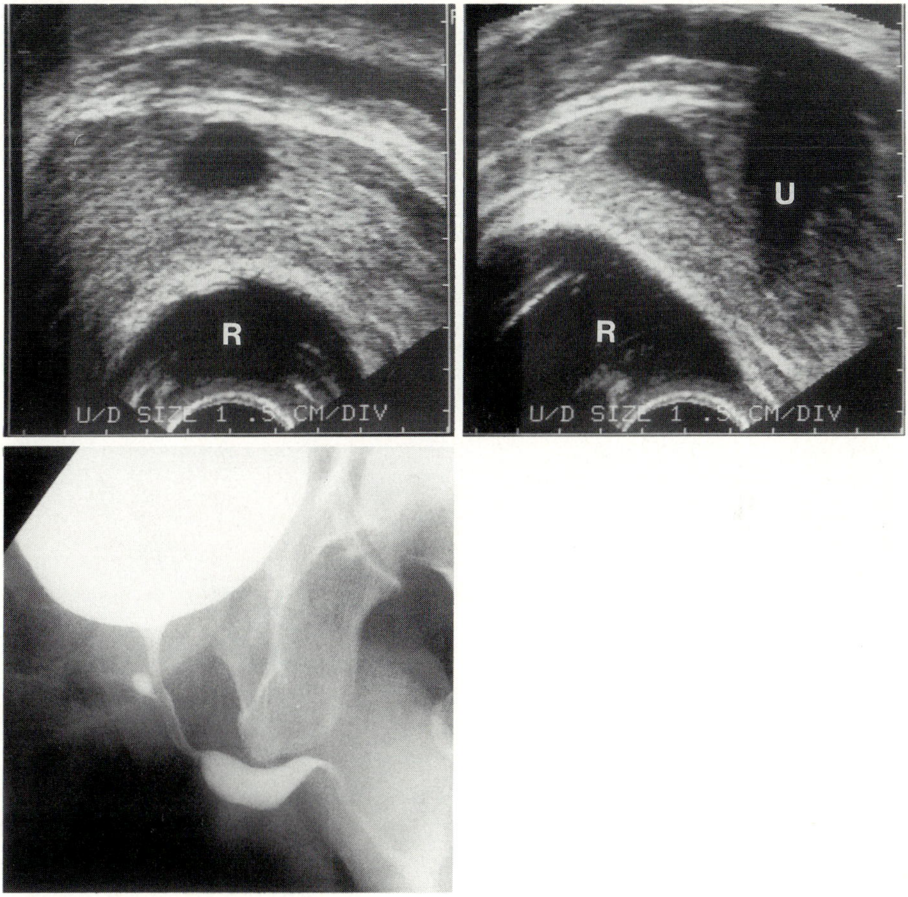

a b

c

Fig. 7.57a–c. Utriculus. TRUS (**a** transverse and **b** sagittal scans) and voiding urethrogram (**c**). Small utriculus (or utricular cyst) presenting as an anechoic structure confined to the gland and a contrast-filled structure behind the urethra. *U*, Proximal prostatic urethra and its surrounding sphincters; *R*, water-filled balloon covering the rectal transducer

to inflammation. When large, these lesions may simulate prostatic utricle and müllerian duct cysts.

7.6.3 Computed Tomography

Only rarely are prostatic cysts demonstrated by CT. Cysts of the seminal vesicles, associated with ipsilateral renal agenesis, can be fairly well depicted on CT. However, it is felt that MRI merits a more important role than CT in the (preoperative) clinical setting of congenital anomalies of the prostate and the seminal vesicles.

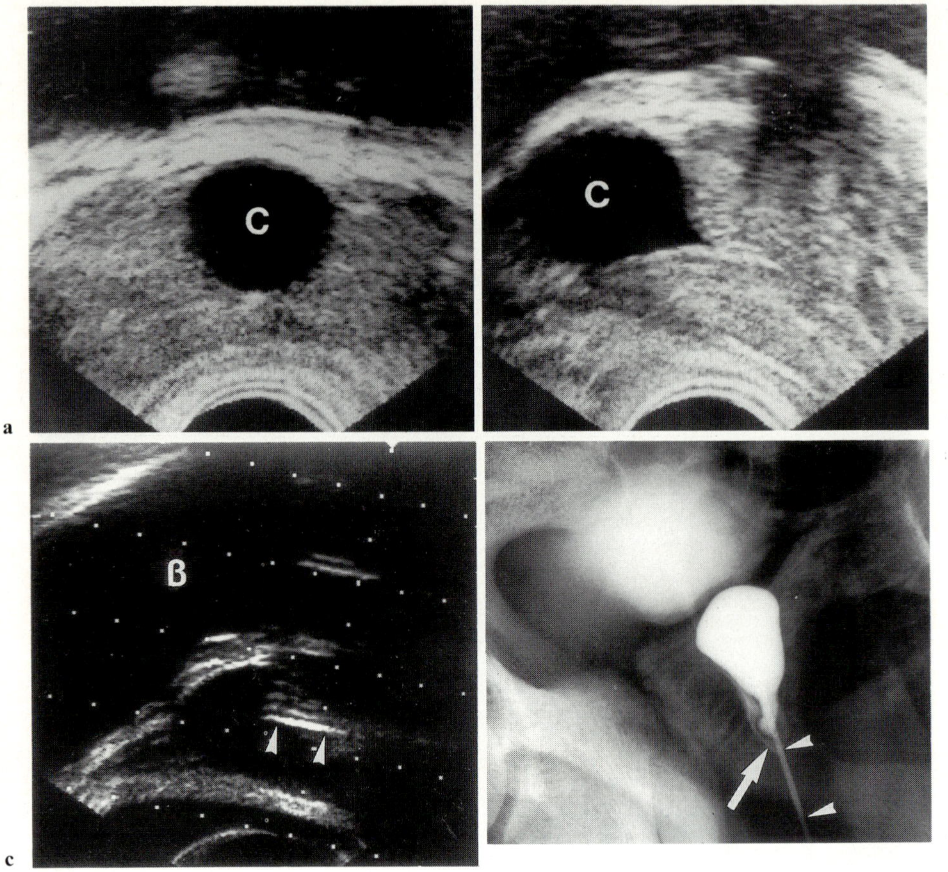

Fig. 7.58a–d. Midline (müllerian duct?) cyst. Midline cyst (**a**) behind the proximal urethra (**b**). This was biopsied under sonographic guidance (**c**; needle indicated by *arrowheads*). The injection of the contrast medium (**d**) shows the connection between the cyst and the urethra (*arrow*). The dye subsequently fills the bladder. *B*, Bladder; *C*, cyst

7.6.4 Magnetic Resonance Imaging

Magnetic resonance imaging is particularly suitable to evaluate the extent of congenital cyst of the prostate and the seminal vesicles because of its capacity for multiplanar imaging. Both prostatic and utricular cysts have a homogeneous high signal intensity on T2-weighted images. Their signal intensity on T1-weighted images depends on the protein content of the cyst fluid: the higher the protein concentration, the higher the signal (THURNHER et al. 1988).

References

Allen KS, Kressel HY, Arger PH, Pollack HM (1989) Age-related changes of the prostate: evaluation by MR imaging. Am J Roentgenol 152:77–81

Amiel J, Chevallier D, Peyrottes A, Benoliel J, Toubol J (1989) Correlations anatomoclinique et biologique dans la pathologie prostatique. A propos de 150 observations. Ann Urol 23:528–530

Aus G, Skude G (1992) Effect of ultrasound guided core biopsy of prostate on serum concentration of prostate specific antigen and acid phosphatase activity. Scand J Urol Nephrol 26:21–23

Ayala AG, Ro JY, Babaian R, et al. (1989) The prostatic capsule: does it exist? Its importance in the staging and treatment of prostatic carcinoma. Am J Surg Pathol 1:21–27

Bain GO, Danyluk JM, Shnikata TK, Jewell LD, Manickavel V (1985) Malignant fibrous histiocytoma of the prostate gland. Urology 26:89–91

Bezzi M, Kressel HY, Allen KS, Schiebler ML, Altman HG, Wein AJ, Pollack HM (1988) Prostatic carcinoma: staging with MR imaging at 1.5 T. Radiology 169:339–346

Billebaud T, Sibert A, Dauge MC, et al. (1990) Intérêt des biopsies systematiques multiples echoguidés dans le diagnostic précoce du cancer de prostate. Ann Urol 24:524–529

Biondetti PR, Lee JKT, Ling D, et al. (1987) Clinical stage B prostate carcinoma: staging with MR imaging. Radiology 162:325–329

Bock E, Calugi V, Stolfi V, Rossi P, D'Ascenzo R, Solivetti FM (1989) Le calcificazioni della prostata: studio con ecografia transrettale. Radiol Med 77:501–503

Brawer MK, Rennels MA, Nagle RB, Soiderer MH, Lee F (1989) Prostatic intraepithelial neoplasia: a lesion that may be confused with cancer on prostatic ultrasound. J Urol 142:1510–1512

Broseta E, Boronat F, Dominguez C, Vidal J, Llopis B, Jimenez-Cruz JF (1989) Modificacion del patron ecografico del carcinoma de prostata tratado mediante agonistas Lh-rh. Arch Esp Urol 42:125–128

Bryan PJ, Butler HE, Nelson AD, et al. (1986) Magnetic resonance imaging of the prostate. AJR 146:543–548

Buonocore E, Hesemann C, Pavlicek W, et al. (1984) Clinical and in vitro magnetic resonance imaging of prostatic carcinoma. AJR 143:1267–1272

Burks DD, Drolshagen LF, Fleischer AC, et al. (1986) Transrectal sonography of benign and malignant prostatic lesions. AJR 146:1187–1191

Butteric JA, Schnitzer B, Abell MR (1971) Ectopic prostatic tissue in urethra: a clinicopathologic entity and significant cause of hematuria. J Urol 105:97–99

Carrol CL, Sommer FG, McNeal JE, et al. (1987) The abnormal prostate: MR imaging at 1.5 T with histopathologic correlation. Radiology 163:521–525

Carroll PR, Sugimura K, Cohen MB, Hricak H (1992) Detection and staging of prostatic carcinoma after transurethral resection or open enucleation of the prostate: accuracy of magnetic resonance imaging. J Urol 147:402–406

Carter HB, Hamper UM, Sheth S, et al. (1989) Evaluation of transrectal ultrasound in the early detection of prostate cancer. J Urol 142:1008–1010

Carter SS, Torp-Pedersen ST, Holm HH (1989) Ultrasound-guided implantation techniques in treatment of prostate cancer. Urol Clin North Am 16:751–762

Catalona WJ, Scott WW (1978) Carcinoma of the prostate: a review. J Urol 119:1–7

Chadwick DJ, Cobby M, Goddard P, Gingell JC (1991) Comparison of transrectal ultrasound and magnetic resonance imaging in the staging of prostate cancer. Br J Urol 67:616–621

Chan TW, Kressel HY (1991) Prostate and seminal vesicles after irradiation: MR appearance. J Magn Reson Imaging 1:503–511

Christiansen E, Purvis K (1991) Diagnosis of chronic abacterial prostato-vesiculitis by rectal ultrasonography in relation to symptoms and findings. Br J Urol 67:173–176

Clements R, Griffiths GJ, Peeling WB, Edwards AM (1989) Transrectal ultrasound in monitoring response to treatment of prostate disease. Urol Clin North Am 16:735–740

Coffield KS, Speights VO, Brawn PN (1992) Ultrasound detection of prostate cancer in postmortem specimens with histopathological correlation. J Urol 147:822–826

Cytron S, Weinberger M, Pitlik SD, et al. (1988) Value of transrectal ultrasonography for diagnosis and treatment of prostatic abscess. Urology 32:454–458

Dahnert WF, Hamper UM, Eggleston JC, et al. (1986) Prostatic evaluation by transrectal sonography with histopathologic correlation: the echopenic appearance of early carcinoma. Radiology 158:97–102

Daniels GF, McNeal JE, Stamey TA (1992) Predictive value of contralateral biopsies in unilaterally palpable prostate cancer. J Urol 147:870–874

de la Rosette JJ, Karthaus HF, Debruyne FM (1992) Ultrasonographic findings in patients with nonbacterial prostatitis. Urol Int 48:323–326

Devine CJ Jr, Gonzalez-Serva L, Stecker JF, Jr, et al. (1980) Utricular configuration in hypospadias and intersex. J Urol 123:407–411

Devonec M, Fendler JP, Monsallier M, Mouriquand P, Mestas JL, Dutrieux-Berger N, Perrin P (1989) Prostatic cancer diagnosis with ultrasonically guided prostatic biopsy: results in 226 cases. Prog Clin Biol Res 303P:35–40

Devonec M, Fendler JP, Monsallier M, et al. (1990) The significance of the prostatic hypoechoic area: results in 226 ultrasonically guided prostatic biopsies. J Urol 143:316–319

Dhom G (1983) Epidemiologic aspects of latent and clinically manifest carcinoma of the prostate. J Cancer Res Clin Oncol 106:210–218

Di Trapani D, Pavone C, Serretta V, Cavallo N, Costa G, Pavone-Macaluso M (1988) Chronic prostatitis and prostatodynia: ultrasonographic alterations of the prostate, bladder neck, seminal vesicles and periprostatic venous plexus. Eur Urol 15:230–234

Doble A, Carter SS (1989) Ultrasonographic findings in prostatitis. Urol Clin North Am 16:763–772

Doble A, Thomas BJ, Walker MM, Harris JR, Witherow RO, Taylor-Robinson D (1989) The role of *Chlamydia trachomatis* in chronic abacterial prostatitis: a study using ultrasound guided biopsy. J Urol 141:332–333

Dooms GC, Hricak H (1986) Magnetic resonance imaging of the pelvis: prostate and urinary bladder. Urol Radiol 8:156–165

Drach GW, Meares EM Jr, Stamey TA (1978) Classification of benign diseases associated with prostatic pain: prostatitis or prostatodynia? J Urol 120:266

Drew JB, Begun FP, Jacobs SC (1989) Doppler-assisted nerve-sparing radical prostatectomy. Urology 33:228–229

Dyke CH, Toi A, Sweet JM (1990) Value of random US-guided transrectal prostate biopsy. Radiology 176:345–349

Egawa S, Carter SS, Wheeler TM, Scardino PT (1989) Ultrasonographic changes in the normal and malignant prostate after definitive radiotherapy. Urol Clin North Am 16:741–749

Egawa S, Greene DR, Flanagan WF, Wheeler TM, Scardino PT (1991a) Transrectal ultrasonography in stage A prostate cancer: detection of residual tumor after transurethral resection of prostate. J Urol 146:366–371

Egawa S, Wheeler TM, Scardino PT (1991b) The sonographic appearance of irradiated prostate cancer. Br J Urol 68:172–177

Egawa S, Wheeler TM, Greene DR, Scardino PT (1992) Unusual hyperechoic appearance of prostate cancer on transrectal ultrasonography. Br J Urol 69:169–174

Epstein JI, Hutchins GM (1984) Granulomatous prostatitis: distinction among allergic, nonspecific and post-transurethral resection lesions. Hum Pathol 15:818–822

Franks LM (1954) Benign nodular hyperplasia of the prostate: a review. Ann R Coll Surg Engl 14:92–106

Friedman AC, Seidmon EJ, Radecki PR, et al. (1988) Relative merits of MRI, transrectal endosonography and CT in the diagnosis and staging of carcinoma of the prostate. Urology 31:530–537

Geller J (1989) Pathogenesis and medical treatment of benign prostatic hyperplasia. Prostate Suppl 2P:95–104

Gevenois PA, Salmon I, Stallenberg B, van Sinoy ML, van Regemorter G, Struyven J (1990) Magnetic resonance imaging of the normal prostate at 1.5 T Br J Radiol 63:101–107

Gleason DF and Veterans Administration Cooperative Research Group (1977) Histologic grading in clinical staging of prostatic carcinoma. In: Tannenbaum M (ed) Urologic pathology: the prostate. Lea & Febiger, Philadelphia, pp 171–197

Grayhack JT, Kozlowski JM (1987) Benign prostatic hyperplasia. In: Gillenwater JY, Grayhack JT, Howard SS, et al. (eds) Adult and pediatric urology, vol 2. Year Book Medical Publishers, Chicago, pp 1062–1125

Greene DR, Egawa S, Hellerstein DK, Scardino PT (1990) Sonographic measurements of transition zone of prostate in men with and without benign prostatic hyperplasia. Urology 36:293–299

Gregg DC, Sty JR (1989) Sonographic diagnosis of enlarged prostatic utricle. Ultrasound Med 8:51–52

Grups JW, Gruss A, Wirth M, Frohmuller HG (1990) Diagnostic value of transrectal ultrasound in tumor staging and in the detection of incidental prostatic cancer. Urol Int 45:38–40

Guercini F, Solivetti FM, Dimitri M, D'Ascenzo R, Micali F (1991) Il color Doppler nella diagnosi delle neoplasie prostatiche maligne. Risultati preliminari. Arch Ital Urol Nefrol Androl 63 (Suppl 2P):29–33

Gustafsson O, Norming U, Nyman CR, Ohstrom M (1990) Complications following combined transrectal aspiration and core biopsy of the prostate. Scand J Urol Nephrol 24:249–251

Hamper UM, Epstein JI, Sheth S, Walsh PC, Sanders RC (1990) Cystic lesions of the prostate gland. A sonographic-pathologic correlation. J Ultrasound 9:395–402

Hamper UM, Sheth S, Walsh PC, Holtz PM, Epstein JI (1991) Capsular transgression of prostatic carcinoma: evaluation with transrectal US with pathologic correlation. Radiology 178:791–795

Hardt NS, Kaude JV, Li KC, Ros PR, Hackett RL (1988) Sonography of the prostate: in vitro correlation of sonographic and anatomic findings in normal glands. Am J Roentgenol 151:955–959

Hendrikx AJ, Doesburg WH, Reintjes AG, Strijk SP, Debruyne FM (1988) Effectiveness of ultrasound in the preoperative evaluation of patients with prostatism. Prostate 13:199–208

Hernandez AD, Smith JA Jr (1990) Transrectal ultrasonography for the early detection and staging of prostate cancer. Urol Clin North Am 17:745–757

Hodge KH, McNeal JE, Terris MK (1989a) Random systematic versus directed ultrasound guided transrectal core biopsies of the prostate. J Urol 142:71–75

Hodge KK, McNeal JE, Stamey TA (1989b) Ultrasound guided transrectal core biopsies of the palpable abnormal prostate. J Urol 142:66–70

Holm L, Forsberg L (1984) Computed tomography and ultrasound studies of prostatic utricle cyst associated with unilateral renal agenesis. Scand J Nephrol 18:87–89

Hricak H, Dooms GC, Jeffrey RB, et al. (1987) Prostatic Carcinoma: staging by clinical assessment, CT and MR imaging. Radiology 162:331–336

Jaeger N, Bockisch A, Hunerman B, et al. (1987) The diagnostic significance of magnetic resonace imaging in prostate tumors. Int Urol Nephrol 19:299–305

Jakobsen H, Torp-Pedersen S, Juul N (1988) Ultrasonic evaluation of age-related human prostatic growth and development of benign prostatic hyperplasia. Scand J Urol Nephrol Suppl 107P:26–31

Jimenez-Cruz JF, Tormo FB, Gomez JG (1988) Treatment of chronic prostatitis: intraprostatic antibiotic injections under echography control. J Urol 139:967–970

Jones DR, Griffiths GJ, Parkinson MC, et al. (1989) Structure and per-rectal ultrasonography of prostatic disease using cadaver specimens. Br J Urol 64:611–617

Kabalin JN, Hodge KK, McNeal JE, Freiha FS, Stamey TA (1989) Identification of residual cancer in the prostate following radiation therapy: role of transrectal ultrasound guided biopsy and prostate specific antigen. J Urol 142:326–331

Kahn T, Burrig K, Schmitz-Drager B, Lewin JS, Furst G, Modder U (1989) Prostatic carcinoma and benign prostatic hyperplasia: MR imaging with histopathologic correlation. Radiology 173:847–851

Kaye KW, Richter L (1990) Ultrasonographic anatomy of normal prostate gland: reconstruction by computer graphics. Urology 35:12–17

Klimas K, Bennett B, Gardner WA (1985) Prostate calculi: a review, Prostate 7:91–96

Kovi J (1983) Carcinoma of the prostate: A disease of black men? J Natl Med Assoc 75:121–122

Larkin BT, Berquist TH, Utz DC (1986) Evaluation of the prostate by magnetic resonance imaging. Magn Reson Imaging 4:53–58

Lee F, Gray JM, McLeary RD, et al. (1985) Transrectal ultrasound in the diagnosis of prostate cancer: location, echogenicity, histopathology and staging. Prostate 7:117–129

Lee F, Gray JM, McLeary RD, et al. (1986) Prostatic evaluation by transrectal sonography: criteria for diagnosis of early carcinoma. Radiology 158:91–96

Lee F, Torp-Pedersen S, Meisleman L, et al. (1988) Transrectal ultrasound in the diagnosis and staging of local disease after I125 seed implantation for prostate cancer. Int J Radiat Oncol Biol Phys 15:1453–1459

Lee F, Torp-Pedersen ST, McLeary RD (1989a) Diagnosis of prostate cancer by transrectal ultrasound. Urol Clin North Am 16:663–673

Lee F, Torp-Pedersen S, Littrup PJ, et al. (1989b) Hypo-echoic lesions of the prostate: clinical relevance of tumor size, digital rectal examination, and prostate-specific antigen. Radiology 170:29–32

Lee F, Torp-Pedersen ST, Siders DB, Littrup PJ, McLeary RD (1989c) Transrectal ultrasound in the diagnosis and staging of prostatic carcinoma. Radiology 170:609–615

Lee F Jr, Bronson JP, Lee F, et al. (1991) Nonpalpable cancer of the prostate: assessment with transrectal US. Radiology 178:197–199

Lee F, Siders DB, Torp-Pedersen ST, et al. (1991) Prostate cancer: transrectal ultrasound and pathology comparison. A preliminary study of outer gland (peripheral and central zones) and inner gland (transition zone) cancer. Cancer 67:1132–1142

Lee JKT, Heiken JP, Ling D, et al. (1984) Magnetic Resonance Imaging of abdominal and pelvic lymphadenopathy. Radiology 153:181–188

Lee JKT, Rholl KS (1986) MRI of the bladder and prostate. AJR 147:732–736

Ling D, Lee JKT, Heiken JP, et al. (1986) Prostatic carcinoma and benign prostatic hyperplasia: inability of MR imaging to distinguish between the two diseases. Radiology 158:103–107

Littrup PJ, Kane RA, Williams CR, et al. (1991) Determination of prostate volume with transrectal US for cancer screening. Part II. Accuracy of in vitro and in vivo techniques. Radiology 179:49–53

Lovett K, Rifkin MD, McCue PA, Choi H (1992) MR imaging characteristics of noncancerous lesions of the prostate. J Magn Reson Imaging 2:35–39

Lytton B (1983) Interracial incidence of benign prostatic hypertrophy. In: Hinman F Jr (ed) Benign prostatic hypertrophy. Springer, New York Berlin Heidelberg, pp 22–26

Martin JF, Hajek P, Baker L, Gylys-Morin V, Fitzmorris-Glass R, Mattrey RR (1988) Inflatable surface coil for MR imaging of the prostate. Radiology 167:268–270

McNeal JE (1969) Origin and development of carcinoma in the prostate. Cancer 23:24–34

McNeal JE (1981) The zonal anatomy of the prostate. Prostate 2:35–49

McNeal JE (1983) The prostate gland: morphology and pathobiology. In Stamey TA (ed) Monographs in urology, vol 4. Burroughs Wellcome, Research Triangle Park, N.C., pp 3–33

McNeal JE (1988) Normal anatomy of the prostate and changes in benign hypertrophy and carcinoma. Semi Ultrasound CT MR. 9:329–334

McNeal JE, Redwine EA, Freiha FS, et al. (1988) Zonal distribution of prostatic adenocarcinoma. Correlation with histologic pattern and direction of spread. Am J Surg Pathol 12:897–906

McSherry SA, Levy F, Schiebler ML, Keefe B, Dent GA, Mohler JL (1991) Preoperative prediction of pathological tumor volume and stage in clinically localized prostate cancer: comparison of digital rectal examination, transrectal ultrasonography and magnetic resonance imaging. J Urol 146:85–89

Mirowitz SA, Hammerman AM (1992) CT depiction of prostatic zonal anatomy. J Comput Assist Tomogr 16:439–441

Mirowitz SA, Brown JJ, Heiken JP (1993) Evaluation of the prostate and prostatic carcinoma with gadolinium-enhanced endorectal coil MR imaging. Radiology 186:153–157

Moerman P, Fryns JP, Godderis P, Lauwerijns JM (1984) Pathogenesis of the prune-belly syndrome: a functional urethral obstruction caused by prostatic hypoplasia. Pediatrics 73:470–475

Morgan CL, Calkins RF, Cavalcanti EJ (1981) Computed tomography in the evaluation, staging, and therapy of carcinoma of the bladder and prostate. Radiology 140:751–761

Muldoon LD, Resnick MI (1990) Normal anatomy of the prostate. In Resnick MI (ed) Prostatic ultrasonography. B.C. Decker, Philadelphia, pp 33–39

Myers RP, Goellner JR, Cahill DR (1987) Prostate shape, external striated urethral sphincter and radical prostatectomy: the apical dissection. J Urol 138:543–550

Naito S, Kimiya K, Hasegawa Y, Kumazawa J (1988) Digital examination and transrectal ultrasonography in the diagnosis of prostatic cancer. Eur Urol 14:3

Neal DE Jr, Clejan S, Sarma D, Moon TD (1992) Prostate specific antigen and prostatitis. I. Effect of prostatitis on serum PSA in the human and nonhuman primate. Prostate 20:105–111

Nghiem HT, Kellman GM, Sandberg SA, et al. (1990) Cystic lesions of the prostate. Radiographics 10:635–650

Nielsen KK, Klarskov P, Nordling J, Andersen JT, Holm HH (1990) The intraprostatic spiral. New treatment for urinary retention. Br J Urol 65:500–503

Orland SM, Hanno PM, Wein AJ (1985) Prostatitis, prostatosis and prostatodynia. Urology 25:439–459

Oyen R, Ameye F, Baert L, Marchal G, Baert AL (1991a) Intrarectal Doppler studies of arterial flow during endo-urethral hyperthermia: preliminary results. Eur Radiol (Suppl) 1:63

Oyen R, Ameye F, Van Poppel H, Baert L, Baert AL (1991b) Accuracy of CT and FNAB in the staging of localized prostate carcinoma and bladder carcinoma. Eur Radiol (Suppl) 1:35

Oyen R, Baert L, Baert AL (1991c) Sonography in the diagnosis and the treatment of prostate abscesses. Eur Radiol (Suppl) 1:35

Oyen R, Baert L, Marchal G, Baert AL (1991d) The significance of a hypoechoic area in the central and peripheral zone of the prostate: a study of 27 cases. Eur Radiol (Suppl) 1:35

Oyen R, Van de Voorde W, Van Poppel H, et al. (1993) Benign prostatic nodules in the peripheral zone of the prostate. Radiology 189:707–711

Papanicolaou N, Pfister RC, Stafford SA, et al. (1987) Prostatic abscess: imaging with transrectal sonography and MR. AJR 149:981–982

Parivar F, Rajanayagam V, Waluch V, Eto RT, Jones LW, Ross BD (1991) Endorectal surface coil MR imaging of prostatic carcinoma with the inversion-recovery sequence. J Magn Reson Imaging 1:657–664

Partin AW, Carter HB, Chan DW, et al. (1990) Prostate Specific Antigen in the staging of localised prostate cancer: influence of tumor differentiation, tumor volume and benign hyperplasia. J Urol 143:747

Perrin P, Maquet JH, Bringeon G, et al. (1991) Screening for prostate cancer. Comparison of transrectal ultrasound, prostate specific antigen and rectal examination. Br J Urol 68:263–265

Phillips M, Kressel H, Spritzer C, et al. (1987) Prostatic disorders: MR imaging at 1.5 T. Radiology 164:386–392

Pollack HM (1991) Imaging of the prostate gland. Eur Urol 20 (Suppl 1P). 50–58

Polse S, Edelbrock H (1968) Prostatic utricle enlargement as a cause of vesicle outlet obstruction in children. J Urol 100:329–330

Poon PY, McCallum RW, Henkelman MH, et al. (1985) Magnetic resonance imaging of the prostate. Radiology 154:143–149

Poon PY, McCallum RW, Henkelman RM, et al. (1988) MRI of periprostatic venous plexus in staging of early prostatic carcinoma. J Can Ass Radiol 39:111–114

Poon PY, Bronskill MJ, Poon CS, McCallum RW, Henkelman RM (1991) Optimization of prostatic magnetic resonance imaging technique. J Can Ass Radiol 42:423–430

Quint LE, Van Erp JS, Bland PH, et al. (1991) Carcinoma of the prostate: MR images obtained with body coils do not accurately reflect tumor volume. Am J Roentgenol 156:511–516

Rifkin MD, Choi H (1988) Implications of small, peripheral hypo-echoic lesions in endorectal US of the prostate. Radiology 166:619–622

Rifkin MD, McGlynn ET, Choi H (1989) Echogenicity of prostate cancer correlated with histologic grade and stromal fibrosis: endorectal US studies. Radiology 170:549–552

Rifkin MD, Zerhouni EA, Gatsonis CA, et al. (1990) Comparison of magnetic resonance imaging and ultrasonography in staging early prostate cancer. Results of a multi-institutional cooperative trial. N Engl J Med 323:621–626

Rifkin MD, Alexander AA, Helinek TG, Merton DA (1991) Color Doppler as an adjunct to prostate ultrasound. Scand J Urol Nephrol Suppl 137P:85–89

Rifkin MD, Sudakoff GS, Alexander AA (1993) Prostate: techniques, results and potential applications of color Doppler US scanning. Radiology 186:509–513

Ryan PG, Peeling WB (1990) Perineal prostatic tumor seedling after 'Tru-Cut' needle biopsy: case report and review of the literature. Eur Urol 17:189–192

Schiebler ML, Tomaszewski JE, Bezzi M, et al. (1989) Prostatic carcinoma and benign prostatic hyperplasia: correlation of high-resolution MR and histopathologic findings. Radiology 172:131–137

Schnall MD, Imai Y, Tomaszewski J, Pollack HM, Lenkinski RE, Kressel HY (1991) Prostate cancer: local staging with endorectal surface oil MR imaging. Radiology 178:797–802

Schröder FH, Hermanek P, Denis L, et al. (1992) The TNM classification of prostate cancer. Prostate Suppl 4:129–138

Seymour MA, Oesterling JE (1992) Anterior rectal wall hematoma: complication of transrectal ultrasound-guided biopsy of prostate. Urology 39:77–181

Shinohara K, Scardino PT, Carter SS, Wheeler TM (1989) Pathologic basis of the sonographic appearance of the normal and malignant prostate. Urol Clin North Am 16:675–691

Siders DB, Lee F (1992) Histologic changes of irradiated prostatic carcinoma diagnosed by transrectal ultrasound. Hum Pathol 23:344–351

Sloan JB (1991) Prostate balloon dilatation monitored by transrectal ultrasound. Urology 38:20–25

Smith BH, Dehner LP (1972) Sarcoma of the prostate gland. Am J Clin Pathol 58:43–50

Sneller ZW, Hop WC, Carpentier PJ, Schroder FH (1992) Prognosis and prostatic volume changes during endocrine management of prostate cancer: a longitudinal study. J Urol 147:962–966

Spigelman SS, McNeal JE, Freiha FS, et al. (1986) Rectal examination in volume determination of carcinoma of the prostate: clinical and anatomical considerations. J Urol 136:1228–1230

Stamey TA, Yang N, Hay AR, McNeal JE, Freiha FS, Redwine E (1987) Prostate-specific antigen as a serum marker for adenocarcinoma of the prostate. N Eng J Med 317:909

Stamey TA, McNeal JE, Redwine EA, et al. (1988) Morphometric and clinical studies on 68 consecutive radical prostatectomies. J Urol 139:1235–1241

Tannenbaum M (1975) Sarcomas of the prostate gland. Urology 5:810–824

Terris MK, Stamey TA (1991) Determination of prostate volume by transrectal ultrasound. J Urol 145:984–987

Terris MK, McNeal JE, Stamey TA (1992a) Detection of clinically significant prostate cancer by transrectal ultrasound-guided systematic biopsies. J Urol 148:829–832

Terris MK, McNeal JE, Stamey TA (1992b) Transrectal ultrasound imaging and ultrasound guided prostate biopsies of residual carcinoma in clinical stage A carcinoma of the prostate. J Urol 147:864–869

Thickman D, Miller GJ, Hopper KD (1990) Prostate cancer: comparison of preoperative 0.35 T MRI with whole-mount histopathology. Magn Reson Imaging 8:205–211

Thornhill BA, Morehouse HT, Coleman P, et al. (1987) Prostatic abscess: CT and sonographic findings. AJR 148:899–900

Thurnher S, Hricak H, Tanagho EA (1988) Müllerian duct cyst: diagnosis with MR imaging. Radiology 168:25–28

Torp-Pedersen S, Lee F, Littrup PJ, Siders DB, Kumasaka GH, Solomon MH, McLeary RD (1989) Transrectal biopsy of the prostate guided with transrectal US: longitudinal and multiplanar scanning. Radiology 170:23–27

Towfighi J, Sadeghee S, Wheller JE, et al. (1972) Granulomatous prostatitis with emphasis on the eosinophilic variety. Am J Clin Pathol 58:630–641

Vallancien G, Prapotnich D, Veillon B, et al. (1991a) Seminal vesicle biopsies in the preoperative staging of prostatic cancer. Eur Urol 19 : 196–200

Vallancien G, Prapotnich D, Veillon B, et al. (1991b) Systematic prostatic biopsies in 100 men with no suspicion of cancer on digital rectal examination. J Urol 146 : 1308–1312

Van Poppel H, Baert L, Aswarie H, Oyen R (1991) Experience with the intraprostatic spiral. Br J Urol 68 : 604–607

Van Poppel H, Ameye F, Oyen R, et al. (1992) Radical prostatectomy for localized prostatic cancer. Eur J Surg Oncol 18 : 456–462

Veneziano S, Pavlica P, Querze R, Nanni G, Lalanne MG, Vecchi F (1990) Correlation between prostate-specific antigen and prostate volume, evaluated by transrectal ultrasonography: usefulness in diagnosis of prostate cancer. Eur Urol 18 : 112–116

Villers A, McNeal JE, Freiha FS, et al. (1989) The role of perineural space invasion in the local spread of prostatic adenocarcinoma. J Urol 142 : 763–768

Villers A, Terris MK, McNeal JE, Stamey TA (1990) Ultrasound anatomy of the prostate: the normal gland and anatomical variations. J Urol 143 : 732–738

von Eschenback AC, Johnson DE (1978) Adenocarcinoma of the prostate. Compr Ther 4 : 18–26

Wang JH, Chang T (1991) Tuberculosis of the prostate: CT appearance. J. Comput Tomogr 15 : 269–270

Wasserman NF, Kapoor DA, Zhang G, et al. (1991) Ratio of prostatic weight to prostate specific antigen: usefulness in selection of patients for US-guided biopsy. Book of Abstracts RSNA p 242

Wasserman NF, Kapoor DA, Hildebrandt WC, et al. (1992a) Transrectal US in evaluation of patients after radical prostatectomy. Part I. Normal postoperative anatomy. Radiology 185 : 361–366

Wasserman NF, Kapoor DA, Hildebrandt WC, et al. (1992b) Transrectal US in evaluation of patients after radical prostatectomy. Part II. Transrectal US and biopsy findings in the presence of residual and early recurrent prostatic cancer. Radiology 185 : 367–372

Weber JP, Oesterling JE, Peters CA, Partin AW, Chan DW, Walsh PC (1989) The influence of reversible androgen deprivation on serum prostate specific antigen levels in men with benign prostatic hyperplasia. J Urol 141 : 987

Wheeler TM (1989) Anatomic considerations in carcinoma of the prostate. Urol Clin of North Am 16 : 623–634

Wilson JD (1970) Embryology of the genital tract. In: Harrison JH, Gittes RF, Perlmutter AD, et al. (eds) Campbell's urology, vol 2. W.B. Saunders, Philadelphia, pp 1469–1482

8 Progress in Surgery for Benign Prostatic Hyperplasia

STUART D. BOYD

CONTENTS

8.1 Introduction

Over the last century, surgical correction of bladder outlet obstruction secondary to benign prostatic hyperplasia (BPH) has become a commonly accepted procedure. The surgery has been performed either as an open enucleation of the prostate (retropubic, suprapubic, perineal) or as a transurethral resection or incision of the prostate (TURP, TUIP). The choice between the various procedures is usually based on the size of the prostate and the discretion of the surgeon (Fig. 8.1). In the United States, 90% of prostatectomies for BPH are performed transurethrally and approximately 400 000 TURPs are performed annually. The procedure is considered relatively free of life-threatening complications, and in most patients a satisfactory outcome is achieved, though significant problems can occur.

The American Urologic Association, in a 1987 survey of all American urologists, found that prostate surgery accounts for 38% of their major surgeries (HOLTGREWE et al. 1987). According to the United States Medicare Health

STUART D. BOYD, M.D., Associate Professor, Department of Urology, University of Southern California, School of Medicine, 1200 North State Street, #5900, Los Angeles, CA 90033, USA

Petrovich/Baert (Eds.)
Benign Prostatic Hyperplasia

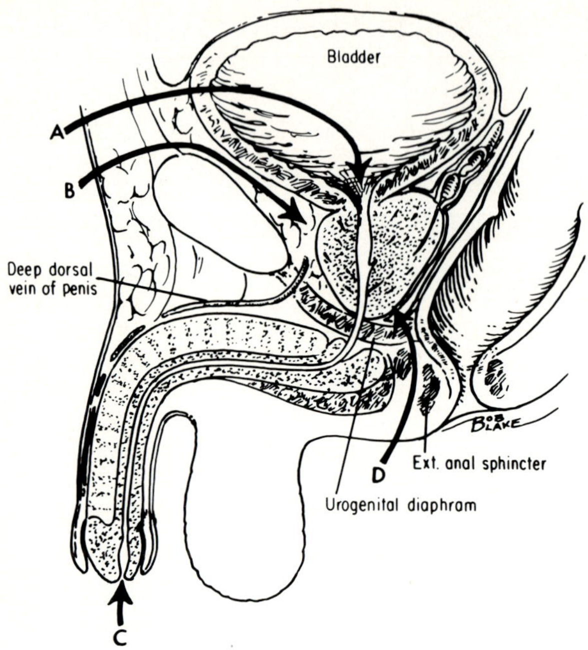

Fig. 8.1. Surgical approaches to the prostate: *A*, suprapubic; *B*, retropubic; *C*, transurethral; *D*, perineal. (Adapted from Paulson 1984).

system, prostate surgery is the second most common reimbursed procedure behind cataract extraction, and it represents a multibillion dollar health care cost. The future of this procedure, however, is currently being called into question. Nonsurgical alternatives for the treatment of BPH are presently receiving much attention in the media. The purpose of this chapter is to present the history and techniques involved in the surgical treatment of the prostate. The article is meant to be an objective state-of-the-art overview while recognizing that the treatment of BPH is presently in a continuing state of evolution.

8.2 Historical Background

The earliest dilation of prostate obstruction probably occurred incidentally during lithotomists' attempts to remove stones from the bladder via perineal urethrostomies. As early as 1575, a French surgeon, Pare, reported the use of a sound to stretch the prostate in order to approach bladder stones (Murphy 1992). It was not until 1806, however, that Sir William Blizard introduced a double gorget, or knife, to be used specifically to incise the prostate through a perineal urethrotomy (Murphy 1972). Due to infection, bleeding, and incontinence, this instrument never achieved wide acceptance. The next advance did not occur until 1834, when Guthrie introduced a sound with a concealed blade to attempt to incise the prostate and bladder neck. Variations of this instrument achieved some popularity throughout Europe over the next 40 years.

The credit for the first partial prostatectomy is generally given to Amussat of Paris, who in 1827 found what he described as a large nut-like obstruction at the bladder neck, which he removed during a perineal lithotomy (Murphy 1972). The patient survived with his symptoms relieved. An actual planned, blind, finger enucleation of the prostate via a median perineal urethrotomy was first described by Gouley in 1873 (Gouley 1983). In contrast to this intraurethral approach, an alternative extraurethral perineal approach was developed by Billroth around 1876 (Murphy 1972). A semicircular incision was made in front of the anus, the rectal urethralis muscle was divided, and the prostate was partially removed. The first complete enucleation of the prostate under vision through a perineal incision was performed by Proust in 1901 (Proust 1901). It was Young's description, however, of a similar procedure in 1908 that became the classic perineal prostatectomy. By 1911, Young reported doing 450 of these operations with a mortality of 3.7% (Young 1903). Young's perineal approach has remained virtually unchanged to this day.

The history of the suprapubic prostatectomy began in 1887, when McGill of Leeds performed three successful suprapubic operations to partially excise obstructing tissue (McGill 1887). In 1890 Belfield reviewed the experience in 88 cases and concluded that when the operation was not successful, this was almost always due to incomplete removal of the adenoma. In 1895, Fuller of New York described six complete enucleations and over the next 10 years performed more than 300 suprapubic prostatectomies (Fuller 1905). In 1901 Freyer of London achieved great notoriety as he claimed to have perfected the operation (Ashley et al. 1971). His operation, however, was still basically a blind removal of the prostatic tissue. Development of a more precise open operation really did not begin until the 1920s. By 1933, Harris of Australia showed that this operation could be performed with a mortality of 2.7% (Harris 1933–1934). Harris' technique emphasized four points: scrupulous aseptic care of the catheter, intraurethral enucleation of the gland, hemostasis after removal of the gland, and partial closure of the prostatic cavity. Harris' contribution was a landmark in the evolution of the safety of the operation.

Retropubic prostatectomy is historically credited to Van Stockem of Rotterdam, who first performed an extravesical suprapubic prostatectomy in 1909 (Murphy 1972). Maier and Merringas of Athens in 1923 completed the important steps of the retropubic prostatectomy, including closure of the capsule and urethral drainage following the surgery (Murphy 1972). It is Millin, however, who is considered the father of the retropubic prostatectomy. His description of this operation in 1947 led to a rapid and popular acceptance of this approach (Millin 1947). His precise description of the operation is still the standard one employed by urologists today.

Endoscopic prostatectomy dates back to early attempts to deal with prostatic obstruction by instruments passed up the urethra. Guthrie's bladder neck incisor, introduced in 1834, was not an endoscopic instrument but paved the way for eventual visual incising devices. Desormeaux is generally regarded as the father of endoscopy and he introduced the first practical endoscope in Paris in 1853 (Desormeaux 1853). In 1877 Bottini of Pavia developed a cauterizer to both coagulate and destroy prostatic tissue (Bottini 1877). Thomas Edison developed the incandescent lamp in 1879. The next major advance in cystoscopes came in 1889, when Nitze introduced a cystoscope with both distal lighting and a lens system (Braasch 1918). The first effective transurethral instrument to remove prostatic tissue was Young's cold punch, which he introduced in 1909. Though more effective than previous methods, this instrument was still used blindly with no means of controlling bleeding. In 1918, Braasch added direct vision to the cold punch and in 1927, Bumpus added a flexible electrode (Braasch 1918; Bumpus 1927).

The first formal resectoscope was introduced by Stern in 1926 (Stern 1926). It relied on several previous discoveries. In 1910, Beer introduced electric current that could achieve coagulation (Beer 1910). In 1911 Wappler found that bipolar current was even more effective. The cutting current was developed by Bovie in 1920 (McLean 1929). The Bakelite sheath was introduced by Walker of London in 1925 (Walker 1925). The culmination of this development was the Stern-McCarthy resectoscope in 1931 (McCarthy 1931). Resectoscopes have markedly evolved since that time but all of the newer resectoscopes are only variations on the theme of the original Stern-McCarthy instrument.

The concept of TUIP again dates back to Guthrie's instrument from 1834. In 1961 Keitzer was the first to actually introduce endoscopic incision of the bladder neck and prostate (Keitzer et al. 1961). He constructed a small cold cutting knife to fit the universal resectoscope. Orandi popularized this procedure in 1973 and has championed its use ever since (Orandi 1973). Today, TUIP is a widely accepted method for the treatment of intravesical obstruction secondary to small prostate glands (less than 20–30 g). The use of the laser to perform these prostate incisions has evolved in the last 2 years. It appears that prostates of every size, with and without median lobes, are amenable to treatment with the laser. As the technology evolves and because of the potential for liver complications, the laser prostatectomy may become the surgical procedure of choice in the future.

8.3 Indications for Surgery

As more and more men have been operated on for prostatic obstruction in recent years, the criteria for prostatic surgical intervention have come under increased scrutiny. What is becoming clear, unfortunately, is that there are no clear indications for treatment. There appear to be wide variations in the rates of surgical treatment in different health care systems. Much of the problem is related to the fact that there is no consensus as to what constitutes prostatic obstruction. Obstruction secondary to BPH has not been shown to correlate with any single parameter such as symptoms, digital prostate examination, estimation of prostate size, cystoscopy, or maximum uroflow (see Chap. 6). The indications for surgery become increasingly strained when one tries to define the goals of surgery. For example, is the goal of surgery to relieve obstruction or to prevent urinary retention and renal failure? Since the patient usually seeks help for relief of his symptoms, is it justified that the primary goal of treatment be directed towards the patient's wishes? Unfortunately, it is difficult to identify which patients will benefit from surgery and which will have a poor postoperative outcome. It is well known that approximately 75–80% of patients improve following surgery but the rest of the patients often are not better or may even be made worse by the operation. Since prostate surgery, however, is still considered the gold standard when comparing various alternative treatments for bladder outlet obstruction, some indications need to be identified.

The best absolute indications for surgical intervention appear to be refractory urinary retention, azotemia, recurrent gross hematuria, recurrent infections, and bladder calculi. It is estimated that only about 10% of patients with prostatism will develop acute retention. The precipitating cause is often felt to be prostatic infarction. When acute retention is treated by transient catheter drainage, 70% of cases recur within 1 week and at least 90% recur within 1 year (Breumd 1982). Therefore acute retention definitely seems to be an indication for intervention.

The risk of patients developing azotemia secondary to BPH is low. Deterioration of renal function secondary to BPH is often a silent phenomenon. Patients may present with weakness or malaise and the diagnosis may be made on routine laboratory determination. Stabilization of renal function often can occur with catheter drainage but long-term correction needs to be achieved with definitive treatment of the prostate. Unfortunately, definitive treatment may not lead to a complete return of renal function.

Gross hematuria is usually secondary to inflammation or rupture of small superficial blood vessels on the surface of the enlarged prostate. Obviously, it is imperative that other causes of hematuria be ruled out, e.g., renal, bladder, or prostatic cancer. Acute bacterial cystitis with urosepsis can occur in patients with prostatic obstruction and large residual urine volumes. While a single asymptomatic urinary tract infection may not necessitate surgery, most urologists would agree that recurrent or severe urinary tract infections are fairly uncontroversial indications for prostate surgery. Bladder calculi are usually due to urinary stasis. Small calculi may pass spontaneously or be treated endoscopically. When a large calculus is noted, however, it is usually advantageous to plan a surgical approach on the prostate in conjunction with removal of the calculus.

Strong indications for surgical intervention may include severe obstructive and irritative voiding symptoms. The decision to perform a TURP based on the patient's symptoms, however, is probably one of the most controversial topics in urology today. Obstructive symptoms include decreased force of stream, hesitancy, postvoid fullness, postvoid dribbling, and straining. Irritative symptoms include frequency, urgency, dysuria, and nocturia. Symptom scales have been developed by the American Urologic Association in an attempt to quantify these symptoms and increase the objectivity of their use for preoperative selection of patients and for postoperative evaluation of treatment success (see Chap. 6). While there is little question that symptoms improve in about 80% of patients following surgery, there is debate as to whether alternative forms of therapy might demonstrate similar efficacy.

The presence of significant nocturia is often the symptom that brings patients to the urologist. Unfortunately no direct correlation has been proven between symptoms such as nocturia and the degree of obstruction. One cannot identify which patients are at risk for developing acute retention solely on the basis of their symptoms. Symptom scores also cannot be used to predict ultimate postoperative outcome. It has been shown that patients with low symptom scores may do as well postoperatively as those with higher scores. In conclusion, the subjective nature of symptoms makes them unreliable as the sole criterion for deciding which patients would benefit from a surgical intervention. Reality also must figure in this equation. The symptoms of prostatism such as nocturia, urgency, urgency incontinence, and postmicturition dribbling may significantly impair quality of life. Patients may actually demand treatment, based on the severity of these symptoms.

Two other objective parameters frequently figure in the indications for surgery. Maximum urinary flow rate is a parameter that has received much attention as a predictor of prostatic obstruction. It is generally agreed that maximum flow rates greater than 15 cc/s are reasonably normal and maximum flow rates of less than 10 cc/s are indicative of market obstruction. It has been shown that patients with higher preoperative flow rates (> 12 cc/s) appear to have lower postoperative success rates (see Chap. 6).

Measurable serial postvoid residuals greater than 100 cc are often used as another objective parameter of obstruction. It has been postulated that the etiology of increased postvoid residual in patients with an obstructing prostate is due to fatigue of the detrusor muscle fibers of the bladder during the prolonged voiding contraction that occurs at increased intravesical pressures with decreased flow. Unfortunately there is no clear linear relationship between an increase in postvoid residual and the severity of symptoms or a decrease in urine flow rate. Serial determinations of postvoid residual significantly above 100 cc, however, can be one indication when selecting patients for treatment and is used by most urologists in selecting therapy (see Chap. 6).

8.4 Surgical Techniques

8.4.1 Transurethral Resection of the Prostate

Transurethral resection of the prostate is the standard therapy for BPH in the United States. It is performed with a resectoscope that currently is produced by numerous endoscopic companies worldwide. The resectoscope can be used under direct vision or via video. Fiberoptic light sources are used whenever possible. The resectoscope utilizes a sheath that typically is 24, 26, or 28 French. The cutting or sculpting of the prostatic tissue is done by a cutting loop. A minimum of three or four cutting loops should be available at the time of a procedure. The finer the wire from which the cutting loop is constructed, the less will be the tissue binding to the loop after completion of the cut. The thinner loops, however, generate less heat and consequently may not coagulate as well as loops of heavier gauge wire.

The choice of electrical surgical units should be at the discretion of the surgeon. Newer units have built-in warning systems that detect inadequate current flow. Three types of electrocurrents are used in the electroresection of the prostate: cutting, coagulation, and blended. These currents are bipolar and high frequency, and they ensure safe passage of electrical energy through the body. The cutting current has an undamped current with a wave form of equal amplitude. Cutting is accomplished by dissolution of tissue at the active electrode. Coagulation is accomplished with a highly dampened spark-gap current with no cutting qualities and is adapted solely for coagulation. The effect of the coagulating current is to desiccate tissue and blood. Blended current combines the coagulating properties of the highly dampened spark-gap current with the cutting properties of the undampened oscillator current. The two currents may be blended in any proportion. The grounding electrode should be placed beneath the patient, preferably in an area close to the operative field. The grounding electrode should be large enough to minimize any localized heat effect.

The TURP needs to be performed under continuous flow of fluid. The irrigating fluid should be clear, sterile, nontoxic, and delivered at body temperature. In addition, the fluid should have a low coefficient of electrical conductivity. When solutions of high conductivity, such as physiologic saline, are used, cutting and coagulation become difficult or impossible. The fluid should be iso-osmolar to blood, however, as during the resection there is considerable hazard of introduction of the irrigating fluid into the bloodstream through venous channels opened by the resection. Introduction of nonisotonic solution into the bloodstream will produce hemolysis and the potential for renal dysfunction. The most widely used irrigating solutions contain sorbitol or glycine.

The patient is anesthetized and placed in the lithotomy position. The patient should first be cystoscoped so that the bladder, prostate, and intraurethral landmarks can be examined and familiarized. The urethra should then be dilated to a size 2 French larger than the size of the resectoscope sheath. Only then should the resectoscope be introduced. The bladder should be reinspected to again familiarize the landmarks, especially the ureteral orifices. The bladder should be closely inspected for the presence of diverticuli, stones, or lesions. The prostatic urethra is inspected to evaluate the extent and configuration of the anatomic obstruction. The length of the prostatic urethra should be determined. Particular attention should be paid to the presence and visibility of the verumontanum. Using the verumontanum as the distal landmark of resection will preserve the distal longitudinal and circular fibers that constitute the distal urethral continence mechanism.

The procedure is usually initiated by resecting the median lobe if it exists. A large median lobe may obscure the trigone and the ureteral orifices. One must be careful, however, not to over-resect the bladder neck at the beginning of the procedure. Perforation of the bladder neck early on will greatly complicate the resection. It is helpful, however, that the bladder neck is sufficiently resected without perforating so that it is well opened and fluid and tissue can easily flow through it into the bladder.

Hemostasis during resection is achieved by electrocoagulation. Hemostasis should not be deferred but bleeding points controlled as they are encountered. Widespread indiscriminate coagulation should be avoided as this will produce a large amount of tissue damage, giving rise to delayed sloughing and secondary hemorrhage. Excess coagulation at the bladder neck may also increase the risk of postoperative bladder neck contracture.

During transurethral resection, the surgeon should establish a routine pattern and attempt to adhere to this pattern during resection. Once the bladder neck is sufficiently opened, the resectoscope should be brought back to the level of the verumontanum. The lateral lobes are then resected. This is usually best performed by beginning the resection on the roof of the prostate, removing the adenomatous tissue from 12 o'clock down to 6 o'clock on each side. Usually one lateral lobe is completely resected before the other lobe is approached. As much tissue as possible should be removed with each excursion of the resectoscope loop. This will minimize the number of cuts and facilitate the speed of the procedure. During each resected cut of the lateral lobes, the sheath should remain as stationary as possible at the level of the verumontanum. With the development of a smooth resecting stroke, correct sculpting of the prostatic fossa will be possible. The appearance of the true prostatic striations will indicate the limits of the capsule and the limit of the resection.

In respect of the size of the gland, at the completion of removal of the lateral lobes, a rim of tissue usually remains at the apex. All apical tissue surrounding the verumontanum may be resected without damaging the continence mechanism. At the end of the resection, direct vision from the verumontanum into the bladder should be possible. A general survey of the prostatic cavity should be made and arterial and venous bleeders meticulously coagulated. Any overlooked residual prostatic adenoma should be carefully trimmed away.

All prostatic fragments need to be irrigated out of the bladder. This may be performed with a piston syringe or an Ellik evacuator. The resectoscope should not be removed until the surgeon is completely satisfied that all chips have been removed and hemostasis is secure. Once the resectoscope is removed, a large-bore catheter is inserted. This is typically a three-way 24-French Foley catheter with a 30-cc balloon. The bladder should irrigate clear easily with only light traction on the catheter. If heavy bleeding is still noted, it is best to remove the catheter, reinsert the resectoscope, and identify and control bleeding points.

Acute complications of the procedure include excessive hemorrhage necessitating transfusion, perforation of the prostatic capsule with extravasation of large volumes of irrigating fluid, overabsorption of the irrigating fluid into the general circulation, and urinary tract infection and sepsis. The reabsorption of large amounts of irrigating fluid (TUR syndrome) can produce significant hyponatremia and the symptom complex of agitation, restlessness, nausea, vomiting, and confusion. This is secondary to cerebral edema caused by osmolar fluid shifts from the hypotonic extracellular fluid compartment to the relatively hypertonic intracellular spaces. Cerebral edema produces an increase in intracranial pressure with an elevation of blood pressure, slowing of the pulse, agitation, nausea, vomiting, headaches, convulsion, and coma. Most clinical reactions occur when the serum sodium drops lower than 120 mEq/l. Seizures may be seen at sodium levels below 102 mEq/l. Treatment of post-TUR hyponatremia should include diuretics and hypertonic saline which will permit the body's own homeostatic mechanisms to contribute to the correction of the hyponatremia.

8.4.2 Transurethral Incision of the Prostate

A viable alternative to resection of small prostate glands is transurethral incision of the prostate. This is generally indicated in patients with type I or type II prostates containing less than 20 g of resectable tissue. Type I prostates have a circular or purse-string appearance to the bladder neck with little lateral lobe tissue. Type II prostates have bulging lateral lobes distally with a median bar at the bladder neck. Typically the lateral lobes contain up to 20 g of tissue. With lateral lobes larger than this, a TURP is indicated. TUIP is particularly suitable for poor-risk patients in whom blood loss and fluid absorption is to be avoided, and for those younger patients who wish to minimize the likelihood of retrograde ejaculation. The TUIP is performed with a resectoscope that utilizes an electric knife. Normally two incisions are made at 5 and 7 o'clock beginning at the level of the ureteral orifices and extending back to the verumontanum in the groove between the lateral and median lobes and to the side of the verumontanum. The incisions should be carried down to the prostatic capsule. The procedure is typically performed under anesthesia but usually requires a shorter post-operative stay than the TURP. Typically the patient can have his catheter removed in 1 or 2 days. If patients are selected properly, the results appear very comparable with TURP, and with far fewer complications.

8.4.3 Open Prostatectomy

Open enucleation of the prostate is usually performed on larger glands. Most urologists consider prostate glands over 80 g an indication for open enucleation. Other indications for an open enucleation include one or more bladder diverticula that require excision for satisfactory bladder emptying, bladder calculi that cannot be managed with transurethral litholapexy, stricture disease that precludes transurethral instrumentation, a small bladder capacity that makes transurethral resection difficult, and skeletal disorders that prohibit the lithotomy position. Contraindications to an open prostatectomy include small adenomas which can be exceedingly difficult to enucleate, and suspected prostatic carcinoma. In the presence of carcinoma the cleavage plane around the adenoma is very difficult to obtain and incomplete removal or perforation is common.

Open enucleation is performed via three different routes: retropubic, suprapubic, and perineal. In the United States, most open prostatectomies are performed in either a retropubic or a suprapubic fashion.

8.4.3.1 Retropubic Prostatectomy

The retropubic approach utilizes a lower abdominal incision to expose the bladder and prostate. A catheter is passed per urethrum and the bladder emptied. With the balloon of the catheter inflated, it is easy to palpate the transition between the bladder neck and the prostate. A self-retaining retractor is placed in the pelvis and the anterior prostatic capsule identified. It helps to sweep off the loose fibrofatty tissues overlying the prostatic capsule. Before an incision is made in the capsule, 2-0 chromic sutures are applied in a rectangular fashion in the capsule, outlining the area to be incised. These sutures help with hemostasis. The prostatic capsule is incised in a transverse fashion with electrocautery. When the incision is carried down to the adenoma, the cleavage plane between the capsule and the adenoma becomes readily apparent due to the differing textures of the fibrous capsule and the smooth, bland adenoma. The cleavage plane inferior, superior, and lateral to the capsulotomy is developed initially by spreading Metzenbaum scissors. A finger is then introduced to extend the plane behind the adenoma on each side and to isolate the urethral mucousa at the apex of the adenoma. The urethral catheter is removed and the urethra is divided under direct vision with scissors. The anterior plane of dissection is then extended superiorly with the finger to enter the lumen of the bladder. The adenoma is grasped with a tenaculum and delivered through the capsulotomy. Residual mucosal attachments at the posterior bladder outlet are divided with scissors. The prostatic fossa is examined to identify and remove any retained nodules of hyperplastic tissue. The prostatic fossa is examined very closely for hemostasis. The trigone and ureteral orifices are also inspected and identified. If the bladder outlet is snug to the index finger, a wedge of tissue is excised from the posteromedial lip to help prevent contracture of the bladder neck. The inferior vesicle arteries are secured with 2-0 chromic sutures that encompass the full thickness of the bladder neck at the 4 and 8 o'clock positions. The mucosa of the posterior outlet is anchored down into the prostatic fossa with interrupted 2-0 chromic sutures. A three-way 24-French Foley catheter with a 30-cc balloon is introduced per urethrum into the bladder. The balloon is typically filled with 45 cc of water. The capuslotomy is closed with 2-0 chromic suture. The bladder is irrigated clear of any clots. A Penrose drain is placed in the retropubic space and brought out through a separate stab wound in the lower abdomen before the incision is closed. The urethral catheter is generally removed on the fifth seventh postoperative days and the pelvic drain removed the following day.

8.4.3.2 Suprapubic Prostatectomy

Suprapubic prostatectomies are generally indicated when there is an accompanying large bladder stone or when there is an extremely large median lobe. The patient is again placed in the supine position and a lower abdominal midline incision made. A Foley catheter is introduced per urethrum and the bladder filled with 200–300 cc of sterile saline. Exposure is maintained with a self-retaining retractor.

The coarse fibers of the bladder muscle are exposed by sweeping the peritoneum from the anterosuperior aspect of the bladder, and the prevesicle space is developed to expose the bladder outlet and the base of the prostate. A 2-0 chromic suture is applied to the midline of the bladder about 2 cm above the base of the bladder. A transverse cystotomy incision is made with electrocautery. The bladder outlet is identified and the ureteral orifices are noted. The ureters must be well identified and their relationship to the median lobe well established. The bladder mucosa is then incised around the base of the median lobe and bladder neck, taking care to maintain a distance from the ureteral orifices. An index finger is introduced into the prostatic urethra and thrust anteriorally to "crack" the adenoma. The plane between the adenoma and the prostatic capsule is developed laterally, posteriorly, and inferiorly with blunt finger dissection. The urethral mucosa at the apex of the adenoma is divided with scissors. The adenoma is delivered into the bladder and removed. Chromic sutures again are applied to the bladder outlet at the 4 and 8 o'clock positions to secure the inferior vesicle arteries. If significant bleeding still occurs, additional suturing of the bladder neck may be required. Before closing, the bladder outlet should be further anchored to the posterior capsule with 2-0 chromic sutures to bring the trigone down towards the floor of the prostate. A three-way 24-French Foley catheter with a 30-cc balloon is introduced per urethrum into the bladder. A large-caliber suprapubic cystostomy catheter is also placed. The bladder is closed and a Penrose drain placed through a separate stab wound in the pelvis to drain the retropubic space. The abdominal incision is finally closed. The urethral catheter is generally removed on the third postoperative day and the suprapubic catheter removed in 5–7 days as long as the patient demonstrates that he can void satisfactorily. The pelvic drain usually can be removed on the day after the suprapubic catheter is removed.

8.4.3.3 Perineal Prostatectomy

Perineal prostatectomy is utilized infrequently. Most urologists feel that exposure and hemostasis are harder to obtain using this technique. The patient is placed in an exaggerated lithotomy position. A curved Lowsley tractor is passed per urethrum into the bladder to help expose the prostate to the perineum. A semilunar incision is made above the anus in the perineum. The ischiorectal fossa is developed on each side perpendicular to the plane of the perineum using the index finger. The central tendon is isolated by gentle finger dissection, being carefully separated from the underlying rectum. Once the central tendon is divided, the rectum is displaced posterioraly and the anal sphincter can be identified. The prostate can then be visualized. Once the rectourethralis is further identified and sharply divided, the rectum can be displaced further posteriorly and the prostate well isolated. An incision is made in the prostatic capsule and the adenoma enucleated both sharply and bluntly and sutures placed in the bladder neck at the 4 and 8 o'clock positions. A three-way 24-French Foley catheter is passed per urethrum into the bladder and the prostatic capsule closed. The wound is drained with a Penrose drain. The most common acute complication after perineal prostatectomy is inadvertent injury to the rectum. This should be corrected prior to closure. The most common complication after open prostatectomy in general is hemorrhage necessitating transfusion.

8.4.4 Laser Prostatectomy

The newest surgical technique for prostatectomy involves the use of the laser (Costello et al. 1992). Two different laser prostatectomy techniques have been introduced and will be discussed in detail in Chap. 11. Both techniques utilize the neodymium:YAG laser. Transurethral laser-induced prostatectomy (TULIP) utilizes a laser fiber positioned at the bladder neck via the use of ultrasonography. The laser is then used to oblate the prostatic tissue back to the verumontanum in a radial fashion. Although TULIP remains experimental and long-term results are lacking, the technique appears to be safe in that injury to adjacent organs has not been reported. More recently, direct-vision right-angle laser fibers have been introduced to be utilized through a standard cystoscope. This allows direct-vision incision of the prostate perpendicular to application of the laser. Total treatment time is normally less than 15 min. The disadvantages include the need to become proficient in a new technique, the possibility of complications with laser, and the possibility of ineffectual treatment of larger prostates. A catheter must also be left indwelling for 1-2 weeks to allow the gradual dissolution of the prostatic adenoma.

8.4.5 Prostatic Stents

One further future surgical treatment of the prostate involves the use of prostatic stents (Oesterling 1991). These are not currently approved by the FDA but have been used in Europe for the past few years (see Chap. 9). Spiral stents made of either stainless steel or titanium can be visually placed in the prostatic fossa and expand the prostatic urethra to a diameter as large as 42 French. Custom-length stents can be made to reside from the bladder neck back to the verumontanum. The stent is placed in the operating room with the patient under anesthesia. The stent should not protrude into the bladder proximally or beyond the verumontanum distally. Postoperatively an indwelling urethral catheter need not be left in place and the patient typically can be discharged the same day or the following morning. The prostatic fossa gradually epithelializes over the stent but a permanent channel is maintained. Initially this procedure was used only for poor surgical risk patients but recently it has been more widely applied. Complications have been few but most subjects have irritative voiding symptoms for up to 6 weeks after stent placement.

8.5 Results of Surgical Treatment

Despite the large number of patients who have undergone TURPs, data on results have been reported in only a limited number of patients. Approximately 75%–80% of patients will have long-term improvement in their obstructive and irritative symptom scores. A similar number of patients will have a demonstrable improvement in their maximum uroflow rates and in their postvoid residuals. Nielsen et al. (1989) demonstrated that these results are fairly durable over at least 7 years. There was some drop in patient satisfaction, however, between the 3- and 7-year interval. Open prostatectomies appear to give fairly similar results, as does the TUIP procedure for smaller prostates.

The long-term complications following these surgical interventions may be extensive. These complications may include bleeding requiring transfusion (6%), erectile dysfunction (5%–40%), incontinence (1%), urinary tract infection (5%), retrograde ejaculation (greater than 50%), urethral stricture (5%), and death (1%). Reoperation rates for these procedures vary from 1% to 2% per year. Roos and associates reported in 1988 that patients undergoing TURP are at a greater risk of cardiovascular death than individuals undergoing open prostatectomy (Roos et al. 1989). The relative risk for death after TURP was approximately 1.3 times greater. This same group also reported that the reoperation rate for TURP was approximately 3 times greater than the reoperation rate for open prostatectomy. Both of these points have recently been refuted at the 1992 American Urologic Meeting in Washington, D.C. (Lim et al. 1992).

8.6 Conclusions

Prostatectomy currently represents the most established and effective treatment for BPH. Absolute indications for surgery include refractory urinary retention, renal insufficiency, recurrent gross hematuria, recurrent urinary tract infection, and bladder calculi. Patients with extremely large median lobes are probably also best treated with surgery. The vast majority of individuals seeking urologic treatment for BPH do not have absolute indications for intervention. Most patients present because of moderate to severe obstructive and irritative voiding symptoms. It is under these conditions that indication for surgery becomes less certain. It is in these patients that alternative nonsurgical forms of treatment may become increasingly commonplace. These patients are being treated for quality of life problems. If good nonsurgical treatment alternatives are available, it is most likely that patients will opt for these techniques rather than surgery. This has already been clearly demonstrated in the field of urology when one considers the current treatment of stone disease. Open surgery for stones has almost disappeared and been totally replaced by electro-shock wave lithotripsy and various endoscopic procedures.

As noted in the other chapters in this book, the treatment of BPH is evolving and will continue to do so as a more comprehensive understanding of the relative efficacy and morbidity of surgical and nonsurgical alternatives is developed. Prostatectomy still represents the most definitive treatment for BPH but probably will continue to play a diminishing role in the future. Minor surgical procedures such as inserting prostatic stents and nonsurgical alternatives such as microwave therapy, alpha blockade, hormonal therapy, and balloon dilation will become increasingly popular over the next decade as patients increasingly demand nonsurgical approaches. The challenge for physicians in the future will be to identify the best indications for each procedure so that the most effective treatment can be advocated for any combination of symptoms and physical findings.

References

Ashley JSA, Howlett A, Morris JN (1971) Case-fatality of hyperplasia of the prostate in two teaching and three regional board hospitals. Lancet II: 1308–1311

Beer E (1910) Removal of neoplasms of the urinary bladder. JAMA 54: 1768–1769

Belfield WT (1890) Operations on the enlarged prostate, with a tabulated summary of cases. Am J Med Sci 100: 439–452

Bottini E (1877) Radicale Behandlung der auf Hypertrophie de la Prostata beruhenden Ischurie. Arch Klin Chir 21: 1–24

Braasch WF (1918) Median bar excisor. JAMA 70: 758–759

Breumd, Klavsov P, Munck LK, et al. (1982) Significance of acute urinary retention due to intravesical obstruction. Scand J Urol Nephrol 16: 21–25

Bumpus HC (1927) Punch operation for prostatic obstruction. Surg Clin North Am 7: 1473–1478

Costello AJ, Bowsher WG, Bolton DM, et al. (1992) Laser ablation of the prostate in patients with benign prostatic hypertrophy. Br J Urol 69: 604–605

Desormeaux AJ (1853) De l'endoscope. Bull Acad Med

Fuller E (1905) The question of priority in the adoption of the method of total enucleation, suprapubically, of the hypertrophied prostate. Ann Surg 41: 520–534

Gouley JWS (1983) Diseases of the urinary organs. William Wood, New York

Harris SH (1933-1934) Prostatectomy with closure: five years' experience. Br J Surg 21: 434–452

Holtgrewe HL, Mebust WK, Dowd JB, et al. (1987) Transurethral prostatectomy: practice aspects of the dominant operation in American urology. J Urol 141: 248–258

Keitzer W, Cervantes L, Demaculangan A, et al. (1961) Transurethral incision of bladder neck for contracture. J Urol 86:242–244

Lim R, Bolkier M, Levin DR (1992) Prognostic correlations between patients treated for BPH by transurethral resection (TURP) and transabdominal resection (retropubic or suprapubic). J Urol 147:366

McCarthy JF (1931) A new apparatus for endoscopic plastic surgery of prostate, diathermia and excision of vesical growth. J Urol 26:695–696

McGill AF (1887) Suprapubic prostatectomy. Br Med J II:1104–1105

McLean AJ (1929) The Bovie electrosurgical current generator. Arch Surg 18:1863–1873

Millin T (1947) Retropubic urinary surgery. Livingstone, Edinburgh

Murphy LTJ (1972) The history of urology. Charles C. Thomas, Springfield. ILL.

Nielsen KT, Christensen MM, Madsen PO, Bruskewitz RC (1989) Symptom analysis and uroflowmetry 7 years after transurethral resection of the prostate. J Urol 142:1251–1253

Oesterling JE (1991) The obstructive prostate and the intraurethral stent. Contemp Urol 3:61–72

Orandi A (1973) Transurethral incision of the prostate. J Urol 110:229–232

Paulson DF (1984) The prostate. In: Paulson DE (ed) Genitourinary surgery. Churchill Livingstone, New York

Proust R (1901) Technique de la prostatectomie perineale. Assoc Fr Urol Procr Verb 5:361–388

Roos NP, Wennberg JE, Malenka DJ, et al. (1989) Mortality and reoperation after open and transurethral resection of the prostate for benign prostatic hyperplasia. N Engl J Med 320:1120–1124

Stern M (1926) Resection of obstruction at the vesical orifice: new instruments and a new method. JAMA 87:1726–1729

Walker KM (1925) Perurethral operations for prostatic obstruction. Br Med J I:201–204

Young HH (1903) Conservative perineal prostatectomy: presentation of new instruments and technic. JAMA 44:999–1009

9 The Use of Endoprostheses in the Management of Benign Prostatic Hyperplasia

HENDRIK VANDEURSEN, HEIN VAN POPPEL, and LUC BAERT

CONTENTS

9.1 Introduction

Infravesical obstruction to urine flow related to enlargement of the prostate or bladder neck is the single most common cause of male urologic complaints. Operative prostatectomy by either open or transurethral access is a well-established treatment technique for benign prostatic hyperplasia (BPH) caused by infravesical obstruction. Treatment results are generally very good but serious morbidity and occasional mortality are associated with conventional surgery, especially in the elderly and unfit patients. Debilitated patients with BPH who have multiple contraindications to surgical removal of bladder outlet obstruction may be treated with long-term indwelling bladder catheterization. The treatment, however, is often accompanied by multiple sequelae including urinary tract infection, sepsis, and renal insufficiency.

HENDRIK VANDEURSEN, MD, PhD, Professor, and HEIN VAN POPPEL, MD, PhD, Professor, Department of Urology, St. Pieter's Hospital, Catholic University of Leuven, Brusselsestraat 69, 3000 Leuven, Belgium

LUC BAERT, MD, PhD, Professor and Chairman, Department of Urology, St. Pieter's Hospital, Catholic University of Leuven, Brusselsestraat 69, 3000 Leuven, Belgium and Clinical Professor of Urology and Radiation Oncology, University of Southern California, School of Medicine, Los Angeles, CA 90033, USA

Petrovich/Baert (Eds.)
Benign Prostatic Hyperplasia

Table 9.1. The role of endoprostheses

Vascular
Coronary arteries
Peripheral (iliac, femoral, popliteal) arteries
Renal artery
Gastrointestinal
Biliary tract
Urologic
Urethral strictures
Detrusor–external sphincter dyssynergia
Renal artery stenosis
Benign prostatic hyperplasia

Providing a simple minimally invasive but still effective treatment for prostatism is an important goal. The concept of placing a stent across a stenotic lumen after dilation has been investigated for the past two decades in many areas of the human anatomy. Sites which have been treated with stents include the respiratory tract, arteries, and the gastrointestinal tract. More recently, the lower male urinary tract has also been under investigation as the site for the use of endoprostheses in the management of detrusor–external sphincter dyssynergia and urethral stricture in elderly and debilitated patients suffering from obstructive benign hyperplasia (Table 9.1). The notion of implanting a device transurethrally to open up the prostatic urethra is inherent to basic urologic management of prostatic obstruction. Currently available intraprostatic stents include devices for temporary implantation such as the intraprostatic spiral (ProstaKath) and intraurethral catheters (Angiomed), while the Urolume Wallstent (American Medical Systems) and the ASI titanium stent (Advanced Surgical Intervention) are intended for permanent implantation.

9.2 Temporary Implantation of Urethral Stents

9.2.1 Intraprostatic Spiral

The urologic spiral was first introduced by FABIAN (1980) for effective treatment of urinary retention without the need for an indwelling urethral catheter in elderly, surgically unfit patients. This spiral represents a single wire of surgical-grade stainless steel and is coated with 24K gold to increase tissue acceptance and inhibit bacterial colonization and encrustation. The Prostakath (Engineers and Doctors AS, Copenhagen, Denmark) does not become epithelialized.

The design of this endoprosthesis requires placement of several spiral loops to open up the prostatic urethra (Fig. 9.1). The proximal end is tapered to allow easy insertion into the prostatic urethra and extends across the bladder neck, protruding into the bladder. Distal to the spiral loops in the prostatic urethra

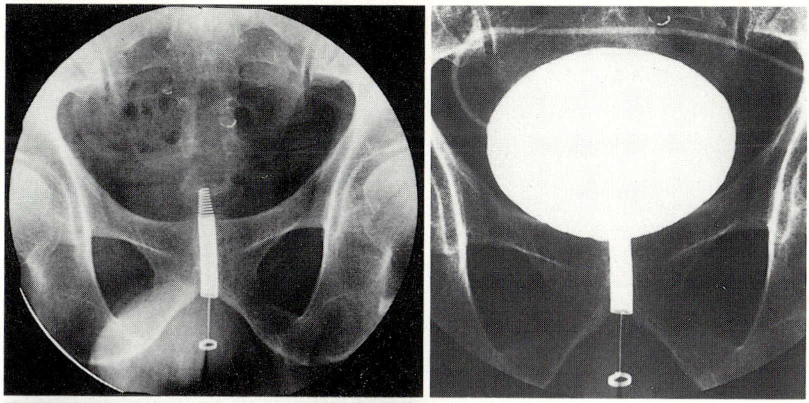

a b

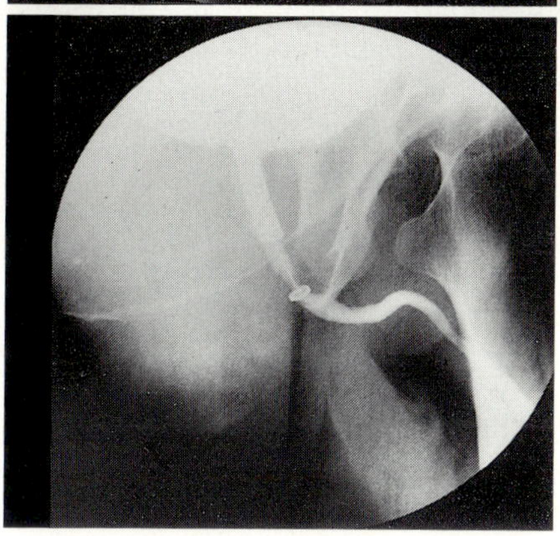

c

Fig. 9.1. **a** Plain x-ray, **b** cystogram, and **c** voiding cystogram in a patient with an intraprostatic spiral

a 2-cm segment of straight wire traverses the external urinary sphincter. Distal to the continence zone a two spiral loop segment is located in the proximal bulbar urethra to prevent migration of the device and to facilitate its repositioning. The outside diameter of the Prostakath is 21 French and it is available in 4.5-,5.5-, 6.5- and 7.5-cm lengths according to the length of the prostatic urethra. The length of the prostatic urethra is determined sonographically or endoscopically.

The Prostakath is inserted under local anesthesia with either sonographic or endoscopic guidance. Repositioning or withdrawal is feasible with grasping forceps through a 21-French cystoscope. Caution is needed as pulling the stent down the urethra may unravel the spiral, damaging the urethra and finally resulting in stricture formation.

Complications associated with the Prostakath include failed insertion, hematuria, urinary tract infection, and stent dislodgment. Urgency and urge incontinence occur as a consequence of irritation but these complaints are transient. Anticholinergic and antispasmodic medications are highly effective in controlling these transient problems. Although initial short-term results were quite good, increasing experience with longer follow-up revealed that the use of these spirals is unsatisfactory due to their frequent displacement.

In our experience, the intraprostatic spiral represents a valid alternative to transurethral bladder catheterization in patients with acute urinary retention. This spiral can be used for a limited period only. It is not indicated in large prostates, in patients with irritative voiding disorders, or in those with longstanding infravesical obstruction and chronic urinary retention (VAN POPPEL et al. 1991). The Porges Urospiral is similar in design to the Prostakath; the indications, techniques of application, and treatment results are likewise similar.

9.2.2 Intraurethral Catheters

Polyurethane stents (Angiomed) intended for intraprostatic insertion are also available. The indications for their use are similar to those of intraprostatic spirals. Their main advantage is lower expense. Treatment results and complications are comparable with the use of either device.

9.3 Permanently Implanted Stents

9.3.1 Self-expandable Stents

Originally, steel mesh stents – in particular, the Urolume Wallstent (American Medical Systems) – were developed for endovascular use. Recently they have been under clinical investigation for the treatment of urethral strictures or bladder outlet obstruction due to BPH or locally advanced prostatic adenocarcinoma in patients in whom more radical surgical intervention is impossible.

The stent is a biocompatible inert prosthesis constructed from surgical-grade stainless steel that is woven into a fine tubular mesh (Fig. 9.2). It is both flexible

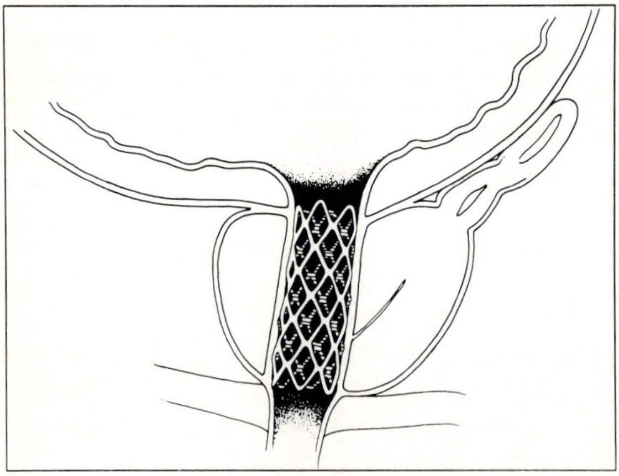

Fig. 9.2. The Urolume stent in the prostatic urethra

and self-expanding. The stent is held compressed in a delivery tool and when fully expanded it reaches an internal diameter of 42 French (1.4 cm). It is available in 2- and 3-cm lengths. In patients with a prostatic urethra length exceeding 3 cm, two or more stents overlapping their ends by 0.5 cm are required.

Prior to the stent implantation, the length of the prostatic urethra and the location of the distal sphincter are determined either sonographically or endoscopically. The device may be inserted under local anesthesia although locoregional anesthesia is preferable. It is implanted by means of a specially designed deployment tool to allow for accurate stent placement under direct endoscopic control with 0° lens. The stent self-expands to create a widely patent prostatic urethra. In our own experience and that of others, one of the keys to successful placement is not to allow the stent to protrude into the bladder proximally or extend onto the verumontanum distally.

Excellent tissue acceptability of these stents is the rule as they become covered by urethral epithelium, and within 4–6 months become fully incorporated

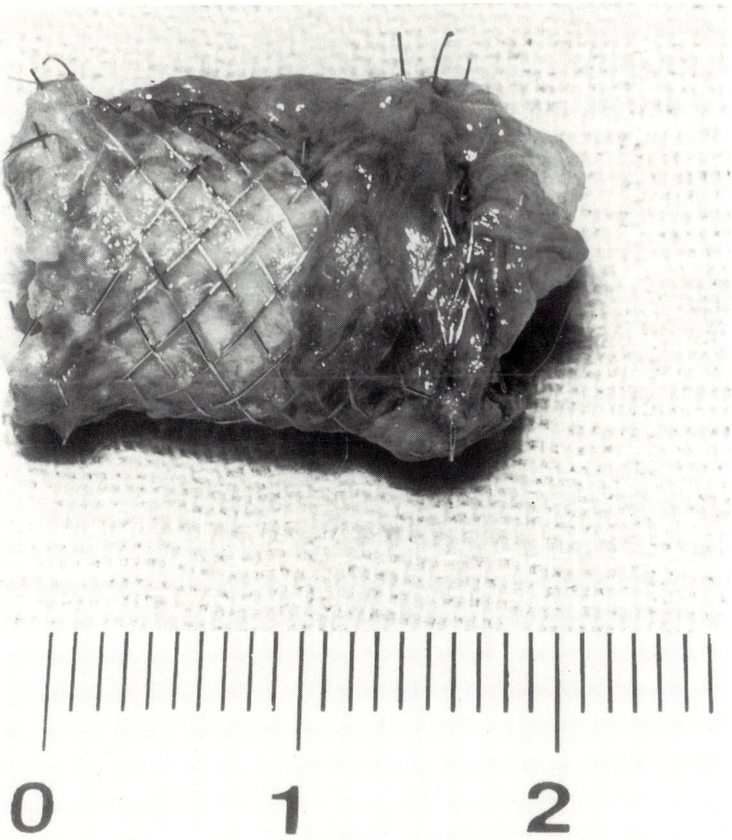

Fig. 9.3. Urolume stent and intrastent fibrosis

into the urethral wall. Initially, patients may complain of irritative voiding disorders which resolve over time and do not require removal of the device. The persistence of obstructive complaints usually results from failure to cover the entire prostatic urethra.

In contrast to the intraprostatic spiral, repositioning of the intraprostatic stent is complex even when performed at the time of insertion. This is due to the design of the stent with its self-retaining margins. If stent repositioning or removal is necessary, the withdrawal is accomplished through a resectoscope sheath to minimize trauma to the urethra. Withdrawal of the stent becomes more difficult once it is covered by epithelium. It requires transurethral resection at low current and extraction of the stent by grasping it with forceps. Pulling of the stent at its distal end facilitates its lengthening and thus the reduction of its diameter, allowing for its withdrawal through the resectoscope sheath.

Encrustation of the stent is rare as the stent is covered by urothelium. Long-term stent patency may be limited due to intrastent fibrosis (Fig. 9.3), as has been reported in patients treated for stricture of the urethra (BAERT et al. 1993).

Preliminary results with the Wallstent in the management of BPH as described by OESTERLING (1991) seem encouraging. In a group of 24 patients, the mean urinary peak flow rate increased from 9.6 ml/s to 20 ml/s and the mean postvoid residual volume decreased from 107 ml to 32 ml. No major side-effects were reported in this series of 24 patients.

In conclusion, the Wallstent offers some important advantages over the spiral devices. The elastic properties and radial force of this endoprosthesis prevent its migration, while epithelial covering enhances tissue acceptance and reduces the risk of encrustation. Assessment of the risk for intrastent fibrosis requires long-term follow-up.

9.4 Balloon-expandable Titanium Intraprostatic Stent

Titanium is characterized by excellent biocompatibility and has a long history of safe use in man. Unlike the Wallstent, the intraprostatic titanium stent (Advanced Surgical Intervention, California, USA) is neither flexible nor self-expanding. Prior to its placement, endoscopic measurement of the prostatic length from the bladder neck to the external sphincter is required. The stent is available in variable lengths from 12 to 65 mm, which permits customization of treatment according to the length of the urethra. This represents the main advantage of this device over other urethral stents as a greater prostatic length can be entirely covered by one device. Stent placement can be achieved under local or locoregional anesthesia depending on the patient's general condition and ability to cooperate. The stent is mounted over a balloon on an insertion catheter (Fig. 9.4). By inflating the balloon to 9 atm for 30 s, the stent will reach a fixed diameter of 33 French (11 mm). The stent is then placed between the

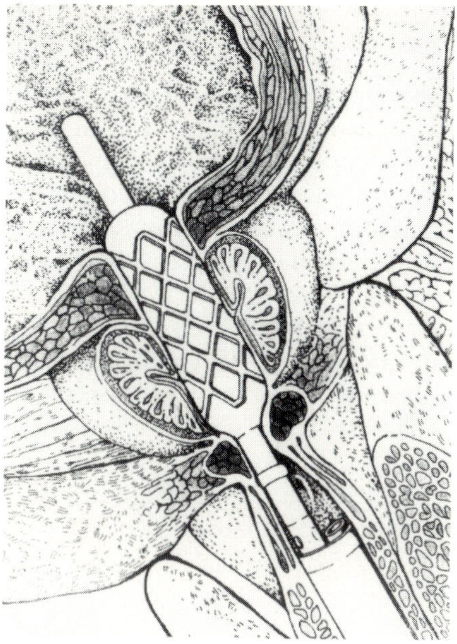

Fig. 9.4. The ASI titanium stent on its balloon delivery system

bladder neck and the external sphincter. Adjustment of the stent is possible using grasping forceps through a cystoscope. KAPLAN and KOO (1990) reported a study of 34 patients who had a minimum follow-up of 12 months. Of the 34 study patients, 29 (85%) showed an improvement in symptom score and peak flow rates.

9.5 Future Urethral Endoprostheses

Biodegradable stents have the advantage of not requiring retrieval of the implanted material, since there is no risk of long-term side-effects related to the presence of implants.

Thermoexpandable stents consist of a titanium–nickel alloy which is characterized by a temperature-dependent form recall. These devices are also being tested in patients with BPH-related infravesical obstruction.

At low temperature, the coil has a soft configuration, but the stent gains stability in the range of body temperature, increasing its internal diameter to 35 French. When the metal is irrigated at a low temperature (15°C), the metal softens and this property allows for its easy introduction and removal under local anesthesia. Different lengths are available, ranging from 20 to 80 mm according to the need of the individual lengths of the prostatic urethra. Early reports on the use of these thermoexpandable stents showed a 50% success rate, with dislodgment as their principal shortcoming (unpublished data).

9.6 Conclusion

Urologists are highly interested in clinical applications of so-called minimally invasive treatment options in selected BPH patients. The search for an alternative to resection of the prostate is especially important in elderly and debilitated patients who often present multiple contraindications to surgery. Therefore, the concept of stenting the prostatic urethra by means of endoprostheses to relieve bladder outlet obstruction secondary to an enlarged prostate is particularly appealing.

The intraprostatic spiral can be applied for a limited period. Additionally, the treatment outcome with the use of this device gauges how a patient will fare after open or endoscopic operative prostatectomy. The use of biodegradable stents might sound attractive but their long-term efficacy, once the stent is resorbed, remains questionable.

Stents intended for permanent implantation in the prostatic urethra offer the advantage of epithelial covering, which reduces complications such as encrustation and dislodgment, but the potential risk of intrastent fibrosis requires long-term follow-up which is not available at present. Properly conducted prospective clinical studies with long-term follow-up are not available for most of the new treatment techniques, thus restricting their widespread clinical use. The significance of many end points for evaluating the efficacy of new treatments remains controversial. Urodynamic studies are routinely being used to assess treatment efficacy, but even a 50% increase in flow rates still may be associated with the presence of infravesical obstruction.

Results obtained in prospective randomized trials with long-term follow-up are required before any of the new treatment techniques is recommended as an alternative to prostatectomy, especially in those patients who are good surgical risks. New, minimally invasive alternative treatments should always be compared to the standard surgical techniques, i.e., transurethral resection of the prostate or open prostatectomy.

The comparison indicates that a new modality should have the following characteristics:

1. Much lower operating time and anesthetic requirements than in traditional treatment techniques
2. Low intraoperative morbidity and short convalescence
3. Easy repositioning and withdrawal of the device
4. Transurethral access through the device
5. One-day single clinic treatment

At present prostatic stents do not represent an alternative to transurethral resection, but rather an alternative to long-term catheterization of the elderly, unfit patient.

References

Baert L, Verhamme L, Van Poppel H, Vandeursen H, Baert J (1993) Long-term consequences of urethral stents. J Urol 150:853–855

Fabian K (1980) Der Interprostatische 'partielle katheter'. Urologe [A] 19:236–238

Kaplan S, Koo H (1990) Prostatic stents. Curr Tech Urol 3:1–8

Oesterling J (1991) The obstructive prostate and the intra-urethral stent. Contemp Urol 3(10):61–72

Van Poppel H, Baert L, Aswarie H, Oyen R (1991) Experience with the intraprostatic spiral. Br J Urol 68:604–607

10 Prostatic Balloon Dilation

MORTEN RIEHMANN and REGINALD C. BRUSKEWITZ

CONTENTS

10.1 Introduction

A brief reflection on the terminology of dilation or dilatation gives no clear idea how to use and distinguish between these words. In the *Oxford English Dictionary*, dilatation is defined as (1) the action or process of dilating, condition of being dilated, enlargement; (2) extension, expansion; (3) amplification, diffuse treatment. Historically both words have been used interchangeably, but today the term dilation seems to be more frequently used than dilatation. This at least seems to be so in the English-written literature. Attempts to distinguish between these two words based on different meanings, i.e. a performance versus a condition, cannot be supported historically either (BLOOM et al. 1992).

In the English-written urologic literature, both terms are used. Since the meaning of the words is arbitrary, it would seem appropriate also in the scientific literature to follow the trend of using dilation instead of dilatation.

MORTEN RIEHMANN, MD, Research Fellow, and REGINALD C. BRUSKEWITZ, MD, Professor of Surgery, Division of Urology, University of Wisconsin, Clinical Sciences Center, 600 Highland Avenue, Madison, WI 53792, USA

Petrovich/Baert (Eds.)
Benign Prostatic Hyperplasia

10.2 Natural History of BPH as It Relates to Balloon Dilation

Benign prostatic hyperplasia (BPH) is a disease of the elderly which actually begins in middle life. At approximately age 35 the first histologic evidence of hyperplastic nodules is noted and the percentage of males with histologically identifiable BPH increases progressively thereafter. Approximately 10–20 years later, discernible enlargement of the prostate as well as the symptoms of prostatism and more objective manifestations of obstruction, such as a decrease in the urinary flow, an increase in voiding pressure, and the development of bladder trabeculation and upper urinary tract deterioration in more extreme cases, is recognized.

Nonetheless, BPH is a process which on the one hand is almost inevitable and on the other hand is distinguished by marked variation from individual to individual in terms of severity of symptoms as well as morphologic and histologic manifestations. Some males have a predominance of epithelial tissue similar to that found in the canine whereas other males have predominately a stromal or a mixed glandular and stromal pattern. Some develop substantial enlargement of the prostate, while others have little in the way of enlargement. As has been noted, the degree of outlet obstruction and voiding symptoms seems to be little correlated with the degree of overall enlargement and may perhaps reflect occlusion of the lumen itself or be associated with dysfunction primarily at the bladder neck level (see Chap. 3 for details).

It is this spectrum of disease, ranging from minimal to significant enlargement and from stromal to epithelial disease, that perhaps has confounded attempts to define the efficacy of balloon dilation of the prostate. Some investigators have claimed outstanding success, albeit with careful patient selection aimed at culling out individuals from within this wide spectrum of disease, while others have noted little in the way of symptom and/or urodynamic improvement following balloon dilation, which some would argue is the result of problems with proper patient selection.

Most of the early investigation of the technique and efficacy of balloon dilation was performed in the canine model, in which radiographic evidence of persistent luminal enlargement was noted following balloon dilation. As a general rule, radiographically demonstrable luminal enlargement has not been recognized in humans and this is perhaps due to the difference in the underlying BPH process. In addition, the early investigations in the dog determined that dilation of the prostate with several or more atmospheres of pressure for 10 min was sufficient. There has been little attempt to investigate the pressure and duration necessary for adequate balloon dilation in the human, although a moderate amount of consideration has been given to different balloon size, shape, or configuration. However, the canine prostate is morphologically different from the human in that it is marked by substantial glandular hyperplasia with little in the way of stromal development or nodular disease. The canine prostate is also not surrounded by capsule that is so readily recognized in humans following the development of BPH.

10.3 History of Balloon Dilation

Prostatic urethral dilation was attempted in the 1840s when investigators such as Mercier designed metal dilators (MERCIER 1850). There were sporadic reports of such crude metal dilators being used during the ensuing century. It was in 1956 that Deisting reported his results in the treatment of 324 males with BPH and symptoms of prostatism using a metal dilator (DEISTING 1956). This device had a movable arm which spread apart from the other opposing arm to disrupt the anterior and posterior prostatic commissures. While these early reports did not include information on objective measurements, Deisting reported global success rates of 48% at 8 years following dilation. Immediately after dilation the success rate was 95%, which dropped to 83% and 74% at 3 and 5 years, respectively. Other investigators during this period reported similar results. It is important to bear in mind that in this epoch, transurethral resection of the prostate was also enjoying favorable reports and increasingly widespread use.

The enthusiasm for prostatic urethral dilation apparently subsided following the reports of Kollberg and Aalkjaer. Kollberg published results showing that in 55 cases only 22% had acceptable results 1–2 years following treatment (KOLLBERG 1959). Aalkjaer, a urologist from the same institution as Deisting, reported results in 296 patients who received either prostatic metal dilation or transurethral resection of the prostate (TURP) (AALKJAER 1965). Follow-up was available out to 7 years. In the TURP treatment group, 18 out of 110 patients required reoperation within 7 years, which is comparable to TURP reoperation rates reported today. Of the remaining 186 patients treated with the Deisting dilator, 14% required nearly immediate TURP to treat persistent acute urinary retention and an additional 38% required redilation within 9 months of the original procedure.

10.4 Contemporary Balloon Dilation

Interventional radiologists can be credited with the development and clinical application of synthetic intravascular balloons used to correct arterial stenosis. These balloons, which were generally directed into the intravascular system through the use of guidewires and a fluoroscopic guidance system, utilized high pressure to dilate stenotic vessels. Initially larger vessels such as the iliac arteries were dilated, but with time and refinement smaller blood vessels, such as coronary arteries, were also routinely treated.

Interventional radiologists were the first to introduce the dilation of the prostate. Six of Quinn and associates' demonstrated widening of the prostatic urethra in 6 dogs, which lasted for more than 8 weeks in five cases (QUINN et al. 1985). Burhenne and associates dilated the prostatic urethra in ten cadavers using a 24-French balloon and a hand-held syringe (Burhenne et al. 1984). Subsequently, Castaneda and his group determined that a 10-min dilation to 60 French (20 mm) was required for long-term radiographically confirmed urethral dilation in dogs (Castaneda et al. 1987, 1989). In humans, 10-min dilation became standard and customary, while balloons larger than 60 French were ultimately utilized. The technique of Burhenne, using a 24-French balloon and a hand-held syringe in cadavers in all likelihood has little bearing on the human clinical condition. Urethras are customarily dilated to 24 French with metal sounds prior to TURP. Although no carefully controlled trial has been performed, it was generally appreciated that this dilation was not sufficient to ameliorate prostatism. In addition, the use of a hand-held syringe implied that little in the way of actual hydraulic pressure, as reflected by higher atmospheric pressures possible with the balloon, was imparted to these cadaverous urethras. Clinical experience would suggest that at the minimum, this higher pressure used with balloons would be necessary for effective treatment.

10.5 Balloon Design

Initially, three placement techniques were employed for prostatic balloon dilation. These included digital, fluoroscopic, and endoscopic positioning of balloons. Initially, considerable energy was devoted to debates about which positioning technique was appropriate. The so-called Dowd balloon, manufactured by Microvasive, Co., had a sufficient length to dilate even the longest of prostates and the bladder neck. A knob distal to the dilating balloon could be palpated through the rectum and, hence, this was called digitally controlled positioning.

Other balloons were manufactured by American Medical Systems, a division of the Pfizer Corporation. This system employed digitally palpated buttons as well as so-called fixation balloons, which were inflated in the bulbous urethra below the external sphincter. These balloons were designed to prevent their migration proximally through the prostate and into the bladder. This, however, did not prove to be the case and they were subsequently renamed positioning balloons. Smaller, 30-French balloons served to partially stabilize the catheters, which can be described as very similar to the Dowd balloons. These balloons could readily be positioned digitally or endoscopically, by passing an endoscope next to the dilating catheter. Fluoroscopic positioning with the use of a guidewire was also easy to accomplish. The Dowd balloons shared these positioning similarities.

In North America, the Advanced Surgical Intervention balloons were the only ones that came in varying lengths, the range being 15–55 mm. There was also a Foley-type balloon in the proximal end which was positioned in the bladder. This proximal balloon was inflated and pulled down against the bladder neck prior to the inflation of the dilating balloon itself. Microvasive and Advanced Surgical Intervention, Inc., championed the development of so-called broad-shouldered balloons. These were designed to dilate and disrupt the apical prostate, but controlled trials to determine whether this occurred were never completed. The Advanced Surgical Intervention balloon was designed to be placed with a specially supplied endoscopic sheath and insertion mechanism.

While controlled trials comparing one balloon against the other were never performed, it is generally believed that balloon size and configuration do not have a substantial bearing on outcome; proponents of balloon dilation appear to emphasize patient selection more than balloon characteristics.

10.6 Patient Selection

Investigators have offered recommendations based on their global clinical experiences as to which patients might benefit most from balloon dilation. Consensus suggests that younger, less symptomatic patients with relatively high peak urine flow rates might be the optimal candidates for this technique. On the other hand, more severe symptoms, older age, reduced peak flow rates, heavy bladder trabeculation, larger prostates and the presence of a median lobe are felt to reduce the chance that balloon dilation would be successful. An explanation for the improvement of less severely afflicted patients might be that the less symptomatic patients tend to have more variability in their symptoms and flow rates, and by a process of regression to the mean, might be expected to improve spontaneously. This hypothesis can be best tested by random assignment of patients in prospective clinical trials to treatment, no treatment, or sham groups.

10.7 Uncontrolled Clinical Trials

The bulk of the literature related to prostatic balloon dilation has been derived from single-institution, uncontrolled trials which have tracked the outcome of patients over relatively short periods. Dowd and Smith reported the results of 50 patients treated with digitally positioned balloons inflated to 90 French at 4 atm for 15 min (Dowd and Smith 1990). The treatment was reported to be well tolerated and only minor complications were noted. While 15 min was not the standard duration of application, this technique demonstrated that 72% of the patients had excellent or acceptable results. This was despite the fact that the patients selected for the above study might be considered to be less likely to respond to treatment: 42% of the patients had complete urinary retention and 62% had failed treatment with an α-blocker. The authors did not find that subsequent redilation of those failing was beneficial. Results of a prospective uncontrolled trial were reported by Wasserman et al. (1990). Seventy-three patients underwent dilation to 25 mm using fluoroscopically positioned balloons of several different designs to between 3 and 5 atm of pressure for 10 min. Dilation was successfully accomplished in 96% of the patients with an average follow-up of 6.2 months. Fifty-four percent exhibited an improvement in their peak urine flow rate while 66% had improvement in symptom score. Median lobe enlargement was associated with symptom improvement in 38%. Symptom score improvements were maintained through 24 months, whereas peak urinary flow rates were maintained for only 12 months. It is important to note that only a small minority of patients were followed for 12–24 months. Unlike the report of Smith and Dowd, these patients did not respond well to a second dilation if the first was unsuccessful. Overall, 68% of the nonresponders were identified in the first 6 months of the study. Of those patients presenting with urinary retention, 28% showed clinical improvement. Only minimal complications were reported.

Another uncontrolled study of 42 patients with both BPH and bladder neck hyperplasia was reported by Goldenberg et al. (1990). A 25-mm, 3-atm balloon, manufactured by Advanced Surgical Intervention, was used to dilate these 42 patients for 10 min. At 6 months, 25% of the patients had an improvement in symptom score and peak flow rates whereas 46% had an improvement in symptoms alone. An additional 21% experienced a 50% improvement in symptom score but without any change in peak flow rates. The authors actually used corrected peak flow determinations; 11% of patients at 1 month had an increase in peak flow rate alone while corrected peak flow rate was seen in 25% of patients. The corrected mean peak flow rate was 24% at 3 months and 28% at 6 months, and remained improved in only 2% of patients at 12 months. Comparison of treatment results obtained in BPH versus bladder neck hyperplasia revealed that 74% of BPH patients but only 58% of bladder neck hyperplasia patients reported a decrease in symptom score at 6 months. These results may suggest that BPH was more responsive to the treatment than bladder neck hyperplasia. A further consideration may be that bladder neck hyperplasia patients had predominantly stromal disease, which is thought to be less responsive to balloon dilation. Complications were mild, including some pain, mild hematuria, and transient urinary retention. This report highlighted a frequent BPH treatment theme whereby improvement in symptom score may be noted with little or no objective change, such as an increase in urine peak flow rates; opinions are divided as to whether this is an acceptable or unacceptable treatment outcome.

In another publication, Wasserman et al. (1990) examined the effects of disease severity on efficacy of balloon dilation. The authors assigned patients to group 1, which included 42 patients with a mean symptom score of 16.8 at baseline (possible range 0–27), or group 2, comprising 49 patients with a mean symptom score of 14.5. The group 1 patients had a higher mean residual urine of 249 ml, as opposed to a mean of 105 ml in group 2, and the mean peak flow rate was lower at 7.9 ml/s as opposed to 10.7 ml/s. Group 1, with more severe manifestations of BPH, had a 43% improvement in their symptom score, while group 2 had an 80% improvement. Mean follow-up was 22 months, ranging from 6 to 48 months. A variety of balloons were inflated from 2.5 to 4.0 atm. They were from 25 to 30 mm in diameter.

10.8 Randomized Trials

Keane et al. (1989) randomized 45 patients to prostatic incision, transurethral resection, or balloon dilation. It should be noted that their mean follow-up was only 4.2 months. The authors concluded that the mean urinary flow rate increased with either incision or resection, but postvoiding residual urine did not change with incision or dilation. No urodynamic changes were noted following balloon dilation. Balloon dilation was not associated with retrograde ejaculation, unlike other procedures. The conclusion of this study was that the role for balloon dilation is probably very limited, perhaps only for infirmed patients.

Lepor and co-workers (1992) conducted a randomized, double-blind study comparing the effectiveness of balloon dilation and cystoscopy, which was viewed as a sham procedure. Thirty-three men with symptomatic BPH were assigned to balloon dilation or cystoscopy under sedation. The sedation was administered so that the patients would not be aware of which treatment they received. Efficacy was adjudged on symptom scores, urinary flow rates, and patient's global assessment. A blinded study nurse supervised the flow rate testing and symptom questionnaires following the procedure. The mean total symptom scores after balloon dilation of the prostate and cystoscopy at 1 month and 3 months were not significantly different, nor was any significant difference found in respect to the peak urinary flow rates. The authors concluded that there was no demonstrated efficacy for balloon dilation. The controversy of this conclusion is reflected by the fact that the editorial comments and reply by the authors following the publication of this study were more lengthy than the paper itself.

A prospective, randomized clinical trial comparing balloon dilation and TURP was prospectively conducted by urologists in Colorado (Kreder et al. 1992). They reported at the 1992 American Urologic Association Meeting that 52 patients aged 45 or older with bladder outlet obstruction secondary to BPH had been enrolled. Both TURP and balloon dilation groups continued to demonstrate a decrease in symptom score; in the TURP group it decreased from a mean of 13.6 to a mean of 6.0 and in the balloon dilation group, from a mean of 14.1 to a mean of 8.6, both reductions being highly statistically significant. The increase in mean peak flow rate was substantial for the TURP group, but there was no change in flow for the balloon dilation group.

10.9 Conclusion

The debate about the efficacy of balloon dilation continues. The two most recent randomized clinical trials have come to very divergent conclusions. The initial investigation of balloon dilation did not include adequate human testing using different time, pressure, and balloon configuration parameters, and certainly did not address the need for randomized trials early on. At this point, evidence regarding efficacy of treatment by balloon dilation is best summed up as inconclusive, and a definitive answer to this question of efficacy awaits further trials.

References

Aalkjaer V (1965) Transurethral resection/prostatectomy versus dilatation treatment in hypertrophy of the prostate. II. A comparison of late results. Urol Int 20: 17–22

Bloom DA, Mory RN, Hinman F Jr (1992) Dilation vs. dilatation: a brief history. J Urol 147: 1682

Burhenne HJ, Chisholm RJ, Quenville NF (1984) Prostatic hyperplasia: radiological intervention. Work in progress. Radiology 152: 655–657

Castaneda F, Lund G, Larson BW, et al. (1987) Prostatic urethra: experimental dilation in dogs. Radiology 163: 645–648

Castaneda F, Isorna S, Hubert JC, et al. (1989) The importance of separation of prostatic lobes in relief of prostatic obstruction by balloon catheter urethroplasty: studies in dogs and humans. AJR 153: 1301–1304

Deisting W (1956) Transurethral dilation of the prostate: a new method in the treatment of prostatic hypertrophy. Urol Int 2: 158–171

Dowd JB, Smith JJ (1990) Balloon dilatation of the prostate. Urol Clin North Am 17: 671–677

Goldenberg SL, Perez-Marrero RA, Lee LM, Emerson L (1990) Endoscopic balloon dilation of the prostate: early experience. J Urol 144: 83–88

Keane FK, Shah JR, O'Donoghue N, Wickham JEA (1989) Resection incision or balloon dilatation for benign hypertrophy. J Urol 141: 254A

Kollberg S (1959) Erfarenheter av transurethral prostatadilatation enlight Deisting. Foredrag vid Med riksstamma, Stockholm

Kreder KJ, Donatucci CF, Crawford DE, Donohue RE, Whitesel J, Yakely R, Berger N (1992) Balloon dilation of the prostate versus transurethral resection: a continuing prospective randomized clinical trial. J Urol 147: 307A

Lepor H, Syperd D, Machi G, Devus J (1992) Randomized double-blind study comparing the effectiveness of balloon dilation of the prostate and cystoscopy for the treatment of symptomatic benign prostatic hyperplasia. J Urol 147: 639–644

Mercier F (1850) Recherches sur les valvules du col de la vessie. Paris

Quinn SF, Dyer R, Smathers R, et al. (1985) Balloon dilatation of the prostatic urethra. Radiology 157: 57–58

Wasserman NF, Reddy PK, Zhang G, Berg PA (1990) Experimental treatment of benign prostatic hyperplasia with transurethral balloon dilation of prostate: preliminary study in 73 humans. Radiology 177: 485–494

11 Laser Therapy in Benign Prostatic Hyperplasia

KEN ANSON and GRAHAM WATSON

CONTENTS

11.1 Introduction

The previous 5 years have seen a large proportion of urologists and prospective patients re-evaluating transurethral resection of the prostate (TURP) and investigating minimally invasive approaches to the prostate. The realisation that new technologies can significantly alter surgical practice is well demonstrated by the impact of extracorporeal shock wave lithotripsy on stone management.

KEN ANSON, FRCS, Research Registrar in Urology, Department of Urology and Minimally Invasive Therapy, Whittington Hospital, Highgate Hill, London N19 5NF, United Kingdom
GRAHAM WATSON, MD, FRCS (Urol), Consultant Urologist, Department of Urology and Minimally Invasive Therapy, Whittington Hospital, Highgate Hill, London N19 5NF, and Senior Lecturer, Institute of Urology, London, United Kingdom

Petrovich/Baert (Eds.)
Benign Prostatic Hyperplasia

Clinicians, in partnership with industry, have subsequently considered the role of all manner of technological devices in the treatment of bladder outflow obstruction secondary to benign prostatic disease. This has not simply been a search for the most pleasing new machine (with the associated benefit for practitioner and manufacturer alike) but has arisen from worries about the risks associated with standard transurethral resection of the prostate (MEBUST et al. 1989; ROOS et al. 1989).

In the United States more than 400000 TURPs are performed annually with vast cost implications for health care institutions (see Chap. 8). The increasing age of the population will inevitably lead to an increased demand for prostatic treatments. The morbidity and mortality associated with TURP is low compared to its efficacy; however, the prolonged in-patient stay, 18% 30-day morbidity (MEBUST et al. 1989) and loss of ejaculation are daunting prospects for the patient. It must also now be considered to exert a significant strain on the myocardium. Any alternative treatment that can offer similar symptomatic improvement but reduce the complications of standard surgery will have an enormous impact on urological practice.

11.2 Historical Background

The interest in the use of lasers for treating prostatic disease initially arose from work by SANDER and BEISLAND (1984), who demonstrated that the neodymium: YAG laser can be safely used to irradiate a resection cavity in cases of localised carcinoma of the prostate. The aim of the treatment was to "sterilise" the capsule and thus irradicate any residual malignant cells. They delivered the laser beam through a conventional fibre angled by means of an Alberran lever. The procedure had to be undertaken after a very complete transurethral resection (performed at a previous session) leaving less than 1 cm thickness of capsule throughout. Further, the laser was delivered via the urethral and suprapubic routes (to treat the apices). Their studies revealed that 14000 J could be safely delivered without injury to surrounding structures (SANDER and BEISLAND 1984). Similar work from MCNICHOLAS and O'DONOGHUE (1991) has confirmed the safety of this procedure but we await the long-term results and comparative studies with radiotherapy before we can establish the efficacy of this procedure.

The use of any laser for the treatment of obstructing benign prostatic tissue was, for some time, considered unsuitable as the volume of tissue that could be vaporised was small. However, the Nd:YAG laser (with a wavelength of 1064 nm) is poorly absorbed and widely scattered in the prostate and this laser can produce efficient coagulative necrosis of larger volumes of prostatic tissue. The necrotic tissue subsequently sloughs, leaving a cavity. Great interest has been generated in this bloodless effect of Nd:YAG laser energy. A number of devices have been developed to deliver the laser energy to the prostate in the hope of forming a large enough cavity to disobstruct the prostatic urethra.

11.3 Transurethral Laser Prostatectomy

In 1991 two centres reported canine prostate feasibility studies using the TULIP (Intrasonix, Burlington, Mass., USA) device (transurethral ultrasound-guided laser-induced prostatectomy) (Assimos et al. 1991; Roth and Aretz 1991). A water-filled balloon is inflated in the prostatic urethra and through this an Nd:YAG laser is delivered via a deflecting prism into the prostate (Fig. 11.1). Transurethral ultrasound transducers are positioned in line with the laser window, allowing sectors of the prostate to be scanned and photo-irradiated from the bladder neck to the verumontanum. The laser and transducers can be moved axially and rotated within the balloon. Significant cavities are formed within the canine prostatic urethra and no major complications have been reported: specifically inadvertent treatment of the distal sphincter mechanism and bladder are avoided.

Clinical trials with this device have shown encouraging early results and the treatment has been rapid and bloodless. Problems arise from exact localisation of the external sphincter as this is poorly seen on transurethral sector scanning. The device is also bulky and expensive.

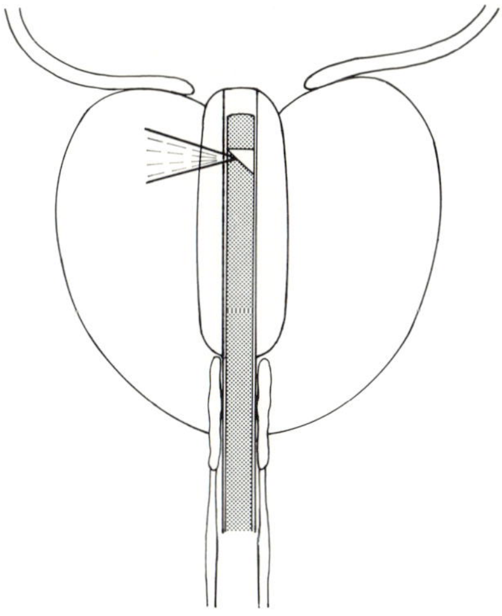

Fig. 11.1. Transurethral ultrasound-guided laser-induced prostatectomy tulip procedure. A sidefiring laser beam can be moved from the bladder neck to the verumontanum within a balloon with simultaneous transurethral ultrasonic imaging

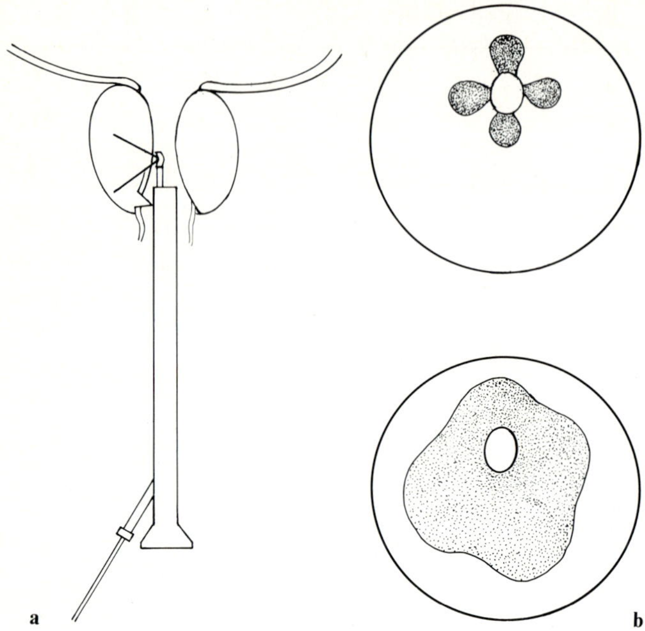

Fig. 11.2. a A sidefiring device delivers the laser beam to the prostatic tissue under cystoscopic control. **b** The zones of coagulative necrosis coalesce. This zone sloughs, leaving a cavity

JOHNSON et al. (1991) described an alternative transurethral approach in which the laser treatment is delivered under direct vision. A sidefiring device, originally developed for endometrial ablation (Lateralase, Trimedyne), is delivered into the prostatic urethra down the instrument channel of a conventional cystoscope (Fig. 11.2a). Laboratory dosimetry and canine experimentation demonstrated that 60 W of Nd:YAG laser treatment delivered for 60 s in four quadrants (Fig. 11.2b) resulted in the formation of a re-epithelialised 2.7-cm cavity within the prostatic urethra 5 weeks after treatment (JOHNSON et al. 1991, 1992). COSTELLO et al. (1992) reported the first clinical experience using this device in 17 patients. The treatment was delivered using the above parameters with an additional 30 s delivered to the bladder neck region in patients with significant middle lobe enlargement. A urethral catheter was inserted for 48–72 h while the oedema settled.

Results at 6 weeks demonstrated a cavity indistinguishable from TURP in ten (59%) patients while seven (41%) patients demonstrated residual occlusive lateral lobe tissue. These procedures were virtually bloodless with no urinary incontinence encountered (COSTELLO et al. 1992).

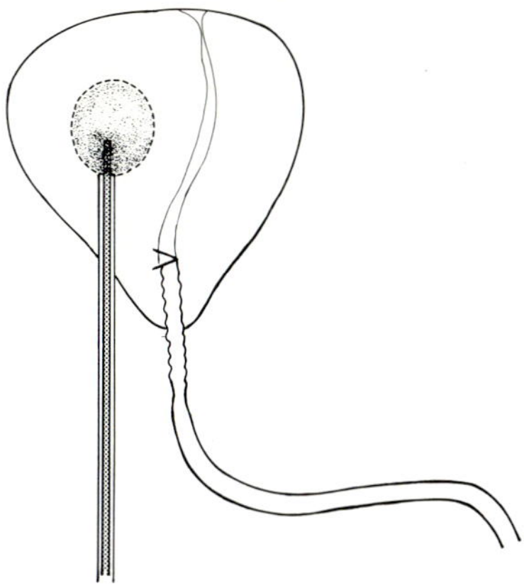

Fig. 11.3. Transperineal interstitial laser fibre placement directly into the substance of the adenoma

11.4 Interstitial Laser Coagulation of the Prostate

An additional approach for delivering laser energy to the prostate is via an interstitial route (Fig. 11.3). In canine experiments the insertion of quartz glass-capped optical fibres into the lateral lobes under transrectal ultrasound control using low-power Nd:YAG (5–10 W for 5–10 min) treatment results in an approximate 20-mm diameter area of coagulative necrosis. Early results in the human suggest encouraging improvements in flow rates (HOFSTETTER et al. 1992). McNICHOLAS et al. (1991) demonstrated a similar effect using multiple bare fibres. This transperineal interstitial approach would preserve the urethra and reduce the passage of necrotic slough that may follow transurethral photo-irradiation.

11.5 Endoscopic Laser Coagulation of the Prostate

The neodymium:YAG laser is the most logical wavelength for causing coagulation of the prostate. Despite the paucity of experimental evidence in the human prostate, extrapolation from studies in the canine and other human tissue suggest that photo-irradiation with Nd:YAG will result in the formation of a sizeable cavity 4–6 weeks after treatment.

We have used this laser to treat 42 patients using two different sidefiring devices (Urolase, Bard, UK; Myriadlase, Myriadlase Inc., Calif., USA).

11.5.1 Patients and Methods

Forty-two patients (mean age of 67; range 52–82 years) with bladder outflow obstruction and palpably benign prostate glands were studied. Eight (19%) presented in acute urinary retention and the rest of the patients had uncomplicated outflow obstruction. Pre-treatment evaluation consisted of the American Urological Association (AUA) symptom score, sexual history and uroflowmetry. Mid-stream urine culture and routine blood tests were performed. The post-micturition residual urinary volumes and upper tracts were assessed with transabdominal ultrasonography. Follow-up clinical evaluations consisted of AUA symptom score, uroflowmetry and post-micturition residual urinary volumetric assessment at 4, 12 and 26 weeks post-operatively.

11.5.2 Operative Methods

Under either spinal or general anaesthesia a preliminary cystoscopic assessment was performed to exclude synchronous bladder pathology. Prostatic urethral length was measured from bladder neck to verumontanum using a graduated 8-Ch ureteric catheter under direct vision. With laser ablation of the prostate there was no prostatic material available for histological assessment and therefore prostatic biopsy was required either before or at the time of surgery. In our first few patients transrectal prostatic biopsies were taken immediately prior to surgery but two patients developed postoperative temperatures and one patient experienced rigors of short duration. All subsequent patients underwent multiple endoscopic transurethral prostatic biopsies (Roth-Miller Endocut needle) (Miller et al. 1990) prior to laser irradiation and there were no further postoperative pyrexias.

A 16-Ch suprapubic catheter was inserted with the Add A Cath introducer and allowed free bladder drainage in the immediate postoperative period. The urethra was dilated to 24 Ch and using a standard 23-Ch cystoscope with a single Albarran deflector the laser fibre was delivered into the prostatic urethral lumen under direct vision.

The deflecting device was positioned midway between the verumontanum and the bladder neck. The tip was kept out of contact with prostatic tissue (contact during laser treatment may destroy the deflector mechanism). Saline was used for irrigation in all cases. Using the Urolase fibre 60 W of energy was delivered for 60 s to areas of obstructing tissue in the 2, 4, 8 and 10 o'clock positions. Any significant middle lobe tissue received a further 60 s of treatment at 60 W. If the prostatic urethra exceeded 4.2 cm in length a second round of treatment was delivered in the same positions closer to the bladder neck region.

In contrast, using the Myriadlase fibre treatment was directed according to surgeon evaluation. An attempt was made to deliver the energy corresponding to the site of the most prostatic tissue. In general 60 W was delivered for 60 s to the areas outlined above. However, shorter treatments of 30 s duration were occasionally delivered to prominent middle lobes or hypertrophic bladder neck regions. All patients presenting in retention were treated with appropriately sized Urospiral (Porges, UK) endoprostatic stents at the time of surgery.

Of the 42 study patients, 24 (57%) were treated with the Myriadlase and 18 (43%) with the Urolase fibre.

The position and duration of treatment was recorded in all cases. Power transmission from the fibre tip was measured pre- and post-operatively at 3 W (using a Coherent power meter) in order to monitor tip deterioration.

All patients were kept in hospital overnight. Twenty-four hours after surgery blood was taken for haemoglobin and electrolyte estimation.

The patients were discharged home intermittently clamping the suprapubic catheters and were seen 7 days postoperatively, when the majority of catheters were removed. All were treated with prophylactic antibiotics at the time of surgery and oral trimethoprim was continued until catheter removal. All prostatic stents were removed as day cases under sedoanalgesia 8 weeks postoperatively.

11.5.3 Results

In the Myriadlase group the mean treatment time was 11 min and in the Urolase group it was 5.15 min. The mean drop in power transmission with Myriadlase was 29.3% and with Urolase, 12%. One Myriadlase fibre burned out.

The laser treatment is effectively bloodless and most of the bleeding encountered was from instrumentation. No patients received postoperative bladder irrigation; however, five (12%) patients required a single bladder washout (three immediately post-operatively and two on the ward). The mean pre- and postoperative haemoglobin, haematocrit and sodium levels are listed in Table 11.1.

Most patients were discharged within 2 days of surgery. Two (5%) patients developed major complications. One (aged 66) underwent a laparotomy 6 days postoperatively for perforated diverticular disease and a second patient (aged 82) had a perforated peptic ulcer oversewn 10 days postoperatively. Both patients subsequently made uncomplicated recoveries.

The mean drop in AUA symptom score, post-micturition residual urinary volumes and improvements in maximum and average flow rates are outlined in Tables 11.2 (Myriadlase) and 11.3 (Urolase).

In the Myriadlase group two patients have been lost to follow-up. Two patients had incidental carcinoma of the prostate diagnosed on biopsy and were subsequently removed from the trial. There were four treatment failures in the Myriadlase group. Three have already undergone transurethral resection. Their results have been excluded from the 6-month follow up.

All patients in the retention group successfully voided after removal of the prostatic stents.

Table 11.1. A comparison of haemoglobin, haematocrit and sodium changes pre-operatively and 24 h postoperatively in 42 patients treated with sidefire

	Haemoglobin (g/l)	Haematocrit (PCV)	Sodium (mmol/l)
Pre-operative	13.68 ± 0.70	0.409 ± 0.026	139.1 ± 3.53
Postoperative	12.78 ± 1.59	0.401 ± 0.05	136.2 ± 3.59

Table 11.2. A comparison of AUA symptom score, flow rate and post-micturition residual volume changes in patients treated with the Myriadlase sidefire device

	AUA symptom score	Residual volume (ml)	Q max. (ml/s)	Q ave. (ml/s)
Pre-op.	24	148	10.15	4.85 ($n = 24$)
4 weeks	11.9	84	13.5	6.72 ($n = 24$)
12 weeks	9	49	14	6.7 ($n = 23$)
26 weeks	13	83	16	9 ($n = 13$)

Table 11.3. A comparison of AUA symptom score, flow rate and post-micturition residual volume changes in patients treated with the Urolase sidefire device

	AUA symptom score	Residual volume (ml)	Q max. (ml/s)	Q ave. (ml/s)
Pre-op.	19.9	226	9.1	4.7
4 weeks	15	113	10.3	5.6
12 weeks	8.7	65	29.4	12.2

11.5.4 Discussion

The sidefiring devices allow safe and rapid photo-irradiation of obstructing prostatic tissue. The use of conventional endoscopic equipment and the visual treatment monitoring make it an attractive alternative to the TULIP device. As the fibre is not in contact with tissue, vascular channels are not exposed, thus effectively eliminating any significant irrigant absorption. There is virtually no bleeding and in our experience any significant haemorrhage is related to instrumentation.

Costello et al. (1992) reported immediate cavity formation during treatment. In our experience this claim appears optimistic as we have witnessed only mild change in the shape of the prostatic urethra and any popcorn effect that may occur rarely results in a significant volume of tissue vaporisation. The treatment is characterised by progressive whitening of irradiated tissue but we rarely encountered vaporisation. At the end of the procedure the prostatic urethra remains obstructed.

11.5.5 Limitations of Endoscopic Laser Coagulation

Worries about irradiation of the distal sphincter mechanism limit the degree of laser irradiation at the apical regions with a sidefiring device. Similarly, middle lobes and the bladder neck region are difficult to treat. These areas can, however, be irradiated using a simple forward-firing bare fibre. There is a theoretical risk of inadvertent bladder mucosal damage using this technique although the degree of beam divergence from a bare fibre is considerable and the risk of significant damage is minimal.

In both our series and that reported by Costello et al. (1992) an unobstructed prostatic cavity was seen at follow-up cystoscopy in some patients but a significant number of patients had residual prostatic tissue. One problem with laser coagulation was that at the time of surgery the size of the eventual cavity could only be imagined. It is logical from the canine studies to assume that in small prostate glands 4 min of laser irradiation at 60 W will produce an adequate cavity; however, in larger glands greater energies are required to produce large enough volumes of coagulation to disobstruct the prostate. At the present time there is insufficient dosimetry information to establish the amount of energy required to coagulate a given volume of human prostatic tissue.

11.5.6 Treatment Toxicity

The postoperative recovery from this procedure is often characterised by a period of frequency of micturition associated with dysuria and occasional frank haematuria (with sterile urine) lasting for up to 8 weeks. Distal penile tip pain at the end of micturition is also a feature of laser coagulation of the prostate in a small number of subjects. Although not disabling, the discomfort can limit normal activity.

Those patients treated with urethral catheterisation or endoprostatic stenting appear to experience less discomfort. The reason for this is unclear but may relate to the reduction of contact of necrotic tissue with urine. Certainly the combination of coagulation and persistent obstruction is associated with significant dysuria.

Flow rate and symptomatic improvement continues for up to 8-10 weeks and this correlates well with the time to maturity of the cavity seen in canine studies.

Despite the shortcomings of the procedure, laser coagulation of the prostate is a quick and bloodless approach to relieving the symptoms of bladder outflow obstruction secondary to benign prostatic disease.

11.6 Endoscopic Laser Vaporisation of the Prostate

More recently great interest has been generated in the vaporisation of prostatic tissue. Much higher energies are required to effect vaporisation of tissue in comparison to deep coagulation. This can be illustrated by considering the difference between heating water to 70°C (at which temperature tissue is coagulated) and boiling water. The energy required to heat 1 cc of water from 37° to 70°C is 138.6 J. The energy to vaporise 1 cc of water is approximately 2600 J.

The use of sapphire contact tips or sculpted fibres results in a higher power density at the fibre end. Vaporisation takes place (via a photothermal effect) when the fibre is placed in contact with tissue. Using the Nd:YAG laser there is a narrow strip of coagulation (approximately 2 mm) deep to the area of vaporisation. This provides reasonable haemostasis but is less haemostatic than deep coagulation. Penetration can be predictably controlled and there is little risk of perforation.

Using a free beam with the Nd:YAG laser, Kandel showed the safety and efficacy of laser vaporisation and coagulation of prostatic tissue in canines (KANDEL et al. 1992). DAUGHTRY and RODAN (1992) published early clinical results using the SLT contact laser system with the Nd:YAG laser at 38–40 W. They performed transurethral laser resection of the prostate in 25 patients who were poor candidates for standard surgery. There was careful patient selection (i.e., small gland volumes and significant bladder decompensation). Of the 25 study patients, 15 (60%) had "good" results with significant improvements in flow rates (> 15 ml per second) and reductions in post-micturition volumes, five (20%) had "fair" results and there were five (20%) failures. There were no significant complications and average estimated blood loss was 100 cc. All patients were treated as day cases and 23 received intravenous sedation only (DAUGHTRY and RODAN 1992). Vaporisation of tissue allows disobstruction of the urethra at the time of surgery by either incisional prostatotomies or the removal of obstructing tissue. The advantage of vaporisation is that what you see at the time of surgery is very nearly what the end result will look like. This is in sharp contrast to coagulation when the size and shape of the eventual cavity are a matter of judgement.

Laser resection of significant volumes of obstructing tissue is slow. A quicker approach is to perform a laser bladder neck incision and prostatotomy to disobstruct the urethra and then coagulate residual tissue with free beam Nd:YAG. Following the incisions a greater area of prostatic tissue is available to be coagulated. This can be performed with either a sidefiring device or a forward-firing bare fibre and is a faster procedure. At the present time the sidefiring devices are being marketed from between $500 and $750. A simple bare fibre costs $100 and is reusable if a simple cleave is performed to produce a fresh fibre surface.

Table 11.4. A comparison of AUA symptom score, flow rate and post-micturition residual volume changes in ten patients (five voiding, five retention) treated with the combination of KTP bladder neck incision and Nd:YAG bare fibre coagulation

	AUA symptom score	Q max. (ml/s)	Q ave. (ml/s)	Residual volume (ml)
Voiding patients ($n = 5$)				
Pre-operative	22.5	7.9	3.3	196.6
4 weeks	13.8	14.2	7.5	112.5
12 weeks	6.6	19.3	9.6	54.5
Retention patients ($n = 5$)				
Pre-operative	–	–	–	–
4 weeks	12.8	18.6	7	102
12 weeks	8	19.7	8	102

11.7 Laser Bladder Neck Incision

Incision of the prostate from the ureteric orifice to the verumontanum can be performed bloodlessly using contact tips with the Nd:YAG laser. One can avoid a contact tip by using a bare fibre and a laser wavelength which is well absorbed by the tissue. The KTP laser (532 nm) delivered via sculpted tips has a similar action to the Nd:YAG laser delivered via contact tips, with slightly less haemostasis. We have also used the holmium:YAG laser (250 μs pulse duration, up to 2 J per pulse at up to 10 Hz) delivered through a bare fibre to incise the prostate.

11.7.1 Laser Bladder Neck Incision and Prostatotomy in Combination with Free Beam Coagulation

We have treated ten patients with laser bladder neck incision and prostatotomy in combination with free beam coagulation. Commonly we have used the Laserscope laser, which allows the simple switch between the KTP and Nd:YAG frequencies. The incisions have been performed with a sculpted fibre using the KTP laser at 30 W. A bare fibre is then used to coagulate residual prostatic tissue using 60–100 W of Nd:YAG. Early results in five voiding and five acute retention patients are outlined in Table 11.4.

11.8 Laser Prostatectomy with Preservation of the Urethra

The discomfort experienced by some patients after laser coagulation and the reduced symptoms in those treated with either a urethral catheter or an endoprostatic stent suggested to us that the contact of urine with necrotic prostatic tissue may, in some part, explain these adverse features.

Use of the Prostatron (Technomed) suggests that the urethra is a sensitive area of the prostate. Urethral cooling during treatment enables a greater energy delivery prior to the onset of discomfort. We have been developing a urethral sparing technique during transurethral laser prostatectomy.

Using either the Nd:YAG laser and a chisel contact tip (SLT, Pennsylvania) or the KTP laser and a contact fibre an incision is made in the prostatic urethra at the level of the verumontanum. A round-ended contact tip is then insinuated into the bulging lateral lobes and a cavity is developed by vaporisation of prostatic tissue. As the process continues the endoscope can be inserted into the cavity and further coagulation of residual adenoma can be performed. Alternatively, a sidefiring probe or just as easily a bare fibre can be used instead of the round-ended contact tip.

The tactile feedback from contact tips enables the prostatic capsule to be identified by an increased resistance to travel of the probe. Perforation of the prostatic capsule has not yet occurred in our experience.

Large cavities in both lateral lobes can be produced by this technique and at the end of the treatment the prostatic urethra is intact and appears viable. It is necessary to insert either a urethral catheter or an endoprostatic stent over a guide wire as the cavities can act as false passages for instrumentation at the end of the procedure.

Seven urethral sparing laser prostatectomies have been performed and early results are encouraging, with improvements in flow rates and reductions in postmicturition residuals. All patients were discharged the day after surgery. There was no significant bleeding in any of the cases. All urethral catheters were removed on the seventh day and all patients voided satisfactorily. Postoperative discomfort was dramatically reduced in all patients.

11.9 Interstitial Laser Coagulation of the Prostate

The improvement of imaging systems (predominantly ultrasound) over the past decade has provided excellent visualisation of organs and abnormal areas of tissue within them. It has also allowed the accurate placement of therapeutic instruments into these abnormal areas for either biopsy or treatment.

The delivery of Nd:YAG laser energy, via fine flexible optical fibres, into tumours to cause thermal tumouricidal effects was first suggested by BOWN (1983). Since then Bown and other workers have investigated this application for a number of tumours including those of the breast, prostate, liver and pancreas. Work from Matthewson, Steger and Hashimoto has shown that lesions of coagulation of up to 15 mm can be caused in a variety of canine and human tissues using between 700 and 1000 J of Nd:YAG laser delivered at low powers (MATTHEWSON et al. 1987; STEGER et al. 1987, 1988; HASHIMOTO et al. 1985).

The success of transrectal ultrasonography (TRUS) in the identification and guided biopsy of small volume prostatic tumours encouraged McNicholas and co-workers to pursue interstitial laser hyperthermia in prostatic carcinoma. They demonstrated that, using low-power Nd:YAG via interstitial fibres in the beagle prostate, small localised early prostatic cancers could be destroyed in situ. The use of multiple interstitial fibres further enhanced the effect, with larger volumes of tissue destroyed. Thermometry measurements showed temperatures of only 36° and 38°C 10 mm from the fibre tip during treatment and these correlated with the margins of the necrotic tissue seen at post-mortem (STEGER and MCNICHOLAS 1990). Having established the feasibility of the technique, both McNicholas and more recently Muschter and Hofstetter have considered the role of interstitial laser coagulation for the treatment of benign prostatic hyperplasia (MCNICHOLAS et al. 1991; HOFSTETTER et al. 1992). The aim has been to induce a sufficiently large volume of necrosis within the gland to disobstruct the prostatic urethra and so provide urodynamically beneficial effects.

In surgically exposed beagle prostate the mean maximal diameter of the area of thermal necrosis following 1200–1500 J measured at 5–14 days after treatment was 16.6 mm. Using a multiple fibre system (two fibres 1.5 cm apart in each lobe) a total of 4020 J produced a 26-mm lesion of necrosis (MCNICHOLAS et al. 1991). The urothelium of the urethra, the external sphincter and the rectum showed no damage.

In 15 patients treated with the Nd:YAG laser (10 W for 5 min via a diffuser probe to each lobe), HOFSTETTER et al. (1992) showed excellent early clinical results with significant falls in obstructive symptoms, an increase in maximal and median flow rates and a decrease in residual volumes. Two (13%) patients experienced mild urinary tract infections but the treatments were otherwise uncomplicated.

In in vitro studies, using the semiconductor laser (DIOMED Cambridge, UK, wavelength 805 nm), we have produced similar sized lesions in animal liver and chicken breast at similar energies. In two patients treated with percutaneous transperineal interstitial laser therapy prior to cystoprostatectomy both the semiconductor and the Nd:YAG laser produced 1.5 × 1.8 cm areas of necrosis within the lateral lobes using 5 W delivered for 10 min. There was no macroscopic evidence of capsular, sphincteric or urethral damage.

Early results suggest that the use of either the Nd:YAG or the semiconductor laser delivered at low powers via an interstitial route can produce significant areas of necrosis within the prostate. The technique of percutaneous insertion of the fibres under TRUS monitoring is safe and could be performed under local anaesthesia. The low powers required can be produced by small laser machines (the Diomed machine can be carried as hand luggage!) and could easily fit into the urologist's office.

The role of interstitial laser coagulation of the prostate in benign prostatic disease has not yet been established; however, it represents the potential for a urethral sparing laser prostatectomy.

11.10 Discussion

The burgeoning of alternative treatments available for symptomatic benign prostatic hyperplasia is well illustrated by the other chapters in this book. The fact that an entire volume is dedicated to innovations in the management of this increasingly common condition further reflects the quest for knowledge in this field.

The range of therapies is wide and many involve the use of highly technical equipment (WATSON 1992). The capital costs of machinery are often considerable and when combined with the additional expenditure on disposables the overall price may be inhibitory. Significant advantages over conventional prostatectomy must be illustrated before these therapies can be fully adopted by the general urologist.

The use of lasers to treat obstructing prostatic tissue has great potential. All treatments are effectively bloodless and offer considerable savings in in-patient costs. The lack of postoperative irrigation saves nursing time and enables early mobilisation of the patient. Blood transfusion is not required and we do not routinely save serum for cross-matching. Many of the treatments could be performed as day cases. The development of local anaesthetic transurethral resection at this institution has taught us that the combination of low levels of sedation and transurethral prostatic injection of local anaesthesia gives a very acceptable operating environment (BIRCH et al. 1990). It is therefore likely that transurethral laser therapy will be equally well tolerated. Our initial experiences suggest that short laser treatments performed under sedoanalgesia are safe and provide comfortable conditions for the patient and surgeon alike. These advances offer the potential for day case, local anaesthetic prostatectomy.

The number of different laser approaches to the prostate allow the surgeon to tailor the treatment to each individual patient. The maintenance of prograde ejaculation is an attractive option for many patients and in our experience this can be achieved with approximately 85% of patients treated with the sidefire device alone. In contrast if combined with bladder neck incision, retrograde ejaculation is likely.

Small glands may be treated with coagulation alone and the larger glands can be effectively disobstructed using a combination of coagulation and vaporisation. We have been assessing the laser treatment in prostate glands larger than the recommended range of 25–35 cc and have used higher energies. Our experience suggests that the 60-W, 60-s regimen will only penetrate to a maximum of 1.5 cm. Logically, to treat to a greater depth, this regimen should be altered to one where longer treatment durations are used.

A number of improvements can be made in tailoring the total energy delivered to each particular gland and at the present time it may be more appropriate to treat only the uncomplicated bladder outflow obstruction in patients with glands of less than 50 cc. Patients with renal impairment are not considered for laser therapy while the technique is still in evolution.

The considerable improvement in flow rates seen after TURP have not always been mirrored in laser prostatectomy. The improvement in symptoms combined with a reduction in post-micturition residual volumes may be all that is required in many patients.

Another approach is to combine laser coagulation with standard diathermy resection. This has the theoretical advantage of a relatively bloodless resection and allows the apical tissue to be resected safely. However, large bleeding vessels are not readily coagulated with Nd:YAG and in our experience this technique simply adds to the operating time and has no advantage over haemostasis performed with electrocautery.

The results from the various forms of microwave hyperthermia, thermotherapy and pharmacotherapy suggest a significant failure rate with a number of patients requiring standard transurethral resection. The laser is one more treatment option lying somewhere between pharmacotherapy and transurethral resection in terms of morbidity. These early results suggest that efficacy is comparable to TURP in the short term. Full urodynamic assessments will be required to make a more meaningful comparison.

Laser prostatectomy is an exciting development in prostatic surgery with great potential but further refinement of the surgical technique followed by clinical comparative trials must be completed before it can be recommended as a viable alternative to transurethral resection.

11.11 Conclusion

There are many different laser approaches to treat an obstructing prostate gland. The strategies include:

1. Tissue may be vaporised providing an immediate channel. This is slow and more suitable for prostatotomies.
2. Tissue may be coagulated rapidly and left to separate, leaving a cavity. This process takes 8 weeks in the human prostate.

In addition:

a) The bladder neck may be spared or incised.
b) Using contact probes the prostatic urethra can be incised and the adenoma vaporised.

c) A transperineal interstitial approach leaves the urethra completely intact.

All laser approaches are associated with minimal bleeding. They can be performed as day cases under sedation with local anaesthetic prostatic block. The free beam or sidefiring approaches delivered cystoscopically can treat the prostate without damaging the bladder neck but many patients suffer temporary prostatitis-like symptoms. Obstruction can persist for 8 weeks following surgery. Flow rate improvements are similar to those with TURP.

Those techniques which divide the bladder neck result in more rapid relief of obstruction but at the cost of retrograde ejaculation. Preservation of the urethra is associated with even less bleeding and less postoperative discomfort.

References

Assimos D, McCullough D, Woodruff R, et al. (1991) Canine transurethral laser – induced prostatectomy. J Endourol 5:145–149

Birch B, Anson K, Miller R (1990) Sedoanalgesia in urology: a safe cost effective alternative to general anaesthesia; a review of 1020 cases. Br J Urol 66:342–350

Bown S (1983) Phototherapy of tumours. World J Surg 7:700–709

Costello A, Bowsher W, Bolton D, et al. (1992) Laser ablation of the prostate in patients with benign prostatic hypertrophy. Br J Urol 69:603–608

Daughtry J, Rodan B (1992) Transurethral laser resection of the prostate. Lasers Surg Med 10:269–278

Hashimoto D, Takami M, Idezuki Y (1985) In depth radiation therapy by YAG laser for malignant tumours in the liver under ultrasound imaging. Gastroenterology 88:1663

Hofstetter A, Hessel S, Keiditsch E, et al. (1992) Hi-tech of the prostate: interstitial laser coagulation of benign prostatic hyperplasia. In: Anderson RR (ed) Progress in biomedical optics. Laser surgery, advanced characterisation, therapeutics, and systems III. The Society of Photo-optical Engineers, Bellingham, USA, pp 25–34

Johnson D, Levinson A, Greskovich F, et al. (1991) Transurethral laser prostatectomy using a right-angle laser delivery system. In: Watson GM, Steiner RW, Pietrafitta JJ (eds) Lasers in urology, laparoscopy and general surgery. The Society of photo-optical instrument Engineers, Bellingham, USA, pp 36–41

Johnson D, Price R, Cromeens D (1992) Histopathological changes occurring in the prostate following transurethral laser prostatectomy. In: Anderson RR (ed) Progress in biomedical optics. Laser surgery, advanced characterisation, therapeutics, and systems III. The Society of photo-optical Engineers, Bellingham, USA, pp 15–18

Kandel L, Harrison L, McCullough D (1992) Transurethral laser prostatectomy in the canine model. Lasers Surg Med 12:33–42

Matthewson K, Coleridge-Smith P, O'Sullivan J, et al. (1987) Biological effects of intrahepatic Nd:YAG laser photocoagulation in the rat. Gastroenterology 93:550–557

McNicholas T, O'Donoghue N (1991) Endoscopic YAG laser coagulation for early prostate cancer. In: Watson GM, Steiner RW, Pietrafitta JJ (eds) Lasers in urology, laparoscopy and general surgery. The Society of Photo-optical Instrument Engineers, Bellingham, USA, pp 56–66

McNicholas T, Steger A, Bown S, et al. (1991) Interstitial laser coagulation of the prostate: experimental studies. In: Watson GM, Steiner RW, Pietrafitta JJ (eds) Lasers in urology, laparoscopy and general surgery. The Society of photo-optical Instrument Engineers, Bellingham, USA; pp 30–35

Mebust W, Holtgrewe H, Cockett A, et al. (1989) Transurethral prostatectomy: immediate and postoperative complications. A cooperative study of 13 participating institutions evaluating 3885 patients. J Urol 141:243–247

Miller R, Birch B, Anson K, et al. (1990) The impact of minimally invasive surgery and sedoanalgesia on urological practice. Postgrad Med J 66 (Suppl 1): S72–S76

Roos N, Wennberg J, Malenka D, et al. (1989) Mortality and reoperation after open and transurethral resection of the prostate for benign prostatic hyperplasia. N Engl J Med 320:1120–1124

Roth R, Aretz H (1991) Transurethral ultrasound–guided laser–induced prostatectomy (TULIP procedure): a canine prostate feasibility study. J Urol 146:1128–1135

Sander S, Beisland H (1984) Lasers in the treatment of localised prostatic carcinoma. J Urol 132:280–281

Steger A, Barr H, Bown S, et al. (1987) Experimental studies on low power interstitial hyperthermia for pancreatic carcinoma. Gut 28:A1382

Steger A , Bown S, Clark C (1988) Interstitial laser hyperthermia: studies in the normal liver. Br J Surg 75:598

Steger A, McNicholas T (1990) Interstitial hyperthermia of the prostate. In: McNicholas TA (ed) Lasers in Urology: principles and practice. Springer, Berlin Heidelberg New York, pp 141–149 (The Bloomsbury in Clinical Science)

Watson G (1992) Minimally invasive therapies of the prostate. J Min Invas Ther 1:231–240

12 The Use of Pharmacologic Agents for Benign Prostatic Hyperplasia

CHRISTOPHER M. DIXON and HERBERT LEPOR

CONTENTS

12.1 Introduction

It is generally accepted that transurethral prostatectomy (TURP) is an effective treatment for bladder outlet obstruction caused by benign prostatic hyperplasia (BPH); however, alternative therapies, in particular medical therapies, have been motivated by patients trying to avoid surgery, pharmaceutical companies expanding into new markets and physicians trying to optimize the treatment of their patients. Beyond these motivations, a critical review of TURP suggests that it is a good procedure but has associated complications in a low but predictable percentage of cases. MEBUST et al. (1989) studied the morbidity following TURP in a cooperative retrospective study of 3885 consecutive patients from 13 institutions. HOLTGREWE et al. (1989) surveyed practicing urologists in the United States with regard to morbidity and mortality. These results are summarized in Table 12.1. Although relatively uncommon, the complications from TURP are significant (see Chap. 8).

Bothersome symptoms represent the primary surgical indication in 90% of TURPs performed in the United States (MEBUST et al. 1989). Other indications

CHRISTOPHER M. DIXON, MD, Assistant Professor, and HERBERT LEPOR, MD, FACS, Professor and Chairman, Department of Urology, New York University, 550 First Avenue New York, New York 10016, USA

Petrovich/Baert (Eds.)
Benign Prostatic Hyperplasia

Table 12.1. Morbidity associated with transurethral prostatectomy

	MEBUST et al. (1989)[a] %	HOLTGREWE et al. (1989)[b] %
Epididymitis	1.2	4.8
Urinary tract infection	2.3	8.4
Impotence	3.5	10.2
Incontinence	0.4	3.3
Transfusion	6.5	10.5
Transurethral resection syndrome	2.0	—
Death	0.2	—

[a] 3885 consecutive prostatectomies at 13 institutions
[b] 35% of practicing American urologists

include increased urinary residual, urinary retention, renal insufficiency, and bladder stones; however, these indications are much less common. Unfortunately, there are limited objective data detailing the symptomatic improvement following prostatectomy but overall it appears that about 80% of patients achieve satisfactory resolution of their symptoms following transurethral surgery (DORFLINGER et al. 1987, 1989; HELLSTROM et al. 1986; LEPOR and RIGUAD 1990; NEAL et al. 1989; ORANDI 1987). There are no available objective data regarding the effectiveness of TURP in improving bladder emptying, reversing renal insufficiency, preventing recurrent infections, or relieving acute or chronic urinary retention despite these accepted indications for the procedure.

Long-term complications after TURP are not well studied. Similarly, the long-term relief of bothersome symptoms is unknown. Approximately 15% of men undergoing TURP will require reoperation within 8 years (WENNBERG et al. 1987). Although prostatectomy is presently the most effective treatment for BPH, the limitations of the procedure and patient interest in nonsurgical alternatives provide a rationale for pursuing medical therapy. Medical management of BPH has become increasingly popular because of the availability of pharmacologic agents that achieve alpha blockade and androgen suppression.

12.2 Alpha Blockade

12.2.1 Rationale

The rationale for alpha blockade in the treatment of symptomatic BPH is based on histologic, pharmacologic, and clinical investigations. Histologically, the cellular elements of the prostate have been quantified using a double immunoenzymatic staining technique and color-assisted image analysis (SHAPIRO et al. 1992b) (see Chap. 5). This technique allows quantification of the prostatic epithelium, smooth muscle, connective tissue, and glandular lumen. In BPH tissue the ratio of stroma to epithelium has been reported to be approximately 5:1 (Bartsch et al. 1979). A significant stromal component is smooth muscle. Shapiro et al. (1992a) have recently used a mouse anti-actin label as a sensitive label for prostate smooth muscle. Double immunoenzymatic staining was performed on 19 biopsy specimens from men with clinical BPH. Quantitative color-assisted computer-assisted image analysis was used to calculate the area densities of smooth muscle (39% $\pm$ 3%), connective tissue (38% $\pm$ 3%), epithelium (12% $\pm$ 1%), and glandular lumen (11% $\pm$ 1%). These studies confirm the presence of smooth muscle as a significant histologic component in BPH tissue.

The pharmacologic rationale for alpha blockade has also been examined. Raz et al. (1973) studied the physiology and pharmacology of the rat prostate and demonstrated its contractility in response to the adrenergic agonist, norepinephrine. Subsequently, Caine et al. (1976, 1978, 1981) made similar observations in the human prostatic adenoma and recognized the clinical usefulness of pharmacologically blocking the smooth muscle contractility in symptomatic BPH patients. Other investigators have subsequently demonstrated that the contractibility of the human adenoma is primarily mediated by the α_1-adrenoreceptors (Heible et al. 1985; Gup et al. 1989; Lepor et al. 1988) and that these receptors are concentrated in the bladder base and prostate but are relatively sparse in the bladder body (Shapiro and Lepor 1987). Taken together, this information suggests that α_1-antagonists could relax the muscle tone of the bladder outlet and prostatic urethra without inhibiting bladder contractility, making these drugs potentially useful in the treatment of BPH.

Two mechanisms of outlet obstruction are generally considered. First, the static component or size of the adenoma obstructing the outlet and secondly, the dynamic component which is related to the smooth muscle tone. Alpha blockade is believed to effect the dynamic component of outlet obstruction by relaxing the smooth muscle. Working under the assumption that the clinical response to alpha blockade should be directly related to the smooth muscle content, Shapiro and Lepor (1992) examined the relationship between the clinical response to terazosin, a selective α_1-blocker, and the percentage area density of smooth muscle in BPH tissue. Prostatic biopsies from 26 men with clinical BPH were examined prior to terazosin therapy (titration to 5 mg daily). Smooth muscle content was quantitated using double immunoenzymatic staining and quantitative color-assisted computer image analysis. A direct relationship between the increase in urinary flow and percent area density of smooth muscle was observed, supporting the proposed mechanism of smooth muscle relaxation by alpha blockade.

12.2.2 Clinical Studies

Alpha blockade for treating BPH is not a new idea and was first reported in 1976 by Marco Caine (Caine et al. 1976). Over the past 15 years, there have been numerous clinical trials that have evaluated alpha blockade for the treatment of

BPH. Although most were deficient in design, almost all of them suggested that alpha blockade was useful in the treatment of BPH. The early studies were done using the nonselective α-blocker, phenoxybenzamine. This drug antagonizes both α_1- and α_2-adrenoreceptors. Although effective in ameliorating the symptoms of prostatism, its nonselective characteristics caused substantial adverse effects, limiting its clinical use.

More recently, selective α_1-antagonists have been developed. Because of their selectivity, the incidence and severity of adverse events is significantly less than with the nonselective drugs. The selective α_1-antagonists include prazosin, alfuzosin, YM617, indoramin, doxazosin, and terazosin. These drugs differ primarily by the duration of their half-lives.

Terazosin is a long-acting selective α_1-antagonist that has been well studied in BPH. The long half-life allows once-a-day dosing, which is likely to improve compliance. The common side-effects of these agents include light-headedness, dizziness, and fatigue. Adverse experiences can be minimized by dose titration and evening administration. There are no significant drug interactions complicating the clinical use of the medication except that concomitant antihypertensive medications, in particular calcium channel blockers, often must be reduced or eliminated. Presently, terazosin is the most thoroughly studied long-acting selective α_1-blocker for the treatment of BPH. The focus of this discussion will center around this drug because earlier agents such as phenoxybenzamine play only a historical role in the medical management of symptomatic BPH and there is a limited clinical database for the other long-acting selective α-blockers.

The clinical study design and outcome assessment parameters of various terazosin studies are summarized in Tables 12.2 and 12.3 respectively. In general, patients with mild to moderate symptoms were enrolled in these studies while those with urinary retention, urinary tract infection, or renal failure were excluded. The primary outcome parameters were improvement in a symptom index (Boyarsky score), urinary peak flow rate (Q_{max}), and the patient's own assessment. From a review of Tables 12.2 and 12.3, the improvement in outcome parameters appears consistent between the investigators.

Recently, the results of a multicenter phase III, double-blind, parallel-group, randomized, placebo-controlled study of a single daily dose of terazosin to patients with symptomatic BPH has been reported (LEPOR et al. 1992). Three-hundred and fourteen patients were treated with placebo or 2, 5, or 10 mg of terazosin in a single daily dose. A statistically significant ($p < 0.05$) improvement from baseline symptom scores was seen in all terazosin treatment groups. The 10 mg terazosin treatment groups also exhibited significantly greater decreases in irritative and total scores relative to the placebo group. The 5 and 10 mg terazosin treatment groups exhibited a significantly greater decrease in obstructive scores relative to the placebo group. The percentage of patients experiencing a greater than 30% improvement in the total symptom score for the placebo and 2, 5, and 10 mg treatment groups was 38%, 54%, 63%, and 70%, respectively. The percentage of patients experiencing greater than 30%

Table 12.2. Study design: terazosin

Author	Enrollment		Follow-up (weeks)	Randomized placebo	Symptom index	Uroflow
	Total	Active				
DUNZENDORFER (1987)	15	15	4	No	Yes	Yes
LEPOR et al. (1989)	22	22	4	No	Yes	Yes
LEPOR et al. (1990)	39	39	8	No	Yes	Yes
FABRICIUS et al. (1990)	52	52	24	No	Yes	Yes
LEPOR et al. (1991)	50	50	4–26	No	Yes	Yes
LEPOR and MACHI (1992)	29	29	4	No	Yes	Yes
LEPOR et al. (1992)	252	192	12	Yes	Yes	Yes
Totals	459	399		1/7	7/7	7/7

Table 12.3. Efficacy assessment: terazosin

Author	Active drug (no.)	Q_{max} (%)	Outcome assessment		
			Symptom index	Subjects improved (%)	Investigators assessment
DUNZENDORFER (1987)	15	+ 31	− 48	–	Yes
LEPOR et al. (1989)	22	+ 63	− 50	89	Yes
LEPOR et al. (1990)	39	+ 42	− 47	91	Yes
FABRICIUS et al. (1990)	52	+ 53	− 55	–	Yes
LEPOR et al. (1991)	50	+ 52	− 53	–	Yes
LEPOR and MACHI (1992)	29	+ 38	− 56	100	Yes
LEPOR et al. (1992)	192	+ 27	− 37	–	Yes
Totals	399	+ 44%	− 49%	93%	7/7

improvement in total symptom score in the 5 and 10 mg treatment groups was significantly greater than in the placebo group.

A statistically significant improvement from baseline was observed in the peak and mean urinary flow rates for all treatment groups. The 10 mg treatment group exhibited a significantly larger increase from baseline in peak and mean urinary flow rates relative to the placebo group.

The relationship between change in urinary flow rate was also a dose-related response. The percentages of patients experiencing a greater than 30% increase in peak urinary flow rate in the placebo and 2, 5, and 10 mg treatment groups were 25%, 36%, 35%, and 58%, respectively. Compared with the placebo group a significantly greater proportion of patients in the 10 mg terazosin treatment group exhibited a greater than 30% improvement in peak urinary flow rate.

Overall, the adverse events in the four treatment groups were minor and reversible. Although a higher incidence of asthenia, flu syndrome, and dizziness were observed in the terazosin treatment groups, the differences from the placebo group were not statistically significant when tested using Fisher's exact test. There was a significantly greater incidence of postural hypotension in the 5 mg terazosin group than in the placebo group. One patient in the 10 mg treatment group developed syncope at the 5 mg dose. The incidence of syncope in the 10 mg treatment group was one out of 79 (1.3%). The incidence of syncope for all terazosin-treated patients was less than 0.5%.

An effort was made to identify clinical or urodynamic factors that would predict a favorable outcome to terazosin therapy. The relationships between percentage change in total symptom score and peak urinary flow rate with baseline, age, prostate size, peak urinary flow rate, mean urinary flow rate, postvoid residual, and total symptom score were examined. No significant association was observed between treatment effect and baseline factors when tested using an analysis of covariance mode with terms for baseline factor, treatment group, and their interaction.

The phase III data support the role of long-acting selective α_1-blockers for the treatment of patients with symptomatic BPH. This study was of short duration and long-term data are necessary to determine the durability of this therapy. A long-term extension study is underway to assess the durability of the clinical response. To date, the response appears to be durable in 150 patients followed for at least 18 months.

12.3 Androgen Suppression

12.3.1 Rationale

Androgen suppression is believed to act on the static component of bladder outlet obstruction. By reducing the adenoma size, outlet resistance is reduced, leading to symptomatic improvement. The observation of prostate regression following androgen suppression is well known, particularly when treating prostatic malignancy. The rationale for treating BPH in this manner is based on the observation that the development and maintenance of BPH requires an intact hypothalamic-pituitary-testes-prostate axis. This is best supported by the failure of BPH to develop in adult Chinese eunuch males castrated before puberty (Wu and Gu 1987). White (1895) published the first report of androgen ablation for the treatment of BPH. One-hundred and eleven men were castrated and were reported to have a decrease in prostate size and substantial improvement. More recently, Peters and Walsh (1987) used morphometric studies to demonstrate a 25% decrease in prostate volume following treatment with a gonadotropin-releasing hormone (GnRH) agonist.

12.3.2 Clinical Studies

For obvious psychologic reasons, as well as the resulting hot flashes and loss of libido, castration for the treatment of BPH is of historical significance only. Medical castration can be achieved by a variety of drugs that act through various mechanisms. These are generally categorized into those that impair androgen production or block the action of androgens and include GnRH agonists, synthetic antiandrogens, progestational hormones, nonsteroidal antiandrogens, and 5α-reductase inhibitors. The primary limitation of many of these drugs that lower serum testosterone is the resulting impotence, loss of libido, and hot flashes. The morbidity associated with most hormonal therapies is often greater than the clinical manifestations of BPH.

Flutamide, a nonsteroidal antiandrogen, has been studied for the treatment of BPH. Caine et al. (1975a) reported improvement in symptoms and flow rates but no change in prostate volume, residual urine, or histology after rebiopsy. This was a placebo-controlled study but a low dose of flutamide was administered and the active treatment period was only 3 months. This may explain the limited clinical response. Stone (1987) reported a 6-month double-blind placebo-controlled study of 84 patients receiving 250 mg three times per day. A 35% improvement in flow rate and a 41% reduction in prostate size were noted in the treatment group. Symptomatic improvement, however, was similar in both groups. Although flutamide monotherapy does not lower serum testosterone, adverse experiences including breast tenderness, diarrhea, and hepatotoxicity have been reported. Drug trials with newer antiandrogens similar to flutamide but with less toxicity have been initiated.

The most extensively studied pharmacologic agent used for androgen suppression is the 5α-reductase inhibitor, finasteride. 5α-Reductase is an enzyme responsible for the intraprostatic conversion of testosterone to dihydrotestosterone, the latter serving as the principal androgen leading to prostate growth. Patients with deficient or defective 5α-reductase, a rare metabolic disorder, have a variety of phenotypic features. For the purposes of this discussion, the most notable features are a very poorly developed prostate but normal external virilization. The observations of the genetic syndrome 5α-reductase deficiency, and in particular the recognition of differential tissue sensitivity to androgens, led to the development of selective inhibition of the 5α-reductase enzyme by the compound finasteride. Since the prostate is sensitive to dihydrotestosterone, blocking production of dihydrotestosterone by inhibiting 5α-reductase should lead to prostate involution. More importantly, this could be accomplished without the undesirable adverse effects seen with other types of androgen suppression.

Human trials with finasteride began in 1986. Early studies confirmed the biochemical efficacy in man, and the suppression of serum and intraprostatic dihydrotestosterone levels. In a 26-week study in patients with BPH, the prostate shrinkage detected was 28% (The Proscar Study Group 1990). The mean increase in the maximum urinary flow rate was approximately 3 ml/s in the drug-treated group, with no change observed in the placebo group. These preliminary studies suggested that reduction in prostate volume resulted in clinically relevant improvement of urinary obstruction.

Recently, a large, multicenter, double-blind, placebo-controlled trial reporting the effect of finasteride in men with BPH has been published (Gormley et al. 1992). This study enrolled 895 men aged 40–83 years with mild to moderate symptoms of prostatism. Inclusion criteria included a peak flow rate $\leq$ 15 cc/s, residual volume $<$ 350 cc, prostate specific antigen (PSA) $<$ 40 μg/l, and the clinical absence of other disorders such as prostatic cancer, prostatitis, or neurogenic bladder. The patients were equally divided into one of three treatment groups: 297 received 5 mg finasteride, 298 received 1 mg finasteride, and 300 received placebo. A single daily dose was administered for 12 months and efficacy assessed monthly. The primary efficacy parameters included a modified symptom score and peak urinary flow rates.

The results indicated that finasteride reduced prostate volume by about 20%, lowered serum dihydrotestosterone by 60%, and lowered serum PSA levels 50%, all confirming the metabolic activity of the drug. The magnitude of improvement in efficacy parameters as compared to placebo was less impressive even in the 5 mg group. The net improvement in the total symptom score was only 1.3 points at 12 months as compared to placebo. Similarly, the net increase in peak flow was only 1.4 cc/s. Although both changes were statistically significant, the clinical significance of such modest improvements can be questioned. A subgroup of these patients (31%) did, however, have a 3 cc/s or more improvement in peak flow.

A clear benefit of this therapy over other available hormonal agents is the lack of adverse effects such as hot flashes or breast tenderness. There does appear to be a slight increase in sexual dysfunction (in particular, decreased libido, decreased ejaculate volume, and impotence), although very few patients withdrew from the study because of these side-effects.

The reduction of PSA in finasteride-treated patients is consistent with its physiologic action but may cause confusion as the use of PSA for the detection of prostatic cancer continues to expand. The interpretation of PSA values after finasteride therapy remains unclear and the clinical guidelines for interpreting PSA values during finasteride therapy have not been established. It would appear that finasteride therapy does not adversely affect the ability to distinguish men with and men without prostatic cancer (GUESS et al. 1993). On the other hand, although the average PSA reduction is about 50% at 12 months (41% at 6 months), the range is rather large (5%–95% range = − 81% to + 20%). Additional data are clearly needed to clarify the interpretation of PSA values during finasteride therapy.

12.4 Combination Treatment

The pathophysiology of bladder outlet obstruction from BPH is thought to be due to dynamic (smooth muscle tone) and static (adenoma size) factors. Since alpha blockade and androgen suppression are believed to act through these independent mechanisms, it seems logical to combine these therapies to further improve the clinical response and optimize medical therapy.

Only one open label pilot study combining alpha blockade and androgen suppression has been reported (LEPOR and MACHI 1992). Twenty-nine males received terazosin therapy alone for 1 month and the combination of 5 mg terazosin and 250 mg flutamide 3 times daily for the subsequent 5 months. The efficacy parameters included change in Boyarsky symptom scores, uroflowmetry, and the patient's assessment of symptom improvement. The efficacy parameters were evaluated at 1 month (terazosin alone) and at either 6 months or the time of early withdrawal from the study (combination therapy). Terazosin alone was associated with statistically significant improvements in total Boyarsky symptom scores (− 57%) and maximum urinary flow rate (+ 38%). Combination therapy resulted in a further reduction of 8% in total symptom scores. Twenty-five percent of subjects exhibited moderate symptom improvement following the addition of the antiandrogen. The differences in the outcome measures between terazosin alone versus combination therapy were not statistically significant. The failure to demonstrate statistical significance was probably related to the small sample size. The majority of subjects in the pilot combination study developed adverse events in response to flutamide which resulted in either dose reduction or premature withdrawal from the study. The mean reduction in prostate volume observed in the 24 evaluable patients receiving combination therapy was 25%, suggesting that adequate androgen suppression was achieved.

A multicenter, randomized, placebo-controlled study has been designed to compare four treatment groups (placebo, alpha blockade with terazosin, androgen suppression with finasteride, and combination therapy with terazosin and finasteride). This study will assess combination therapy but will also directly compare the individual monotherapies using the same entry criteria and outcome assessment parameters. These data are not expected until early 1995.

12.5 Summary

The role of medical therapy in the treatment of BPH is evolving. Alpha blockade is supported by a definite physiologic and pharmacologic rationale as well as the existing peer-reviewed literature. It must be kept in mind that patients enrolled in these studies generally have had mild to moderate symptoms and have been treated for a relatively short period of time. Extrapolation of the use of α-blockers to patients with traditional surgical indications such as urinary retention is not supported by a database. Although our experience has supported the durability of the response for alpha blockade, long-term data are not yet available.

Approximately 60–70% of men will respond favorably to α_1-blockers. Some patients will not tolerate the adverse effects of the drugs and others prefer not to be committed to life-long medical therapy. Terazosin is the best-studied long-acting α_1-blocker for BPH; however, subtypes of the α_1-receptor have been characterized and may ultimately lead to new drugs with improved efficacy and diminished side-effects.

Androgen suppression therapy for BPH has been limited by untoward side-effects; however, newer agents such as finasteride are much better tolerated than earlier drugs. The phase III data for finasteride have been criticized because the sponsoring pharmaceutical company had designed their own symptom score and because the large enrollment statistically overpowered the study. This may have allowed clinically insignificant improvement in outcome parameters to be statistically significant. Nonetheless, there is a rationale for the use of 5α-reductase inhibitors and it has impacted in medical strategies of treating symptomatic patients.

Combination therapy is being actively investigated. The concept is attractive because both mechanisms of outlet obstruction (static and dynamic) are being modified simultaneously. All variations of drug therapy for BPH presently require a life-long commitment by the patient. Long-term efficacy and safety profiles are unknown. There is a much larger safety database relating to alpha blockade because of the use of these agents for treating hypertension.

Studies evaluating the safety and efficacy of medical therapy must be properly designed and should be placebo controlled and randomized. The placebo effect is now well recognized in the treatment of BPH. Symptomatic improvement has been measured with scoring systems that vary from study to study, making comparisons difficult. A validated symptom score has been developed (AUA Symptom Score) and should improve our assessment of this primary outcome parameter.

The optimal patient for medical therapy has not been defined. An accurate diagnosis of symptomatic BPH with the exclusion of related urologic diseases such as prostatic cancer cannot be overstated. Presently, only alpha blockade or finasteride is practical because the other clinically available agents for androgen suppression have side-effects preventing their widespread use. Finasteride and terazosin have been approved by the FDA for treating BPH. In the absence of absolute surgical indications, it would seem appropriate to pursue a course of medical therapy in the majority of patients because of the minimal risk as compared to prostatectomy.

Even though there are many unanswered questions regarding the optimal management of symptomatic BPH, it is clear that medical therapy will have an increasing impact as drug therapy improves and our understanding of this disease progresses.

References

Bartsch G, Muller HR, Oberholzer M, et al. (1979) Light microscopic stereological analysis of the normal human prostate and benign prostatic hyperplasia. J Urol 122: 487–491

Caine M, Perlberg S, Gordon R (1975a) The treatment of benign prostatic hypertrophy with flutamide (SCH 13521): a placebo controlled study. J Urol 114: 564–568

Caine M, Raz S, Ziegler M (1975b) Adrenergic and cholinergic receptors in the human prostate, prostatic capsule, and bladder neck. Br J Urol 27: 193–202

Caine M, Pfau A, Perlberg S (1976) The use of alpha adrenergic blockers in benign prostatic obstruction. Br J Urol 48: 255–263

Caine M, Perlberg S, Mertyk S (1978) A placebo-controlled double-blind study of the effect of phenoxybenzamine in benign prostatic obstruction. Br J Urol 50: 551–555

Caine M, Perlberg S, Shapiro A (1981) Phenoxybenzamine for benign prostatic obstruction: A review of 200 cases. Urology 25: 542–546

Dorflinger T, Oster M, Larsen JF, et al. (1987) Transurethral prostatectomy or incision of the prostate in the treatment of prostatism caused by small benign prostates. Scand J Urol Nephrol 104: 77–81

Dorflinger T, England DM, Madsen PO, et al. (1989) Urodynamic and histological correlations of benign prostatic hypertrophy. Br J Urol 140: 1487–1490

Dunzenndorfer U (1987) Clinical experience: symptomatic management of BPH with terazosin. Urology 32: 27–31

Fabricius PG, Weizert P, Dunzendorger V, et al. (1990) Efficacy of once-a-day terazosin in benign prostatic hyperplasia. Prostate 3 (Suppl): 85–93

Gormley GJ, Stoner E, Bruskewitz RC, et al. (1992) The effect of finasteride in men with benign prostatic hyperplasia. N Engl J Med 327: 1185–1191

Guess HA, Heyse JF, Gormley GJ (1993) The effect of finasteride on prostate specific antigen in men with benign prostatic hyperplasia. Prostate 22: 31–37

Gup DI, Shapiro E, Baumann M, et al. (1989) The contractile properties of human prostatic adenomas are unrelated to the development of intravesical obstruction. Prostate 15: 105–114

Gup DI, Shapiro E, Baumann M, et al. (1990) Autonomic receptors in asymptomatic and symptomatic BPH. J Urol 143: 179–185

Hellstrom P, Lukkarinen O, Kontturi M (1986) Bladder neck incision or transurethral electroresection for the treatment of urinary obstruction caused by a small prostate. Scand J Urol Nephrol 20: 187–192

Hieble JP, Caine M, Zalaznik E (1985) In vitro characterization of the alpha-adrenoceptors in human prostate. Eur J Pharmacol 107: 111–117

Holtgrewe HL, Mebust WK, Dowd JB, et al. (1989) Transurethral prostatectomy: practice aspects of the dominant operation in American Urology. J Urol 141: 248–253

Lepor H, Machi GM (1992) The combination of terazosin and flutamide for symptomatic BPH. Prostate 20: 89–95

Lepor H, Riguad G (1990) The efficacy of transurethral resection of the prostate in men with moderate symptoms of prostatism. J Urol 143: 533–537

Lepor H, Shapiro E (1984) Characterization of alpha$_1$ adrenoceptors in human benign prostatic hyperplasia. J Urol 132: 1226–1229

Lepor H, Baumann M, Shapiro E (1988) The stereospecificity of LY253352 for alpha$_1$ blockade in prostatic hyperplasia. Br J Pharmacol 95: 139–144

Lepor H, Knapp-Maloney G, Wozniak-Petrofsky J (1989) The safety and efficacy of terazosin for the treatment of BPH. Int J Clin Pharmacol Ther Toxicol 27: 392–397

Lepor H, Knapp-Maloney G, Sunshine H (1990) An open-label dose titration study evaluating terazosin for the treatment of symptomatic BPH. J Urol 144: 1393–1398

Lepor H, Henry D, Laddu AR (1991) The efficacy and safety of terazosin for the treatment of symptomatic BPH. Prostate 18:345–356

Lepor H, Auerbach S, Puras-Baez A, et al. (1992) A randomized, placebo-controlled multicenter study of the efficacy and safety of terazosin in the treatment of benign prostatic hyperplasia. J Urol 148: 1467–1474

Mebust WK, Holtgrewe HL, Cockett ATK, et al. (1989) Transurethral prostatectomy: immediate and postoperative complications. A cooperative study of 13 participating institutions evaluating 3,885 patients. J Urol 141: 243–247

Neal DE, Ramsden PD, Sharples L, et al. (1989) Outcome of elective prostatectomy. Br Med J 299: 762–767

Orandi A (1987) Transurethral incision of prostate compared with transurethral resection of the prostate in 132 matching cases. J Urol 138: 810–815

Peters CA, Walsh PC (1987) The effect of nafareline acetate, a luteinizing-hormone-releasing hormone agonist, on benign prostatic hyperplasia. N Engl J Med 317: 599–604

Raz S, Ziegler M, Caine M (1973) Pharmacologic receptors in the prostate. Br J Urol 45:663–667

Shapiro E, Lepor H (1987) Alpha adrenergic receptors in canine lower genitourinary tissues: insight into development and function. J Urol 138: 979–983

Shapiro E, Lepor H (1992) The response to alpha blockade in benign prostatic hyperplasia is related to the percent area density of prostate smooth muscle. Prostate 21: 297–307

Shapiro E, Hartanto V, Lepor H (1992a) Anti-desmin vs. anti-actin for quantifying the area density of prostate smooth muscle. Prostate, 20: 259–268

Shapiro E, Hartanto V, Lepor H (1992b) Quantifying the smooth muscle content of the prostate using double-immunoenzymatic staining and color assisted image analysis. J Urol 147: 1167–1170

Stone MM (1989) Flutamide in treatment of benign prostatic hypertrophy. Urology 34(4): 64–68

The Proscar Study Group (1990) Treatment of benign prostatic hyperplasia (BPH) with Proscar, a 5alpha reductase (5aR) inhibitor. Abstract of workshop conference on androgen therapy: biologic and clinical consequences. January 17, Marco Island, FL

Wennberg JE, Roos N, Sola L, et al. (1987) Use of claims data systems to evaluate health care outcomes: mortality and reoperation following prostatectomy. JAMA 257:933–936

White JW (1895) The result of double castration in hypertrophy of the prostate. Ann Surg 22:1–80

Wu J, Gu F (1987) The prostate 41–65 years post castration: an analysis of 26 eunuchs. Chin Med J 100: 271

13 Physical Principles of Microwave Hyperthermia of the Prostate

MELVIN A. ASTRAHAN and PIOTR S. DEBICKI

CONTENTS

MELVIN A. ASTRAHAN, PhD. Assistant Professor, and PIOTR S. DEBICKI, PhD, Department of Radiation Oncology, University of Southern California, School of Medicine, 1441 Eastlake Avenue, Los Angeles, CA 90033, USA

Petrovich/Baert (Eds.)
Benign Prostatic Hyperplasia

13.1 Microwaves

13.1.1 Introduction

In the beginning...

Had a physicist translated the book of Genesis it might begin:

> ..And God said:
> "Let there be *electromagnetic radiation*!"
> And there was *electromagnetic radiation*. God saw that the *electromagnetic radiation* was good, and He separated the *visible* light from the darkness...

More recently...

More recently, portions of the electromagnetic spectrum outside of visible light have been separated, subdivided and assigned various names. Microwaves are defined to occupy the range 300 MHz to 300 GHz. This range lies between the familiar VHF-TV channels and infrared light as shown in Fig. 13.1. Microwave frequencies are widely used in telecommunications and include the UHF-TV channels, radio-link, cellular phones, and satellite communications. Other applications include civil and military radar, kitchen appliances, and various industrial processes and measurements. Microwave frequencies have found applications in medicine including diathermy, cancer therapy, angioplasty, and now hyperthermia for prostatic disease. Intracavitary applicators introduced via the rectum and/or urethra are presently the most common method of heating the prostate. Microwaves, commonly in the range 433–2450 MHz, are radiated into the tissue surrounding these applicators from an antenna located within the applicator.

13.1.2 Mechanism of Propagation

As microwaves travel through a medium, a time-varying magnetic field (H, amps/meter) may be regarded as generating a time-varying electric field (E, volts/meter) which in turn generates a magnetic field and so on. This concept is illustrated in Fig. 13.2a. In the process, energy is transferred back and forth between the electric and magnetic fields and is propagated across the medium. If part of this energy is absorbed by the medium, the medium is defined to be *lossy*. Tissue is a lossy medium. The fraction of energy absorbed depends on the electromagnetic properties of the medium.

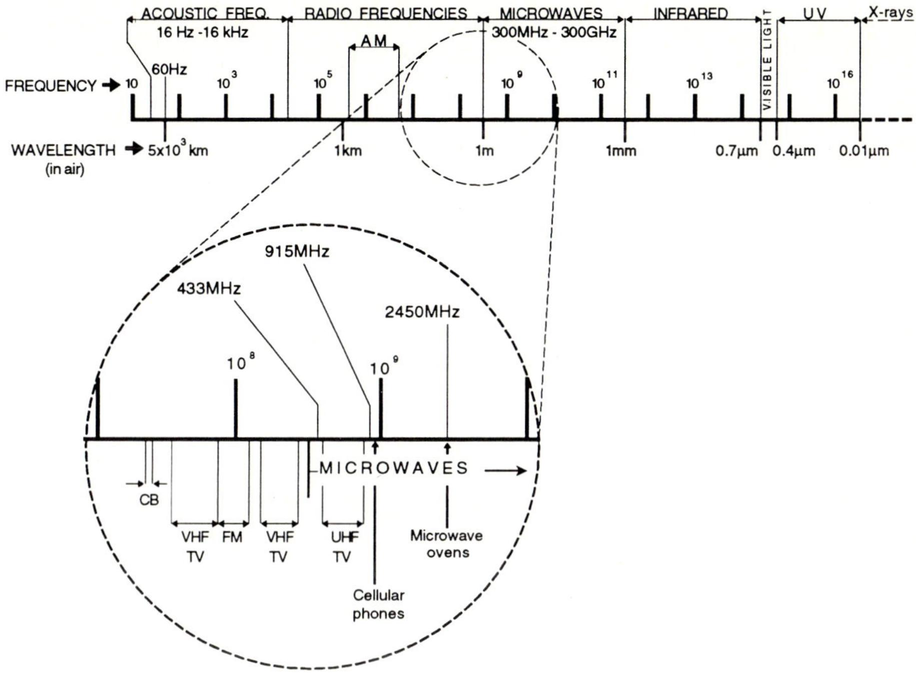

Fig. 13.1. The electromagnetic spectrum from 10 Hz to 10^{17} Hz. The microwave band is defined as the range 300 MHz to 300 GHz, which includes the UHF television channels and kitchen oven frequency of 2450 MHz in addition to the assigned medical frequencies of 433 and 915 MHz. Indicated wavelengths are for air. Wavelength in tissue will be a few times smaller in the enlarged area

13.1.3 Electromagnetic Properties of Tissue

Macroscopically, the magnetic characteristics of a material are quantified by its *permeability* μ. The permeability of tissue (μ_{tissue}) is essentially the same as that of air or vacuum. Therefore the energy associated with the magnetic field of microwaves traveling through tissue, air, or vacuum will be virtually the same. There is no energy loss from the magnetic field in these media.

From the electrical point of view, materials are classified as either *conductors* or *dielectrics*. This classification is related to how easily electrical charges may move within the material. In a good conductor, such as copper, free charges (i.e., electrons) migrate readily from atom to atom under the influence of an electric field. This migration is referred to as an electric *current*. The ratio of the induced current density to the electric field is known as the *conductivity* σ (Siemens/meter) of the material. In a dielectric, the electrons are more strongly bound and cannot be displaced very far from their equilibrium positions. Some dielectrics make good electrical insulators at microwave frequencies and are commonly

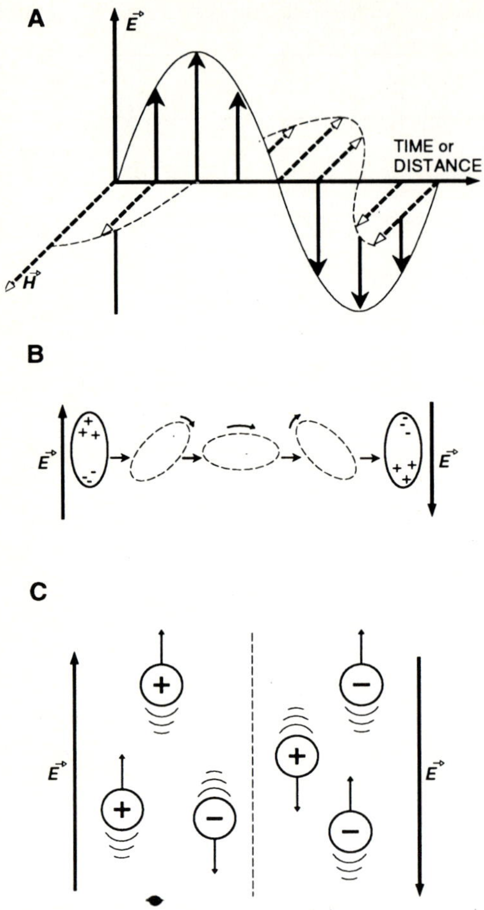

Fig. 13.2. **A** As microwaves propagate through tissue the orientation of the magnetic (***H***) and electric field vectors (***E***) oscillate at the operational frequency. **B** At 2450 MHz (the microwave oven frequency) the dominant mechanism of energy absorption in tissue is the rotation of polarized molecules such as water which try to follow ***E***. **C** At lower frequencies, the displacement of free charges such as electrons and ions by the electric field is the dominant mechanism of energy absorption

used in the construction of prostate applicators. Materials such as Teflon, silicone, and many plastics fall into this category.

Any molecule in which the electron density is distorted with respect to its nuclei, somewhat greater to one side of the molecule for instance, is referred to as an *electrically polarized* molecule and as such constitutes an electric dipole. A dipole may be modeled as two equal but opposite charges separated by a small distance. The water molecule is an example of such a polarized molecule. Under the influence of an electric field, existing molecular dipoles become ordered and additional atomic and molecular dipoles may be induced. In tissue, Cl^- is an example of an anion in which additional polarization may be induced. Induced dipoles can change the conductivity of a material.

At microwave frequencies the conductivity of tissue (σ_{tissue}) is a measure of the current which results not only from the migration of free electrons, but also from the displacement of ions and from the rotation of polarized molecules. The displacement of these molecules and charges requires kinetic energy. From the principle of conservation of energy, this energy may only come from the microwave radiation itself. Thus, electromagnetic energy is absorbed from the wave and converted into molecular kinetic energy, i.e., *heat*. The power density (P, watts/m^3) converted to heat is proportional to the conductivity and the square of the electric field intensity:

$$P = \sigma|\mathbf{E}|^2. \tag{13.1}$$

Since energy is continuously absorbed from a wave as it travels through a lossy medium, the energy (which we will later refer to as the *amplitude*) of the wave decreases as it travels through tissue.

The conductivity of tissue is strongly frequency dependent due to its diverse molecular structure. At the lower end of the microwave band, electromagnetic energy is converted to heat primarily through the displacement of electrons and ions which attempt to follow the oscillating electric field vector. As one moves toward higher frequencies the emphasis gradually shifts to the vibration of polarized molecules, primarily water, which attempt to rotate with the electric field oscillation. These concepts are illustrated in Fig. 13.2b and c.

Tissue demonstrates the properties of both conductor and dielectric at frequencies in the vicinity of 1000 MHz. From an electromagnetic point of view, tissue may be divided into two categories which are related to its water content. The conductivity of tissue with low water content, such as fat and bone, tends to be about an order of magnitude less than tissue with high water content, such as muscle, brain, and most internal organs (including prostate). Among tissue of high water content, the differences in electromagnetic parameters are small.

13.1.4 Plane Waves

In free space, a wavefront is defined to be the surface which is tangent to both the **E** and **H** field vectors. If this surface is a plane, and **E** and **H** have the same value everywhere in that plane, the wavefront is referred to as a "plane wave." When microwaves are launched from a source with a large aperture (such as a waveguide) or when the wavefront is at a great distance from its source, a portion of the wavefront may be considered nearly planar. This is illustrated in Fig. 13.3. The heat absorbed at any location in the tissue will be directly proportional to the energy amplitude of the wave as it passes through that location. The absorbed power density of a plane wave in tissue is plotted in Fig. 13.4 for frequencies between 1 MHz and 10 GHz. The absorbed power density is maximal at the tissue surface and decreases with distance as energy is removed from the wave. As the frequency increases, the rate of absorption increases significantly.

13.1.5 Cylindrical Waves

When microwaves are launched from an intracavitary source of the type commonly associated with prostate hyperthermia the wavefront is nearly cylindrical and it must travel a great distance before a limited portion can be

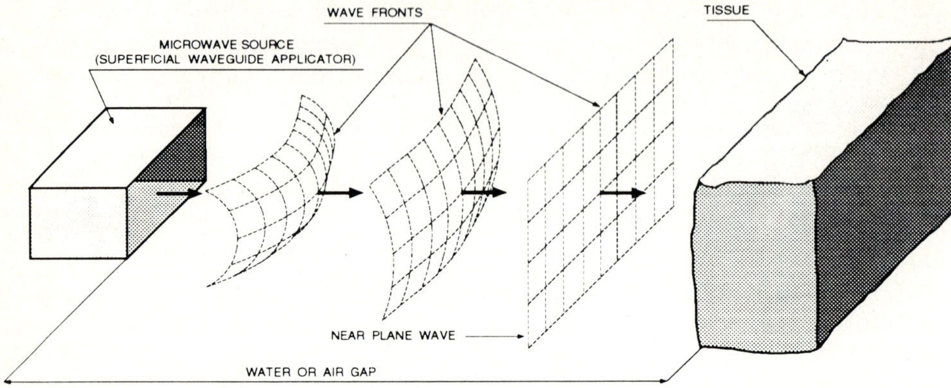

Fig. 13.3. When microwaves are launched from a waveguide applicator into air or deionized water the wave front approaches that of a plane wave

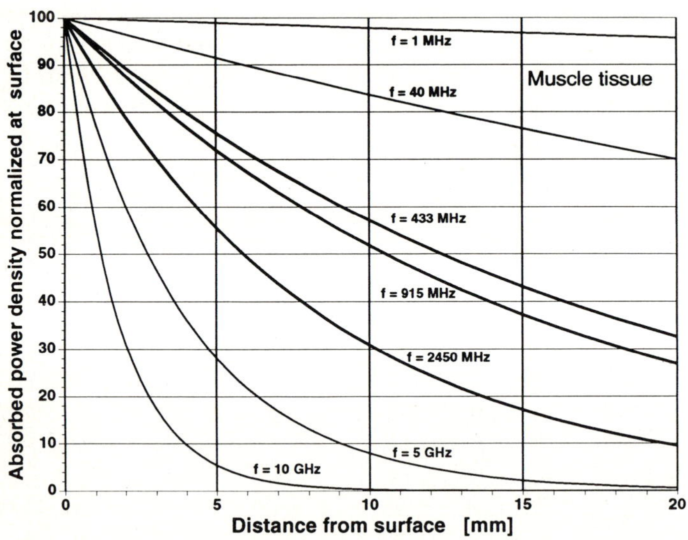

Fig. 13.4. Attenuation of plane waves at various frequencies in muscle tissue

considered "planar." This concept is illustrated in Fig. 13.5. Figure 13.6 illustrates absorbed power density in tissue and in free space for 915-MHz cylindrical waves radiated from applicators of various diameters. For comparison, plane wave curves are also plotted. The absorbed power density is maximum at the applicator–tissue boundary and decreases radially as the energy amplitude of the wave decreases. Note, however, that the absorbed power density decreases more rapidly for the cylindrical wave than the plane wave. This is due to the additional effect of geometric expansion of the wavefront. In free space, for

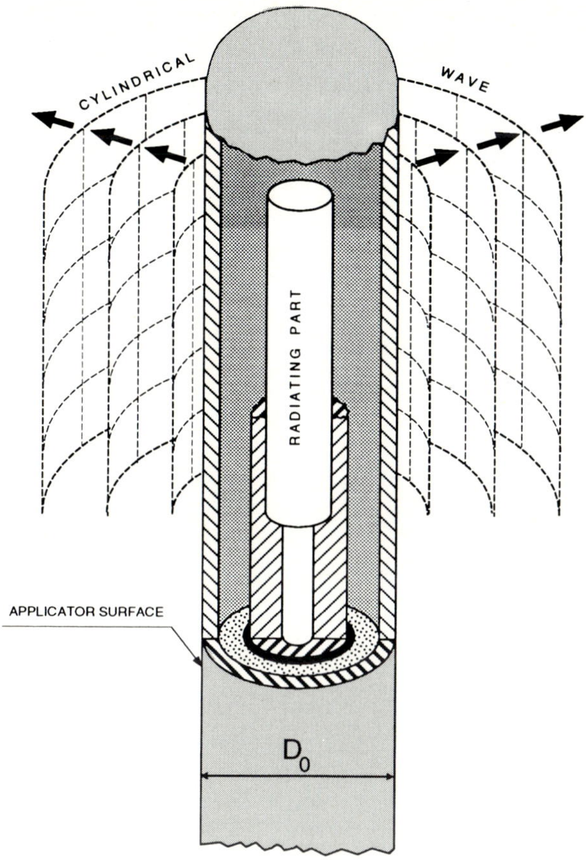

Fig. 13.5. When microwaves are radiated from a symmetrical cylindrical source the wavefront is nearly cylindrical as well

instance, where no energy would be absorbed from the wave, the total energy of the wavefront is constant. The principle of conservation of energy requires that the available energy be distributed over an ever larger wavefront as the wave propagates outward from its source. Thus, the energy amplitude of the wave will decrease with distance from the source independently of tissue absorption. Since the energy amplitude of a cylindrical wave is reduced both by absorption and by geometric expansion, the absorbed power density in tissue will decrease more rapidly for a cylindrical wave than for a plane wave.

As an applicator's diameter approaches infinity, the wave that it produces will more closely approximate a plane wave. Conversely, as an applicator's diameter becomes smaller, the effect of geometric expansion becomes more and more significant until it becomes the dominant cause of absorbed power density decrease in the immediate vicinity of the applicator. This is illustrated in Fig. 13.6, where the influence of geometric expansion is seen as the difference between the plane wave and the cylindrical wave curves. The power density decrease for a particular cylindrical wave resulting from energy absorption in tissue is the difference between the dashed and continuous curves.

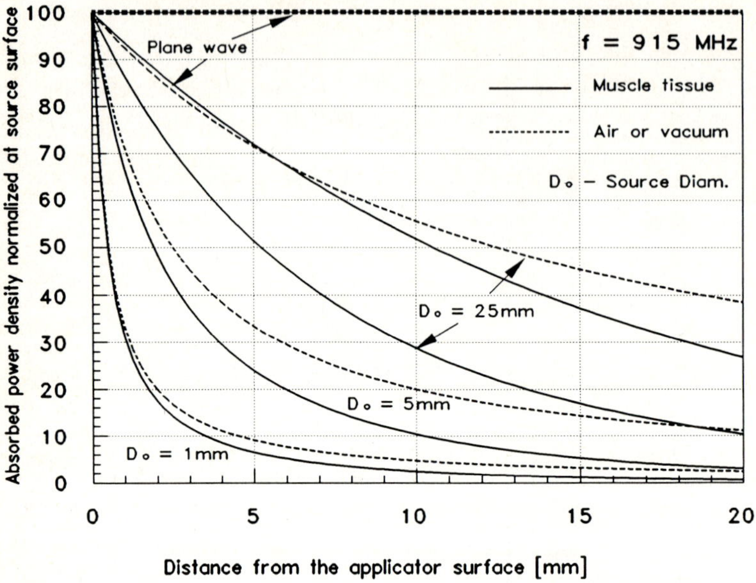

Fig. 13.6. Attenuation of a cylindrical wave in muscle tissue and air for different source diameters. The significance of geometric expansion increases as the source diameter decreases

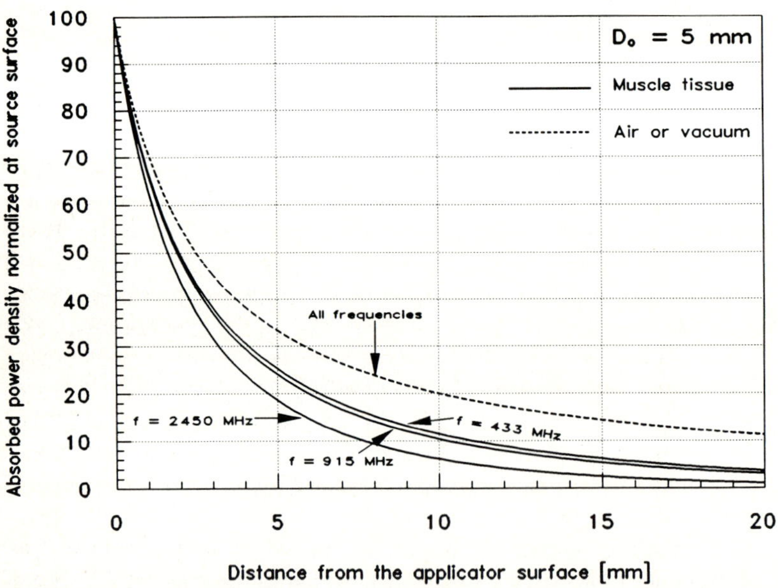

Fig. 13.7. Calculated power density profiles in tissue for a 5-mm-diameter applicator are plotted for frequencies of 433 MHz, 915 MHz and 2450 MHz. For comparison, a curve for air is included. This curve is independent of frequency

Geometric expansion of the wavefront is independent of frequency. Only the absorption characteristics of the tissue are frequency dependent. For a prostate applicator of small diameter, geometric expansion dominates power absorption in the immediate vicinity of the applicator. The heating characteristics of such an applicator are nearly independent of frequency. This is illustrated in Fig. 13.7, in which calculated power density profiles in tissue for a 5-mm-diameter applicator are plotted for frequencies of 433 MHz, 915 MHz, and 2450 MHz.

The rest of the story...

In actuality, the situation is more complicated than modeled above. The microwave applicators used for hyperthermia treatment do not generate ideal plane or cylindrical waves and tissue is certainly not homogeneous. Furthermore, we have ignored microwave scattering and reflections which may occur at tissue boundaries and we have simplified the molecular mechanism of absorption. Nevertheless, the fundamental concepts and conclusions arrived at in the preceding sections are representative of the clinical situation in the prostate.

13.2 Hyperthermia

13.2.1 Temperature and Heat Flow

Temperature is a relative measure of the heat of an object. If there is a net increase in heat, temperature rises. Conversely, if heat decreases, temperature falls. If the temperature is greater in one region of a solid object compared to another, a gradient is created and heat flows from the region of higher temperature to the region of lower temperature. This process is quantitatively described by the Fourier law, which fundamentally states that the rate at which heat flows is a function of the temperature gradient and a property of the material known as the *thermal conductivity*. Thermal conductivity may be constant or may be a function of the local temperature. When the temperature is a function of both time and space, the process of heat flow is known as *transient* conduction as opposed to *steady* conduction, in which temperature is simply a function of spacial location. In tissue, heat transfer is further complicated by blood flow convection in addition to thermal conduction.

During a hyperthermia procedure, the temperature distribution is transient at least until the time at which the prescribed temperature is achieved. If sufficiently high power levels are used, heat will be absorbed far more quickly than it can be conducted away and the transient temperature distribution will closely follow the pattern of heat absorption from the microwaves. If more moderate power levels are used, heat will be absorbed more slowly and thermal conduction will have a greater influence on the transient temperature distribution. When the prescribed treatment temperature has been reached, most hyperthermia systems change to a thermostatic control mode for the remainder of the treatment. As a result, the temperature distribution changes from a transient toward a steady-state condition. This is illustrated in Fig. 13.8.

It is temperature, not simply the amount of heat absorbed from the microwaves, which produces a biologic response. At any particular moment in time the temperature at any spatial location is a complex function of heat absorption, heat flow, blood flow, and even the temperature distribution which existed prior to the treatment.

13.2.2 Thermal Dose

The concept of *dose* is intended to provide a means of predicting and comparing the biologic effect of a given treatment. Thermal dose is a complex topic which is not well defined at this time. Fundamentally, thermal dose is a function of the temperature to which a tissue is exposed and the duration of that exposure. The higher the temperature, or the longer the exposure, the greater the biologic

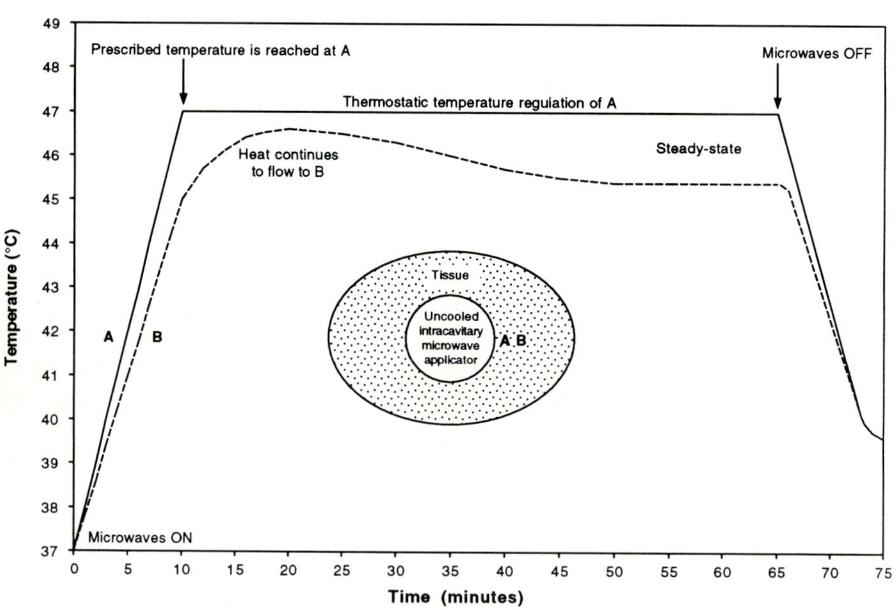

Fig. 13.8. Illustrative model of temperature dynamics during treatment. When the prescribed temperature of 47 °C is reached at thermostatic control location A, the hyperthermia system regulates power to hold A at 47 °C. The temperature at B may continue to rise as heat flows from A, to B, and may later decrease due to physiologic changes. Eventually a nominal steady-state is achieved

response will be. It is the precise relationship between biologic effect and time at different temperatures which is at issue. If hyperthermia were defined to be some specific, constant temperature, then duration of heating would be a simple and reasonable means of expressing thermal dose. In the real situation, however, temperature is never constant, varying both temporally and spatially throughout a treatment.

The obstacles to thermal dosimetry for prostate are thus to: (1) find a method of measuring or estimating temperature as a function of time and space throughout the prostate, and (2) find a means of relating the biologic effect of duration at one temperature to the biologic effect of duration at a different temperature. The first obstacle is a problem of thermometry which can be addressed, at least to some extent, by technical means. The second obstacle is a complex relationship which requires specific biologic dose-response data.

When hyperthermia is used as an adjuvant to cancer therapy, it is generally accepted that to be of significant therapeutic value, a *minimum* temperature of 42 °C is required. This derives from a transition in Arrhenius plots of cell killing at about 42 °–43 °C for many tissues (FIELD and MORRIS 1983) and a complex phenomenon termed thermotolerance (HENLE and DETHLEFSEN 1978) which develops at temperatures below the transition breakpoint (FIELD and RAAPHORST 1990). There is evidence that the breakpoint temperature for some human tumors studied in vitro occurs at 44 °C or higher (HAHN et al. 1989).

SAPARETO and DEWEY (1984) have proposed the concept of a thermal isoeffect dose (TID) which relates time (t) at temperature (T) to equivalent time at some reference temperature according to the formula

$$t_{\text{equiv.}} = tR^{(\mathrm{T}-\mathrm{T_{ref}})}, \tag{13.2}$$

where R is a constant.

At temperatures above the breakpoint, R has a value of approximately 2 both in vitro and in vivo for many tissues (FIELD and MORRIS 1983). At present, the hyperthermic dose-response of normal human prostate, hyperplasic prostate, cancerous prostate, and surrounding tissues are not well documented in the literature.

It would greatly simplify matters if we could achieve a homogeneous temperature distribution in the prostate. This would, presumably, result in a homogeneous biologic response and would also reduce the thermometric requirements since fewer measurements would be needed.

13.3 Principles of Intracavitary Hyperthermia

Since absorbed power density (heating) is greatest in tissue immediately adjacent to an intracavitary applicator's surface and falls off rapidly with distance, it is difficult to deliver a homogeneous hyperthermic dose. For instance, in order to deliver enough heat to raise the temperature of tissue 1 cm from an applicator's surface to a particular level, far more heat must be delivered to the intervening tissue. As a result, the temperature of the intervening tissue may rise to a higher, potentially hazardous level. The problem is not quite as severe, however, as might be expected from the power density profiles of Figs. 13.6 and 13.7. As the temperature of the intervening tissue increases above that of the more distal tissue, a gradient is created and heat flows to the region of lower temperature. The steeper the gradient, the more rapid the flow. Since heat flow is a transient process, the resulting temperature distribution is also transient, depending strongly on the heating rate. Eventually, however, a nominally "steady-state" condition will be achieved during which the temperature distribution will remain nearly constant, as illustrated in Figs. 13.8 and 13.9.

The "effective" therapeutic range of an intracavitary applicator may be defined as the distance over which tissue temperature (T) can be elevated above a critical temperature (typically 42 °C) without exceeding some limiting temperature. By careful choice of applicator design and heating rate, the therapeutic range of a simple applicator can extend to about 1 cm, depending on the temperature tolerance of tissue near the applicator's surface (ASTRAHAN et al. 1989, 1991; PETROVICH et al. 1991). The effective range of an intracavitary applicator may be increased further by actively cooling the applicator's surface. This concept is illustrated in Fig. 13.10a, in which an applicator is cooled by flowing water. By cooling the applicator's surface, heat absorbed by tissue close to the surface is transferred back to the applicator and removed from the environment by the coolant flowing within the applicator. This has the effect of reducing or reversing the temperature gradient in tissue close to the applicator,

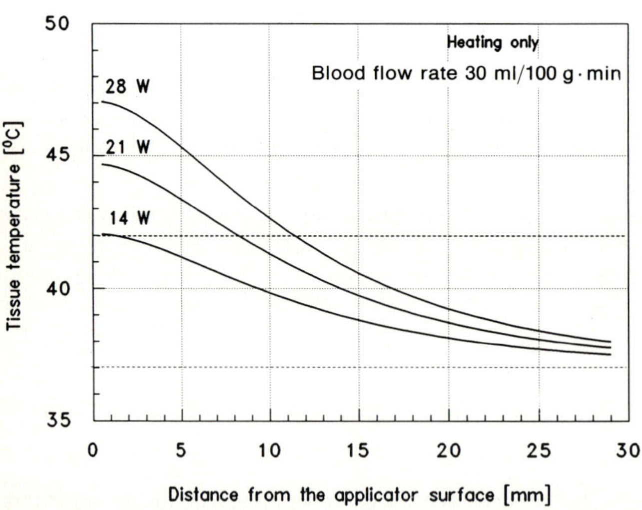

Fig. 13.9. Calculated steady-state temperature profiles for a 25-mm-diameter, 915-MHz directional applicator radiating into muscle tissue of moderate blood flow. These calculations presume the applicator to be a poor heat conductor

displacing the location of maximum temperature outward from the applicator's surface, and increasing the effective range of the applicator by about 50%, as illustrated in Fig. 13.10b. This permits more power to be delivered to, and thus higher temperatures to be achieved in distal tissue without producing hazardous temperatures in tissue adjacent to the applicator. The calculations plotted in Fig. 13.10b, in which a limiting temperature of 47 °C is maintained, illustrate that a change of coolant temperature from 37 ° to 17 °C will produce a 3.5-mm radial shift of the effective range ($T > 42$ °C) of the applicator. Note, however, that this shift also results in a 4-mm-wide layer of tissue adjacent to the

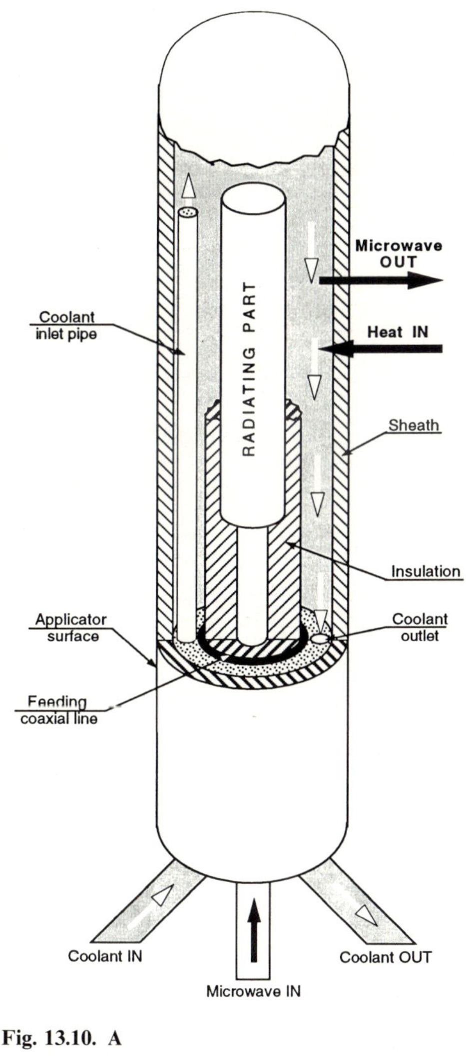

Fig. 13.10. A

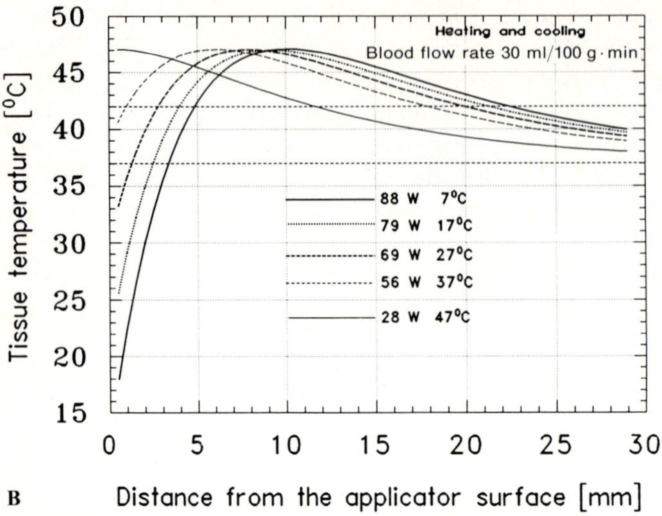

B

Fig. 13.10. **A** Intracavitary applicator actively cooled by flowing water. **B** Calculated steady-state temperature profiles of a 25-mm-diameter, 915-MHz directional applicator radiating into muscle tissue of moderate blood flow for coolant temperatures between 7° and 47 °C. For each coolant temperature, power was selected so as to obtain a maximum temperature of 47 °C

applicator which remains at subtherapeutic levels. Judicious selection of coolant temperature is necessary to achieve optimal results.

The temperature profiles illustrated in Figs. 13.9 and 13.10b were based on a tissue model with constant blood flow. In vivo, however, the situation is far more complicated. Blood flow will vary during a hyperthermia treatment in response to temperature changes. The dynamics of this change are difficult to predict, and can vary dramatically from one treatment to another, even for the same site in the same patient. The influence of blood flow covering a range of rates typically encountered in tissue is modeled in Fig. 13.11. As blood flow increases, the maximum temperature and the temperature gradient decrease significantly in tissue near the applicator for constant microwave power. For instance, if blood flow increases from 30 to 60 ml/100 g · min and power remains constant at 28 W, the calculated tissue temperature close to the applicator will fall from 47 °C to 42.6 °C. Any larger increase in blood flow would result in subtherapeutic temperatures close to the applicator. Decreasing blood flow below 30 ml/100 g could lead to hazardous temperatures adjacent to the applicator.

Note also that temperature changes resulting from variation in blood flow become less pronounced with distance from the applicator. Consider the situation of a prostate hyperthermia procedure in which the location of temperature measurement was 2 cm from the applicator, e.g., temperature measured only in the urethra while using an applicator located in the rectum, or temperature

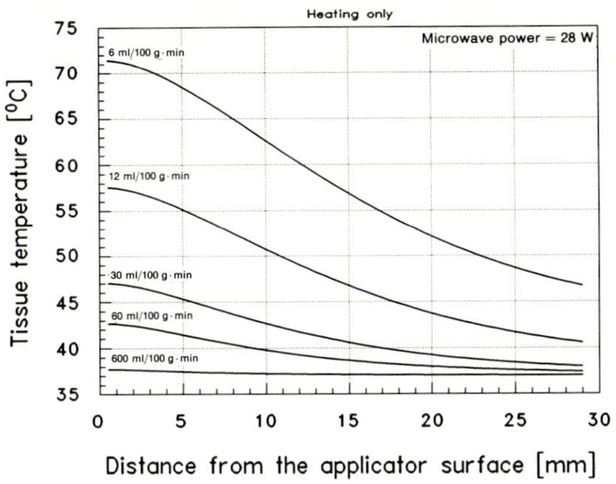

Fig. 13.11. Influence of blood flow rate on temperature profiles. Plotted are calculated steady-state temperature profiles for a 25-mm-diameter, 915-MHz uncooled directional applicator radiating with a constant power of 28 W into muscle tissue of various blood flow rates

measured only on the rectal mucosa while using an applicator located in the urethra. As blood flow changes, only a small temperature change would be measured, even though significant temperature change may be occurring adjacent to the applicator. This illustrates the importance of measuring temperature at as many locations as practical during a hyperthermia procedure.

When an applicator is actively cooled, the temperature profile in tissue close to the applicator surface is strongly influenced by the cooling system. The range of this influence is a function of tissue blood flow, as illustrated in Fig. 13.12. As blood flow increases, the distance to which surface cooling has a calculable effect on the temperature profile decreases due to heat delivered by blood. When microwave power is applied, blood flow modifies the peak temperature which may be achieved, its location, and the gradient in the vicinity of the peak for a particular power level and coolant temperature. Calculated temperature profiles are plotted in Fig. 13.13 for a coolant temperature of 17 °C. For the same blood flow of 30 ml/100 g · min, 69 W is now required to achieve a peak temperature of 47 °C compared to 28 W in the absence of cooling (see Fig. 13.11). The peak shifts from the applicator surface to a distance of 8 mm. Note that in the process, however, subtherapeutic temperatures now extend to a distance of 3 mm from the surface. Figures 13.9 through 13.13 demonstrate the complex interaction of microwave heating, applicator cooling, and blood flow on the prostate temperature distribution.

The intracavitary applicators used for prostate heating may be classified as either transurethral (TU) (Harada et al. 1985; Astrahan et al. 1989, 1991a; Carter et al. 1991; Debicki et al. 1992) or transrectal (TR) (Mendecki et al. 1978; Petrowicz et al. 1982; Yerushalmi et al. 1982; Debicki et al. 1992). For TU applicators, a fairly steep absorbed power gradient is a desirable characteristic since it assures that organs outside the prostate will not be heated. Surface cooling may be applied to TU applicators to increase their range, but this could result in higher temperatures outside of the prostate and makes it difficult to

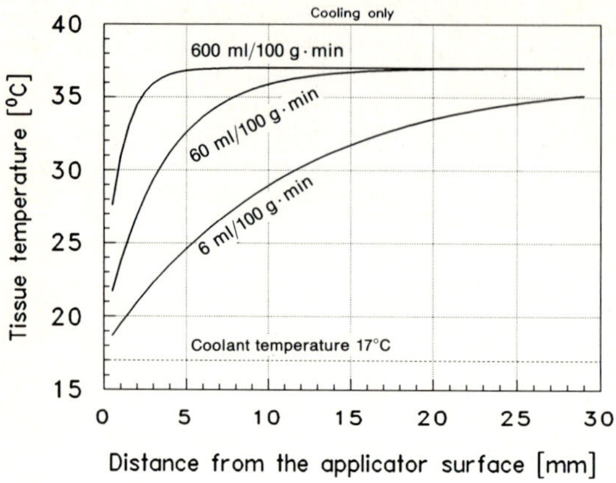

Fig. 13.12. Effect of surface cooling alone for various blood flow rates. Plotted are calculated steady-state temperature profiles in muscle for a 25-mm-diameter applicator actively cooled by 17 °C water

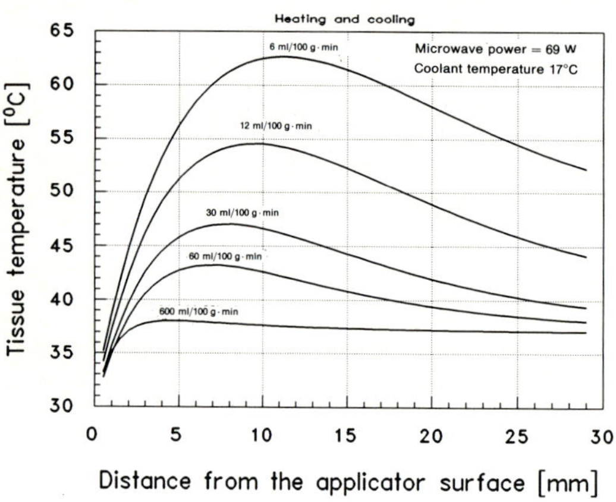

Fig. 13.13. Influence of blood flow rate on temperature profiles for an actively cooled applicator. Plotted are calculated steady-state temperature profiles for a 25-mm-diameter, 915-MHz directional applicator radiating into muscle at a constant microwave power output of 69 W and constant coolant temperature of 17 °C

measure the peak prostatic temperature. Surface cooling is mandatory for TR applicators in order to avoid hazardous temperatures in the intervening rectal mucosa (PETROWICZ et al. 1982).

13.4 Hyperthermia or Thermotherapy?

There has recently appeared in the literature a microwave treatment for benign prostatic hyperplasia (BPH) which has been termed *transurethral microwave thermotherapy* (TUMT) (CARTER et al. 1991). TUMT is a single-fraction heat treatment which employs a cooled TU applicator. *Thermotherapy* is defined as "a minimum of 45 °C for at least 20 minutes in the targeted tissue" and is considered to be different from *hyperthermia*, which is defined as a temperature of "approximately 42.5 °C" (BLUTE et al. 1992). There are several misconceptions of physical and biologic principles in these definitions.

1. Hyperthermia is not simply a temperature of approximately 42.5 °C. It is difficult to achieve a specific homogeneous hyperthermic temperature throughout the prostate using intracavitary microwave devices. Rather, there will always be a range of temperature. In cancer therapy, temperatures > 42 °C are considered necessary for effective therapy, as explained previously. The maximum temperature is usually limited by pain and risk to the tissue in which the peak occurs. For instance, in the case of prostate hyperthermia using an uncooled TR applicator, risk to the intervening rectal mucosa is a treatment-limiting factor.

2. There is no particular significance to the selection of 45 °C for 20 min as a means of distinguishing thermotherapy from hyperthermia. Twenty minutes at 45 °C is a dosimetric prescription and can be considered a thermal isoeffect dose (TID). As such, it can be related to other times and temperatures above the cell-killing breakpoint according to Eq. 13.2. At present, however, the breakpoint and R for human prostate cells are unknown. There is evidence that the breakpoint for some human tumors in vitro may be about 44 °C (Hahn et al. 1989), but in the absence of dosimetric data for BPH, the selection of 45 °C appears to be arbitrary from a physical and biologic perspective.

Consider as well that maximum urethral temperature for TUMT was stated to be 44.5 °C (Blute et al. 1992) in one report and 45.5 °C (Carter et al. 1991) in another. Temperature on the anterior rectal wall between 80 and 100 mm from the anus was reportedly limited to 42.5 °C. For comparison, in reports of *transurethral microwave hyperthermia* (TUMH) by Sapozink et al. (1990), Baert et al. (1990), and Astrahan et al. (1989, 1991a), temperatures in excess of 45 °C for 45 min were also routinely achieved and documented by thermal mapping. Rectal temperature was below 38 °C (Astrahan et al. 1991b). Clearly, 45 °C alone has no significance for differentiating thermotherapy from hyperthermia since both TUMT and TUMH produce a range of temperatures in the prostate, with some locations being greater than, and others being below 45 °C.

As the average temperature increases, however, the time required to achieve a desired biologic effect decreases. Complete destruction of normal canine prostate, for instance, has been reported by Magin et al. (1980) following only 15 min exposure to temperatures above 60 °C. Thus, differences in average treatment temperature would lead to procedural differences between treatment protocols.

3. The definition of TUMT above also refers to "targeted tissue." In the clinical situation, it is difficult enough to define a target volume let alone heat it with great precision. Since the TUMT applicator is cooled, the location of peak temperature is displaced a few millimeters into the prostate. The resulting peak temperature and radial temperature profile will depend on a complex interaction of microwave power, cooling, thermal conduction, and blood flow. Consider a hypothetical treatment in which urethral temperature is 44.5 °C and the radial temperature profile rises to some unknown maximum at some unknown location in the prostate and then falls to 42.5 °C at the rectal mucosa. If we were to define the "target" to be all prostate between the urethra and rectum, thermotherapy is not achieved since not all of the prostate achieved a minimum

temperature of 45 °C. Ironically, therapeutic hyperthermia (i.e., temperatures > 42 °C) is achieved. On the other hand, we could define the "target" to be any tissue which just happens to reach temperatures of 45 °C, in which case thermotherapy would be achieved (somewhere) every time. In this case, however, there will be some uncertainty as to the location of the "target."

4. The fact that the TUMT applicator is cooled is not a valid criteria for distinguishing thermotherapy from hyperthermia since cooling is a common feature of hyperthermia applicators. Neither is fractionation a valid criteria. The thermotherapy protocol calls for a single fraction whereas hyperthermia protocols have historically employed both single and multiple fractions. TUMT could just as well be defined as a single-fraction TUMH procedure.

It should be clear that any difference between thermotherapy and hyperthermia is semantic. There is no physical or biologic rationale for distinguishing between the two.

13.5 Local Hyperthermia and Fractionation

One method of assuring that at least a specified minimum thermal dose will be delivered to a "target" is to heat a tissue volume which includes, but is much larger than, the target volume. *Whole body* and *regional* hyperthermia are examples of this approach. Unfortunately, these techniques produce significant cardiovascular and other stress. *Local* hyperthermia is an approach in which therapeutic temperatures are selectively produced in the target, thereby sparing the surrounding tissue and resulting in far less systemic stress. The deeper the target is located within the body, the more difficult it is to deliver local hyperthermia. Intracavitary TU and TR microwave applicators are examples of devices which deliver local hyperthermia deep within the body.

There are various means of increasing the probability of delivering a specified minimum thermal dose to a target while sparing the surrounding tissues as much as possible. One method is to fractionate treatment so that surrounding normal tissue might have a chance to repair any potential or sublethal damage (Field 1978; Raaphorst 1990) while thermal dose to the target is homogenized as a result of physiologic changes occurring between fractions (Baert et al. 1990). Another method is to design applicators with heating patterns which selectively heat the target volume and/or remove heat outside the target, and to measure temperature as extensively as is practical.

13.6 Applicator Heating Patterns

The rate at which tissue absorbs heat from microwaves is referred to as the specific absorption rate (SAR) measured in W/kg. SAR is related to the absorbed power density by the relation

$$P = \rho \mathrm{SAR}, \tag{13.3}$$

where ρ is tissue density in kg/m^3.

Normalized values of P and SAR are identical if ρ is constant, which may be assumed in the prostate. The heating patterns of microwave applicators are often compared by measuring their SAR distributions (ROEMER et al. 1985) in a static, electromagnetically tissue-like material referred to as a "phantom." SAR distributions in phantom for various 915-MHz TU and TR applicators are illustrated in Fig. 13.14 and 13.15. These data have been normalized to a value of 1 at the point of maximum SAR.

Figure 13.14 plots isoSAR curves measured in a plane tangent (see Fig. 13.15c) to three different uncooled TU applicators. The applicator on the left employs three dipole antennas mounted on the surface of a Foley urologic catheter (ASTRAHAN et al. 1989). These antennas are designed to produce a secondary heating peak near their distal tips. The applicator in the center employs a helical antenna wound on a Foley catheter (ASTRAHAN et al. 1991a). The device on the right is a hybrid of dipole and helical antenna elements (DEBICKI et al. 1992) positioned within a Foley catheter. Using the 0.5 isoSAR curve for

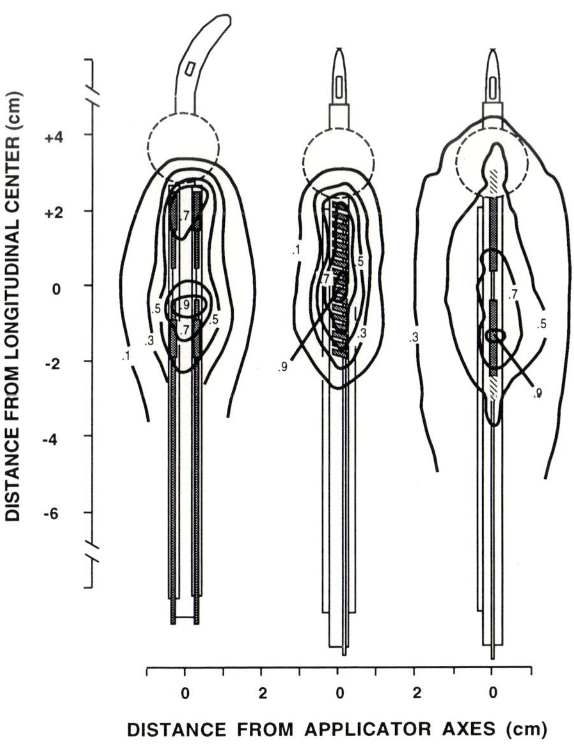

Fig. 13.14. IsoSAR curves measured in a plane tangent to three different uncooled TU applicators. SAR values less than 0.1 are probably irrelevant to clinical hyperthermia. (See text for explanation)

A

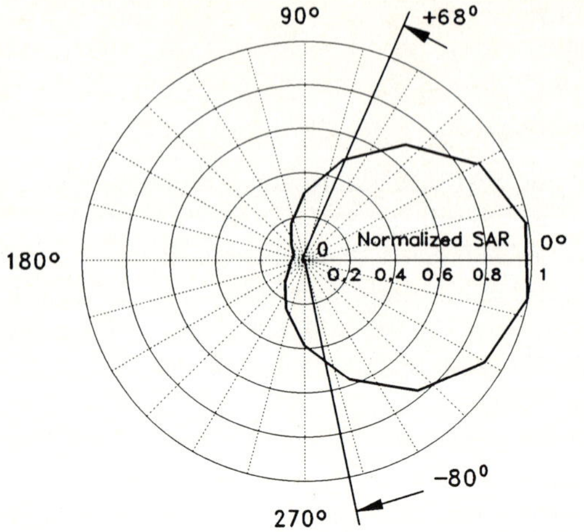
90°
+68°
180°
0
Normalized SAR
0°
0.2 0.4 0.6 0.8 1
-80°
270°

B

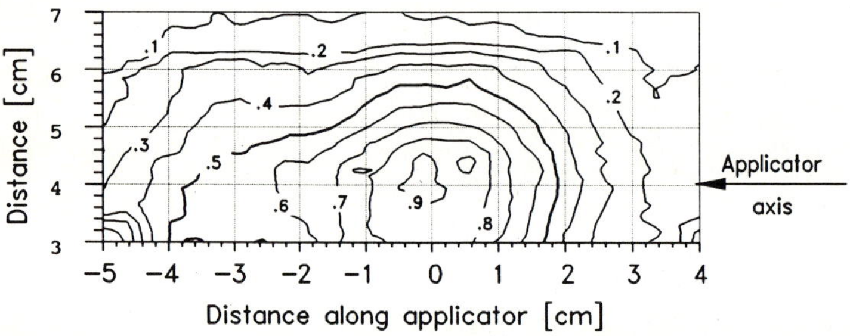
Distance [cm]
Distance along applicator [cm]
Applicator axis
.1
.2
.3
.4
.5
.6
.7
.8
.9

C

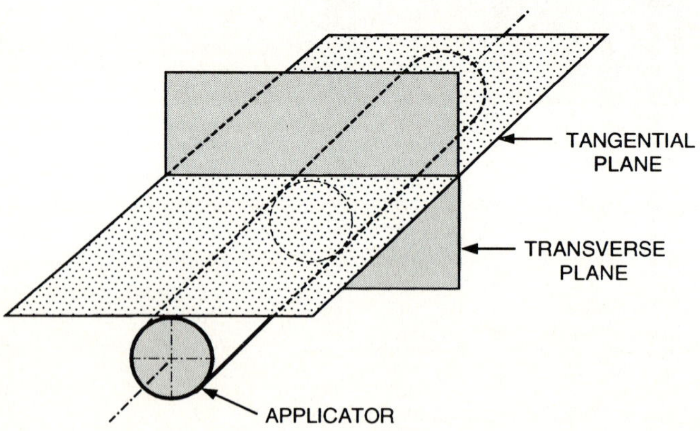
TANGENTIAL PLANE
TRANSVERSE PLANE
APPLICATOR

comparison, these applicators all heat a nominally cylindrical volume of about 4 cm in length to a depth between 0.3 and 1 cm surrounding the antennas. SAR values less than 0.1 are irrelevant to clinical hyperthermia since they are rarely associated with therapeutic temperatures.

Figure 13.15 illustrates SAR characteristics of a 25-mm-diameter directional TR applicator (Debicki et al. 1992). Rectal applicators used to heat the prostate have directional characteristics in order to avoid heating tissue other than the prostate. Figure 13.15a plots the directional pattern transverse to the applicator axis near the longitudinal center of the radiating area. SAR was measured at 1 cm from the surface of the applicator in a liquid phantom. The beam width at the 0.5 level is about 150°. Figure 13.15b plots isoSAR curves in a plane tangent (see Fig. 13.15c) to the applicator surface. The length of the effective radiating area, defined by the 0.5 curve, is about 5 cm.

In order to optimize treatment, it would be advantageous if the effective heating length of prostate applicators were adjustable. It would also be desirable for the beam width of TR applicators to be adjustable as well. This would enable the heating pattern to be customized to the size of individual prostates. We expect these capabilities will be developed in the future.

The SAR distribution defines only the rate at which heat is absorbed. The resulting temperature distribution in vivo is transient and will depend, as explained previously, on many other factors including heat removed by applicator cooling and blood flow dynamics. Since the resulting temperature distribution is difficult to predict, it must be measured during treatment. SAR patterns are useful, however, as a method of comparing applicators. For instance, applicators with similar SAR characteristics (and heat flow characteristics) should produce similar temperature distributions. Applicators which produce multiple SAR peaks, such as the applicator illustrated on the left side of Fig. 13.14, will likely produce temperature distributions with multiple temperature peaks, often termed “hot spots.”

13.6.1 Power Steering

TR applicators can effectively heat the prostate up to about 2 cm from the rectum, whereas uncooled TU applicators selectively heat the periurethral tissue with an effective range of about 0.6 cm. Adding surface cooling to a TU applicator will improve its range somewhat. Neither applicator alone can heat the entire prostate homogeneously.

Fig. 13.15. **A** SAR characteristics of a 25-mm-diameter directional TR applicator directional pattern transverse to the applicator axis. **B** isoSAR curves in a plane tangent to the applicator source. **C** Illustration of the tangential and transverse planes in relation to an applicator. (See text for explanation)

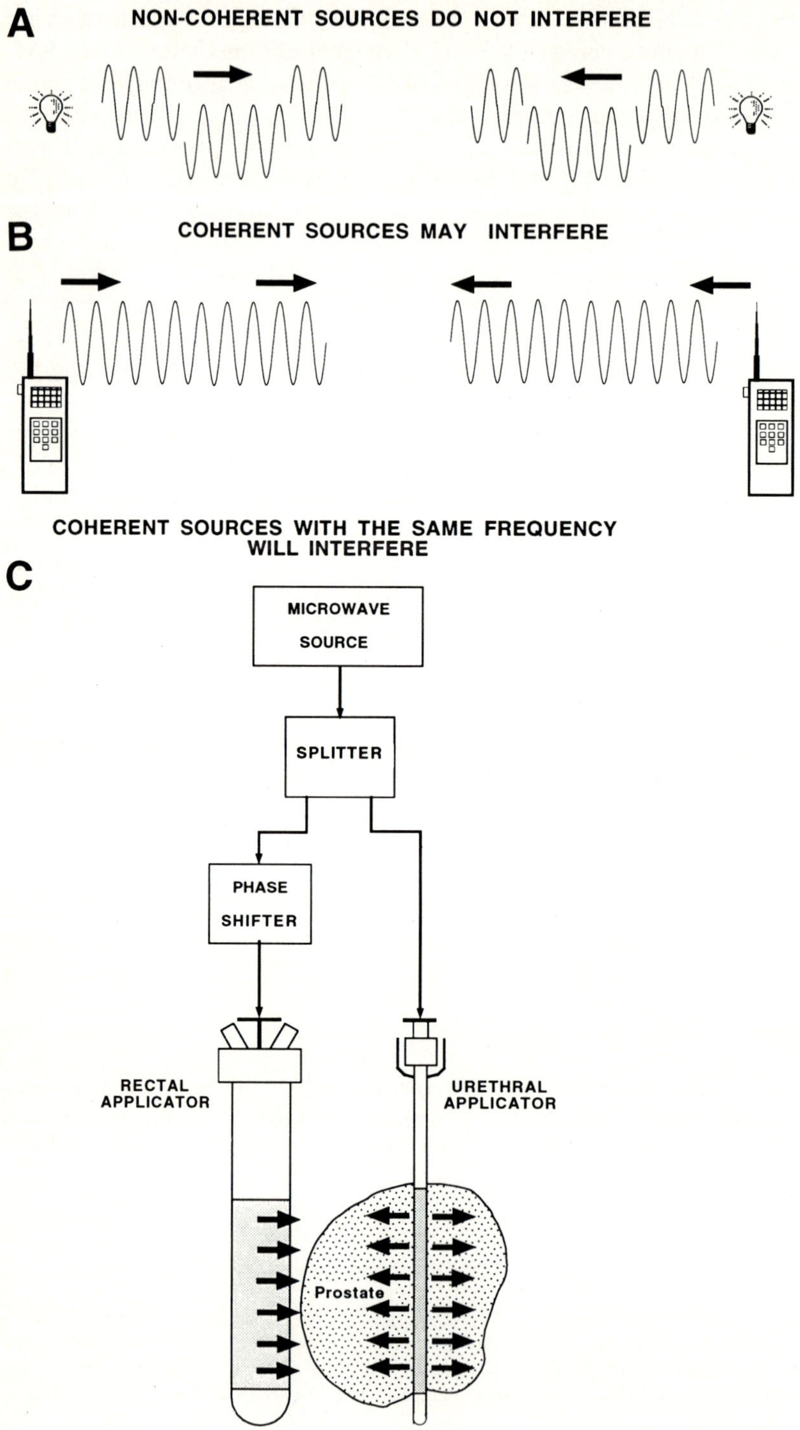
A
NON-COHERENT SOURCES DO NOT INTERFERE
B
COHERENT SOURCES MAY INTERFERE
COHERENT SOURCES WITH THE SAME FREQUENCY
WILL INTERFERE
C
MICROWAVE
SOURCE
SPLITTER
PHASE
SHIFTER
RECTAL
APPLICATOR
URETHRAL
APPLICATOR
Prostate

It is possible to combine TU and TR applicators and thereby change the temperature distribution compared to that of either applicator alone (Debicki et al. 1992). When two applicators are driven coherently and radiate into the same tissue, the microwaves from the two sources will interfere according to the superposition principle. It is important that the two applicators be driven coherently, i.e., that they have a definite phase relationship to one another as illustrated in Fig. 13.16. Two applicators can be driven coherently by splitting the output of a common microwave generator.

Recall that heat absorption from microwaves results from charge displacement in response to an oscillating electric field vector **E**. When the coherent waves from the two applicators arrive at the same point at the same time, the magnitude of **E** will be the vector sum of the contributing vectors from each source, $\mathbf{E}_{TU}$ and $\mathbf{E}_{TR}$. The resulting **E** distribution is referred to as an interference pattern. Both $\mathbf{E}_{TU}$ and $\mathbf{E}_{TR}$ have magnitude and orientation. Thus, if $\mathbf{E}_{TU}$ and $\mathbf{E}_{TR}$ should happen to be of nominally opposite orientation, they will tend to cancel one another and less heat will be dissipated compared to either alone. This is referred to as destructive interference. If, on the other hand, they have approximately the same orientation (at the same time), they will reinforce one another and comparatively more heat will be dissipated. This is referred to as constructive interference. These concepts are illustrated in Fig. 13.17. Since absorbed power is proportional to $|\mathbf{E}|^2$, a moderate change of **E** can result in a significant change in absorbed heat. For instance, if **E** doubles, the absorbed power will quadruple.

The objective of power steering is to improve temperature homogeneity by intentionally creating a situation in which constructive interference (CI) occurs at locations (foci) of low temperature (Debicki et al. 1992). This may be accomplished by adjusting the "phase" between the sources. Phase adjustment permits the field vectors from the sources to be temporally aligned with one another at the point of interest. For example, when a TU or TR applicator is used alone, maximum heating occurs near the applicator surface. If a phase-focus is placed midway between coherent TU and TR applicators, the location of maximum heating will move to the phase-focus. This is illustrated by computer simulation and measurement in phantom in Fig. 13.18 wherein CI produces more homogeneous heating than either applicator alone, and the maximum of the CI curve is located between the applicators.

The main obstacles to temperature homogeneity during hyperthermia are the inhomogeneities associated with power absorption and blood flow. In the future, it may be possible to address these obstacles by using an array of sources

←

Fig. 13.16A–C. The concept of coherent sources. **A** Noncoherent sources such as light bulbs produce wave packets of different phases. **B** Coherent sources produce noninterupted waves which may interfere. **C** Coherent sources with exactly the same frequency will interfere. The best way to produce coherent waves is to split a signal from a common source. A phase shifter may be added to obtain constructive or destructive interference

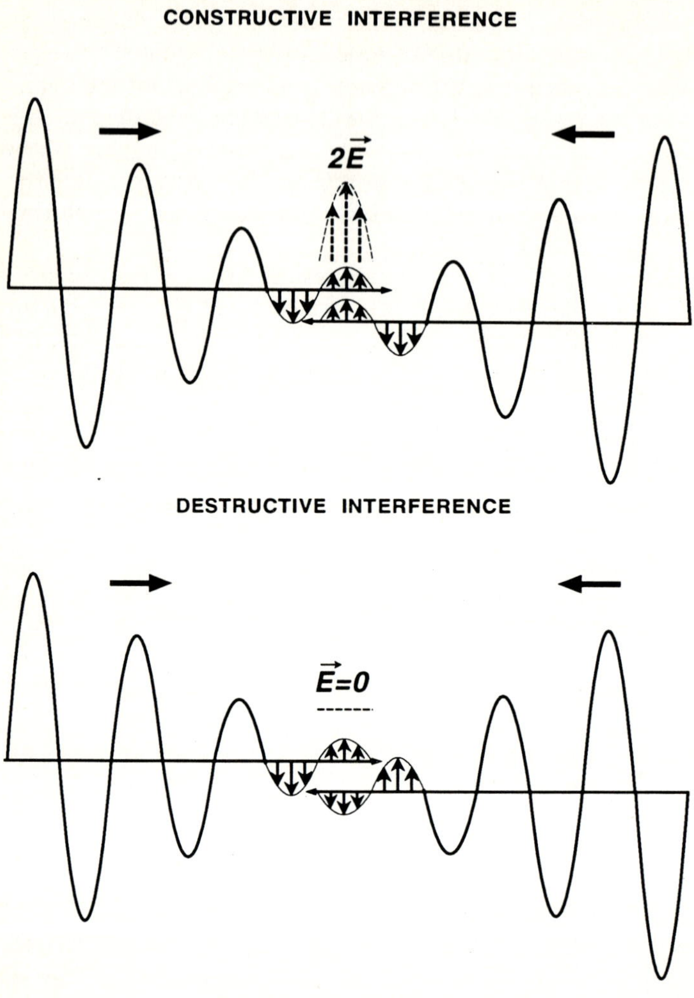

Fig. 13.17. When coherent sources interfere they may produce constructive or destructive interference

and steering a focus of constructive interference throughout the object to be heated. These sources might be microwave applicators (TURNER 1986; DEBICKI et al. 1992; YEH et al. 1992), or perhaps another source of wave energy such as ultrasound transducers (BUCHANAN and HYNYNEN 1992).

The various methods of heating the prostate using intracavitary microwave applicators are summarized in Fig. 13.19. Figure 13.19a illustrates an uncooled TU applicator. The therapeutic zone is a nominally cylindrical region surrounding the prostatic urethra. Figure 13.19b depicts a cooled TU applicator. The therapeutic zone is also approximately cylindrical, but slightly displaced from the applicator surface. Figure 13.19c illustrates a cooled TR applicator. The

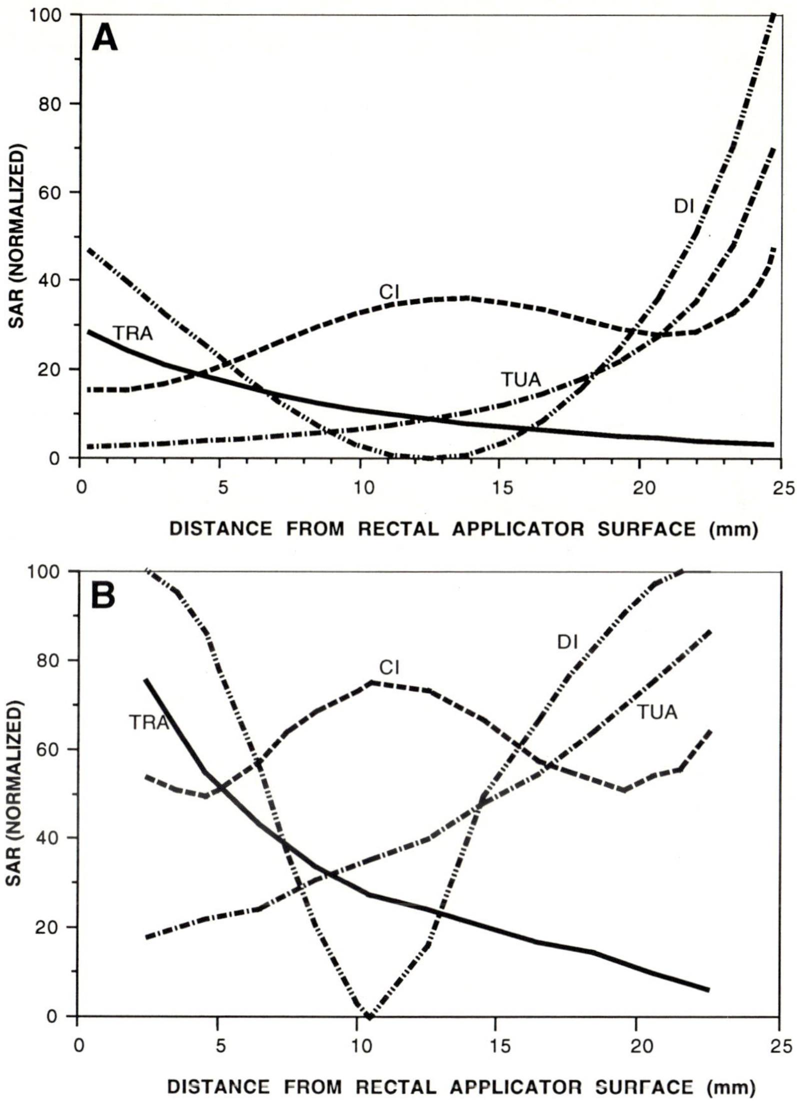

Fig. 13.18A, B. Results of a theoretical and practical investigation of constructive interference (*CI*) and destructive interference (*DI*) using transurethral (*TU*) and transrectal (*TR*) applicators. **A** Computer simulation. **B** Measurements in phantom

therapeutic zone is roughly an ellipsoidal region located between the rectum and urethra. Figure 13.19d depicts combined TU and TR applicators working together with constructive interference (phase steering). The therapeutic zone is potentially larger and more homogeneous than that of either applicator acting alone.

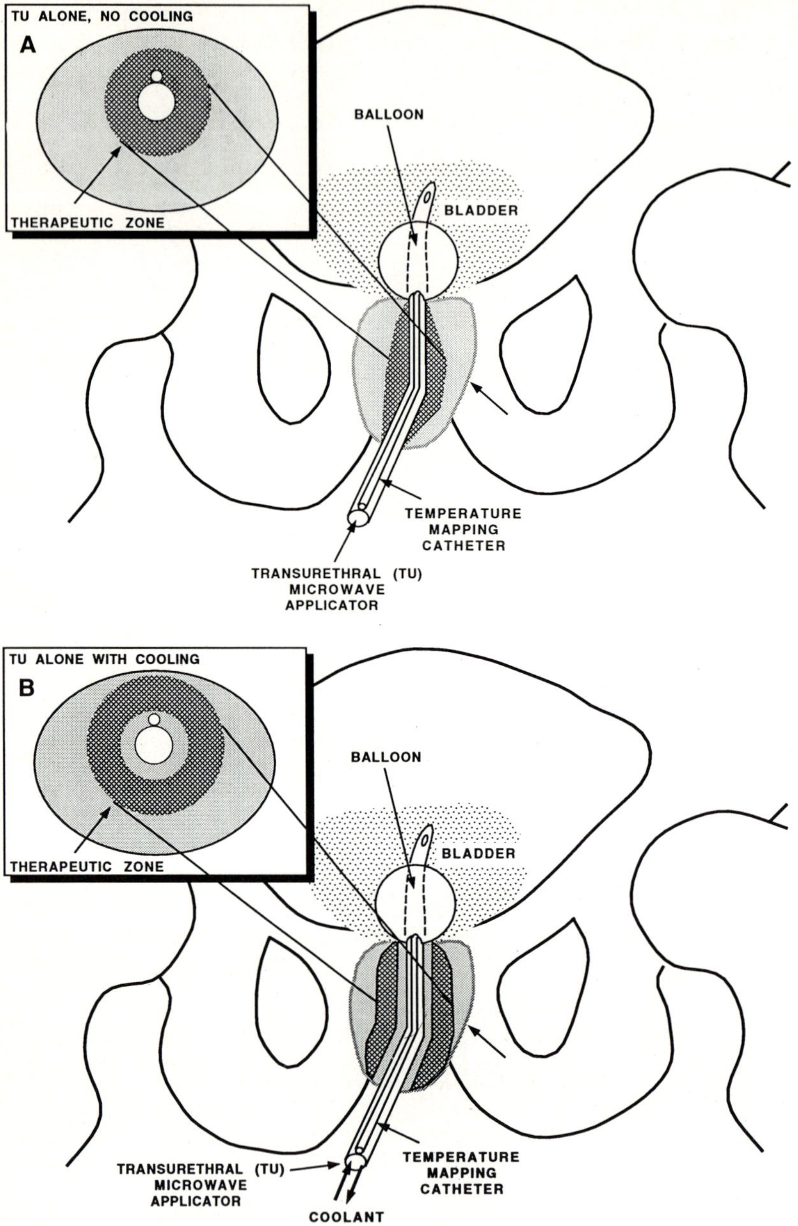

Fig. 13.19A–D. Intracavitary methods of heating the prostate. **A** Transurethral (*TU*) alone without applicator cooling. **B** TU with applicator cooling. **C** Transrectal (*TR*) alone with applicator cooling. **D** Combined TU and TR with phase steering. The therapeutic zones are meant to be illustrative only. They are not drawn precisely to scale (see text for explanation)

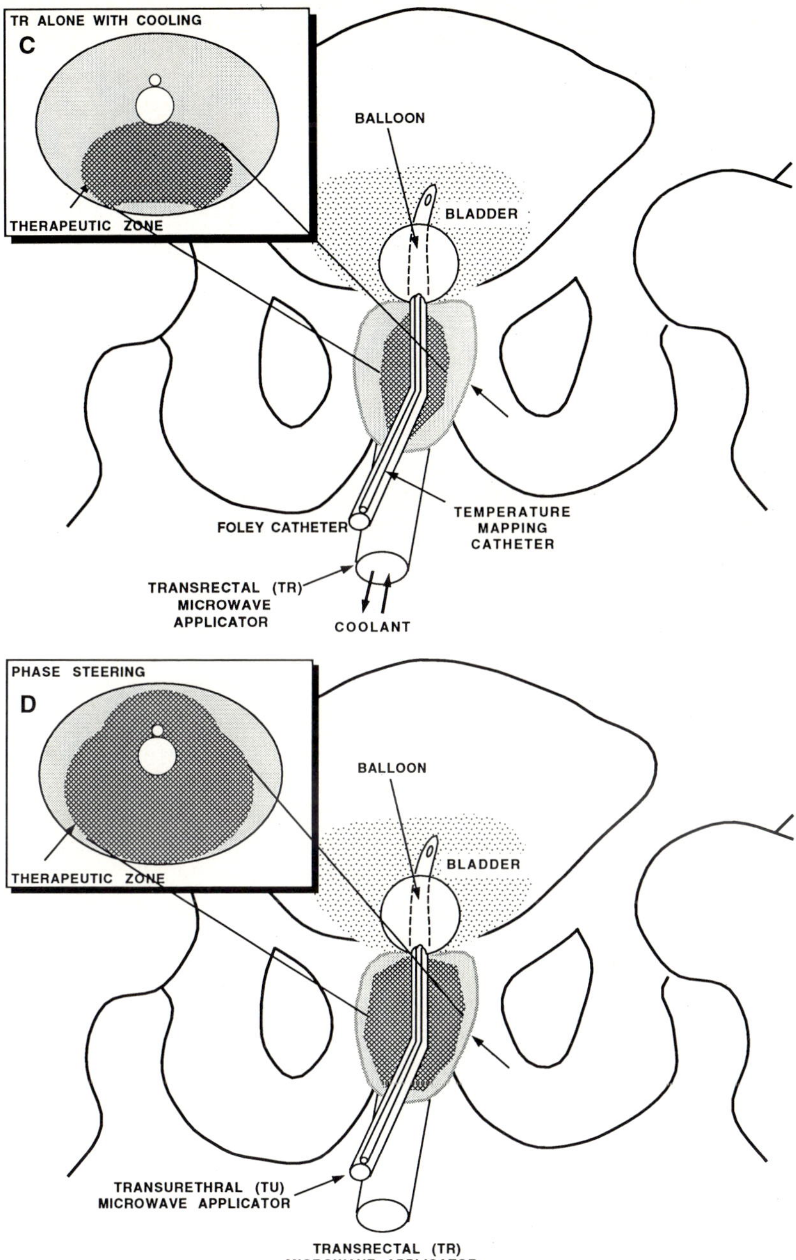
TR ALONE WITH COOLING
C
THERAPEUTIC ZONE
BALLOON
BLADDER
FOLEY CATHETER
TEMPERATURE
MAPPING
CATHETER
TRANSRECTAL (TR)
MICROWAVE
APPLICATOR
COOLANT
PHASE STEERING
D
THERAPEUTIC ZONE
BALLOON
BLADDER
TRANSURETHRAL (TU)
MICROWAVE APPLICATOR
TRANSRECTAL (TR)
MICROWAVE APPLICATOR

Fig. 13.19C, D.

13.7 Thermometry

13.7.1 Why Measure Temperature?

Hyperthermic dose is a function of temperature, and we have seen that blood flow has a significant and complicated influence on temperature distribution. This makes a hyperthermia procedure based on power output or remote temperature measurement unreliable. The hyperthermic dose (and hence the therapeutic benefit) could vary widely and unpredictably among individuals depending on blood flow dynamics. Thus, it is of critical and fundamental importance to measure and document the temperature distribution in the prostate as accurately and extensively as possible in each patient. Present technology does not permit us to noninvasively measure temperature with great precision or spatial resolution. Instead, we depend on miniature sensors, or *probes*, to measure temperature at a few representative locations and then use these data to interpolate or extrapolate temperature throughout the remainder of the heated region. For this reason, it is unwise to suppress pain during a hyperthermia procedure. A patient is capable of sensing temperature changes over a wide region and can communicate this information to the hyperthermia system operator, thereby reducing the risk of complications.

From thermal dosimetry and safety viewpoints, it is desirable to document at least the magnitude and location of the maximum temperature. Most hyperthermia systems use some form of temperature feedback to regulate heating. A common example of this process is a home furnace which is turned on and off by a thermostat. If the feedback sensor does not correctly reflect temperature in the region being heated, the feedback system will be compromised, with potentially hazardous consequences. For instance, heating will not be regulated if the sensor responsible for thermostatic control were to fail or is at a location which is not being heated. This might occur if either the microwave antenna(s) or temperature sensor(s) are not properly positioned with respect to one another. Blood flow can also present a problem. Consider the temperature profiles illustrated in Fig. 13.12. If a feedback temperature sensor were attached to the surface of an actively cooled applicator, the temperature it records will change very little as blood flow changes during treatment. The peak prostatic temperature, however, might change by several degrees, resulting in either subtherapeutic or perhaps hazardous temperatures depending on whether blood flow increases or decreases. Failure to document the maximum temperature decreases the reliability and reproducibility of a hyperthermia procedure by adding uncertainty to the thermal dosimetry and increases the probability of complications.

As depicted in Fig. 13.8 and 13.10, the peak temperature always occurs close to the surface of an uncooled applicator, where it may be easily and reliably measured by a noninvasive surface-mounted sensor. The effective therapeutic range of such an applicator, however, is limited to about 1 cm. By actively cooling an applicator, we can increase its effective range, as illustrated in

Fig. 13.9 and 13.12, but in doing so we sacrifice our ability to noninvasively measure the peak temperature or document its location. In addition, coolant temperature must be properly selected or else subtherapeutic temperatures may extend too far into the tissue. In the absence of invasive temperature measurement, the reliability and reproducibility of treatment using a cooled applicator should be questioned. The advantages and disadvantages of applicator cooling and invasive versus noninvasive thermometry should be carefully considered when developing prostate hyperthermia protocols.

13.7.2 Thermometry Systems

Temperature measurement near an intracavitary microwave applicator is not a trivial task. Since probe sensors actually measure their own temperature, they must be in thermal equilibrium with the surrounding tissue if they are to provide an accurate measurement of the tissue temperature. Temperature measurement is additionally complicated by the steep temperature gradients found near intracavitary applicators. If a sensor is large compared to the gradient, it will sense only an average temperature, while thermal and electromagnetic conduction along its leads could result in measurement error and might even change the temperature profile itself (SAMULSKI et al. 1985). Therefore, the sensors must be located outside of the applicator, in close contact with the tissue to be measured, and yet must perturb the local environment as little as possible.

In addition, if the sensors are electrically conducting, they must be carefully engineered to avoid self-heating in an intense electromagnetic field (CETAS 1990). Various attempts have been made to develop nonmetallic thermometers which exploit thermally sensitive optical properties or which employ radiometric techniques. The most popular methodologies for prostate hyperthermia, however, remain microthermocouples and thermistors owing to their low cost and commercial availability.

Thermocouples are a junction between dissimilar metals in which a current is produced by the thermoelectric effect. Copper and constantan, a copper–nickel alloy, are commonly used in medical applications owing to high sensitivity and probe interchangeability. Thermocouple leads, however, are metallic and thus are both good electrical and thermal conductors. These sensors are susceptible to many sources of error resulting from electromagnetic interference and thermal conduction along the leads. This is particularly true of thermocouple sensors attached to the surface of an actively cooled applicator.

Thermistors are a semiconductor whose resistance varies inversely with temperature. In order to avoid self-heating in the presence of microwaves, it is desirable to use very high resistance thermistors and high resistance leads made of a nonmetallic conductor such as carbon-impregnated Teflon (BOWMAN 1976). The use of nonmetallic leads also minimizes thermal conduction error of the type associated with thermocouples. The disadvantage of thermistor probes is that unless carefully selected, they are not interchangeable and may require periodic recalibration.

13.7.3 Temperature Mapping

One of the main reasons for interest in prostate hyperthermia is to provide a nonsurgical alternative for treatment of prostatic diseases such as BPH. Thus, it is desirable for a hyperthermia system to measure temperature by the least invasive means possible and yet document the temperature at as many locations as possible. A compromise is to attach one or more small catheters to the surface of urethral (see Fig. 13.19a) and/or rectal applicators and to move a thermometry probe in small increments along those catheters so as to "map" the temperature profile along the catheter (ASTRAHAN et al. 1989, 1991a, b; SAPOZINK et al. 1990). Alternatively, multisensor probes consisting of an array of sensors at fixed spacing along a single probe may be used (ASTRAHAN et al. 1989b), or an array of sensors may simply be built into the applicator itself (CARTER et al. 1991). In either case, the more locations at which temperatures are measured, the more reliable a hyperthermia treatment will be and the less risk it will entail.

When a sensor is attached to the surface of an applicator, it is influenced by the radiative, conductive, and convective properties of the applicator in addition to the surrounding tissue. If an applicator is actively cooled, surface measurements lose significance since the probe senses an average of the applicator and tissue temperature. More extensive and more accurate measurement of prostate temperature profiles may be obtained using small, interstitially implanted probes at the expense of making the procedure more invasive (ASTRAHAN et al. 1991b). Once a device can be shown to produce a reliable and predictable temperature distribution, interstitial measurements might be bypassed without compromising safety.

13.8 Quality Assurance

Prostate hyperthermia systems fundamentally consist of an intracavitary applicator, a microwave source and power amplifier, power and temperature-measuring subsystems, and possibly an applicator cooling subsystem. A microcomputer is used to integrate and coordinate these subsystems. In order to assure safe, reliable, and reproducible treatment it is obvious that these systems must be properly maintained. Our experience suggests that the applicator and power components of a hyperthermia system are generally reliable and change slowly with time. It is generally sufficient to test and calibrate these subsystems on an annual basis. The thermometry system, on the other hand, is the most clinically critical component and tends to be the least reliable due to physical abuse during treatment. It is generally recommended that hyperthermia thermometry systems should maintain an accuracy of about 0.1 °C. The thermometry system should be tested prior to each treatment, and calibration checks performed at periodic intervals. A calibration test prior to treatment can be as simple as placing the probe in an object of known temperature, or intercomparing probes (on the assumption that it is improbable several probes will simultaneously drift or fail in the same manner). The periodic calibration interval and method of calibration will depend on the particular thermometric technology employed.

13.9 Conclusion

The fundamental task of prostate hyperthermia is to heat the prostate to a prescribed temperature for a prescribed period of time. At present, the most common method of heating the prostate is an intracavitary microwave applicator which is located within either the urethra or the rectum.

The physical properties which describe the interaction of microwaves with tissue indicate that applicators which operate at frequencies near 1 GHz are well suited to heating the prostate. In the vicinity of 1 GHz, the applicators have effective heating radii of 0.5–2 cm and the wavelength in tissue is comparable to the dimensions of the prostate. This enables the future development of phase-steered applicators which employ both urethral and rectal elements. At lower frequencies the wavelength becomes too long to confine phase focusing to within the prostate and applicator dimensions become progressively larger. At higher frequencies attenuation limits heating to the immediate vicinity of an applicator's surface.

Although prostate hyperthermia is conceptually simple, it is difficult to achieve in the clinic. Blood flow dynamics and thermal conductivity strongly influence the resultant temperature distribution, making it difficult to deliver effective hyperthermia in the absence of direct temperature measurement. The most critical aspects of prostate hyperthermia are the selective delivery of heat to the prostate and the accurate mapping of prostate temperature. Failure to fulfill either of these requirements will produce ineffective or hazardous results.

References

Astrahan MA (1989) Thermal mapping with multisensor probes. Strahlenther Onkol 165: 746–750

Astrahan MA, Sapozink MD, Cohen D, Luxton G, Kampp TD, Boyd S, Petrovich Z (1989) Microwave applicator for transurethral hyperthermia of benign prostatic hyperplasia. Int J Hyperthermia 5: 283–296

Astrahan M, Imanaka K, Jozsef G, Ameye F, Baert L, Sapozink MD, Petrovich Z (1991a) Heating characteristics of a helical microwave applicator for transurethral hyperthermia of benign prostatic hyperplasia. Int J Hyperthermia 7: 141–155

Astrahan M, Ameye F, Oyen P, Willemen P, Baert L, Petrovich, Z (1991b) Interstitial temperature measurements during transurethral microwave hyperthermia, J Urol 145: 304–308

Baert L, Ameye F, Willemen P, Vandenhove J, Lauweryns J, Astrahan M, Petrovich Z (1990) Transurethral microwave hyperthermia for benign prostatic hyperplasia: preliminary clinical and pathological results, J Urol 144: 1383–1387

Blute ML, Tomera KM, Hellerstein DK, Atkinson EJ, Patterson DE, Segura JW (1992) Transurethral microwave thermotherapy for prostatism: early Mayo Foundation experience. Mayo Clin Proc 67: 417–421

Bowman R. (1976) A probe for measuring temperature in radio frequency heated material. IEEE Trans Microwave Theory Tech 24: 43–45

Buchanan MT, Hynynen K (1992) An electrically focused intracavitary ultrasound system for the induction of hyperthermia (abstract). In: Gerner EW (ed) Proceedings of the 6th international congress on hyperthermic oncology, Tucson, Arizona. Hyperthermic Oncology 1992, volume 1, summary papers, 272

Carter S St. C, Patel A, Reddy P, Royer P, Ramsay JWA (1991) Single-session transurethral microwave thermotherapy for the treatment of benign prostatic obstruction. J Endourol 5: 137–144

Cetas TC (1990) Thermometry. In: Field SB, Hand JW (eds) An introduction to the practical aspects of clinical hyperthermia. Taylor & Francis, Philadelphia, pp 423–477

Debicki P, Astrahan MA, Ameye F, Oyen R, Baert L, Haczewski A, Petrovich Z (1992) Temperature steering in prostate by simultaneous transurethral and transrectal hyperthermia. Urology 40: 300–307

Dickson JA, Calderwood SK (1980) Temperature range and selective sensitivity of tumors to hyperthermia: a critical review, Ann N Y Acad Sci 335: 180–205

Field SB (1978) The response of normal tissues to hyperthermia alone or in combination with X-rays. In: (ed) Cancer therapy by hyperthermia and radiation. Proceedings of the 2nd international symposium, Essen, 1977. Urban & Schwarzenberg, Baltimore, pp 37–48

Field SB, Morris CC (1983) The relationship between heating time and temperature: its relevance to clinical hyperthermia, Radiother Oncol 1: 179–183

Field SB, Raaphorst GP (1990) Thermal dose, In: Field SB, Hand JW (eds) An introduction to the practical aspects of clinical hyperthermia. Taylor & Francis, Philadelphia, pp 69–76

Hahn GM, Ning SC, Elizaga M, Kappa DS, Anderson RL (1989) A comparison of thermal responses of human and rodent cells. Int J Radiat Biol 56: 817–825

Harada T, Etori K, Kumazaki T, Nishizawa O, Noto H, Tsuchida S (1985) Microwave surgical treatment of diseases of prostate. Urology 26: 572–576

Henle KJ, Dethlefsen LA (1978) Heat fractionation and thermotolerance: a review. Cancer Res 38: 1843–1851

Magin RL, Fridd CW, Bonfiglio TA, Linke CA (1980) Thermal destruction of the canine prostate by high intensity microwaves. J Surg Res 29: 265–275

Mendecki J, Friedenthal E, Botstein C, Sterzer F, Paglione R, Nowogrodzki M, Beck E (1978) Microwave induced hyperthermia in cancer treatment: apparatus and preliminary results. Int J Radiat Oncol Biol Phys 4: 1095–1103

Petrovich Z, Astrahan M, Baert L (1991) Transurethral microwave heating without urethral cooling: theory and experimental results. Proc. lasers in urology, laparoscopy, and general surgery, SPIE 1421: 14–17

Petrowicz O, Scheiblich J, Crucius A, Erhardt W, Wriedt-Lübbe I, Ultsch B, Blüemel G (1982) High-frequency transmitter for the localized heat treatment of the prostate gland. Natl Cancer Inst Monogr 61: 473–476

Raaphorst GP (1990) Fundamental aspects of hyperthermic biology. In: Field SB, Hand JW (eds) An introduction to the practical aspects of clinical hyperthermia. Taylor & Francis, Philadelphia, pp 10–54

Roemer RB, Fletcher AM, Cetas TC (1985) Obtaining local SAR and blood perfusion data from temperature measurements: steady state and transient techniques compared. Int J Radiat Oncol Biol Phys 11: 1539–1550

Samulski TV, Lyons BE, Britt RH (1985) Temperature measurements in high thermal gradients. II. Analysis of conduction effects. Int J Radiat Oncol Biol Phys 11: 963–971

Sapareto SA, Dewey WC (1984) Thermal dose determination in cancer therapy. Int J Radiat Oncol Biol Phys 10:787–800

Sapozink MD, Boyd SD, Astrahan MA, Jozsef G, Petrovich Z (1990) Transurethral hyperthermia for benign prostatic hyperplasia – preliminary clinical results. J Urol 143:944–950

Turner P (1986) Interstitial equal-phased arrays for EM hyperthermia. IEEE Trans Microwave Theory Tech 34:572–578

Yeh MM, Douple EB, Trembly BS, Jonsson E, Heaney JA, Paulsen KD, Eaton WL (1992) Multiple microwave antenna system for prostate cancer hyperthermia (abstract). In: Gerner EW (ed) Proceedings of the 6th international congress on hyperthermic oncology, Tucson, Arizona, Hyperthermic Oncology 1992, volume 1, summary papers, 269

Yerushalmi A, Servadio C, Leib Z, Fishelovitz Y, Rokowsky E, Stein JA (1982) Local hyperthermia for treatment of carcinoma of the prostate: a preliminary report. Prostate 3:623–630

14 Biologic Effects of Local Microwave Hyperthermia on Prostatic Tissues

FILIP AMEYE and LUC BAERT

CONTENTS

FILIP AMEYE, MD, Department of Urology, St. Pieter's Hospital, Catholic University of Leuven, Brusselsestraat 69, 3000 Leuven, Belgium
LUC BAERT, MD, PhD, Professor and Chairman, Department of Urology, St. Pieter's Hospital, Catholic University of Leuven, Brusselsestraat 69, 3000 Leuven, Belgium and Clinical Professor of Urology and Radiation Oncology, University of Southern California School of Medicine, Los Angeles, CA 90033, USA

Petrovich/Baert (Eds.)
Benign Prostatic Hyperplasia

14.1 Introduction

Hyperthermia (HT) in the range of 42°–45 °C has been under intensive study, particularly during the two past decades, as a treatment for malignant neoplasms. HT has found its greatest applicability as a potentiating adjuvant to radiation and chemotherapy with a selective effect against certain tumor cell subpopulations (DICKSON and CALDERWOOD 1980).

The technical means of producing, measuring, and controlling temperatures in vivo have been refined. Many clinical phase I studies have now been completed for a variety of HT techniques and tumor sites. Phase II studies are currently being conducted, allowing for the further optimization of HT (OLESON et al. 1980). Major efforts have been directed to the definition of many biologic and physiologic mechanisms such as molecular, cellular, and vascular effects of HT (STREFFER and VAN BEUNINGEN 1987; VAUPEL and KALLINOWSKI 1987). Increased understanding of these biologic effects will be used to optimize the clinical applications of HT in the future.

Localized microwave HT in multiple sessions, with therapeutic temperatures between 43 °C and 45 °C, has been introduced recently as a new treatment modality for prostatic diseases. MENDECKI et al. (1980) reported on the use of transrectally applied 2415-MHz microwaves in the treatment of carcinoma of the prostate (CaP). The assumption that hyperplastic prostatic tissues react in the same way to local prostatic heating as do neoplastic tissues, with subsequent shrinking of obstructive tissues, led to the application of microwave HT for benign prostatic hyperplasia (BPH). Transrectal hyperthermia (TRHT) for BPH was first described by YERUSHALMI et al. (1985), followed by several groups using various treatment modalities. Transurethral hyperthermia (TUHT), using 915-MHz microwave applicators, was tested in several clinical phase I studies (SAPOZINK et al. 1990; BAERT et al. 1990). Preliminary and short-term results are promising (BAERT et al. 1991); however, longer follow-up is required to prove long-term efficacy. Recently, new single-session techniques such as transurethral thermotherapy (TUMT), with therapeutic temperatures between 45 °C and 55 °C, and transurethral frequency (TURF), with lower applied frequencies of 0.5–1 MHz, have been introduced.

Better understanding of the thermophysics and biophysical mechanisms of prostate heating can optimize HT treatments for prostatic diseases. However, reports on biologic and pathologic effects of HT on prostatic cells and tissues are scarce. This paper reviews the reported biologic effects in prostatic tissues after prostate HT and compares them with the well-studied HT effects in various normal and malignant tissues. Basic knowledge of these biologic mechanisms can further elucidate possible working mechanisms and optimize HT applications for prostatic diseases in the future.

14.2 Biologic and Physiologic Effects of Hyperthermia on Normal Tissue and Malignant Tumors

14.2.1 Introduction

Study of HT effects on tissue is difficult and complex. Additionally, some HT effects may be organ specific. Normal prostate and benign hyperplastic tissues are morphologically different from malignant tissue. There is a higher heat sensitivity in the latter group. Effects in cell cultures cannot simply be extrapolated to animal or human tissues because of the lack of a normal physiologic and vascular microenvironment in the former. In vivo effects of HT are due to complex interactions at the molecular, cellular, vascular, and tissue levels, finally leading to cell death. Enhancement of response of HT is related to the mitotic cycle, energy status of the cell, hypoxic and acidotic conditions, and vascular changes. The response of the tissue is determined by variable dose-effect relationships dependent upon optimum temperature, fractionation of HT, sequencing of HT in multimodal therapy, and other local tissue variables. Thermotolerance induction and decay effects may further contribute to variation in responses in HT. In presenting the following data, all these variables have to be taken into account.

14.2.2 Molecular and Cellular Effects of Hyperthermia on Normal and Tumor Cells

The molecular and cellular effects of HT in different tissues have been reviewed by Oleson et al. (1980). Heat is an entropic, disordering agent which can disrupt highly ordered structures and processes in cells. Denaturation of intracellular proteins or membrane proteins, lipids, and nucleic acids is suggested to induce an initial multistep cascade response. Specific cell membrane proteins and receptors, such as insulin receptors or phospholipases, mitochondrial electron transports chains, and RNA molecular complexes are all prone to heat damage. The changes in the cytoskeleton and cytoplasmatic matrix, especially by interaction with the intermediate filament structures, alter inter- and intracellular interactions and correlate well with alterations in cell survival.

Advances have been made in understanding the secondary biochemical events in cells after this initial phase of reaction to HT. A wide range of membrane enzymes, receptors, and transport systems have been investigated as targets for HT. The insulin receptor is inactivated by heat with similar kinetics to cell inactivation. Inhibition of sodium-dependent amino acid transport appears to be correlated with inhibition of growth in lymphoid lines. A number of enzymes involved in transmembrane signal transduction are stimulated by heat. HT causes an increase in cyclic adenosine monophosphate (c-AMP) levels and phospholipases A_2 and C, giving rise to cascade responses involved in all aspects of cellular regulations. Especially the activation of the latter enzyme may be of great importance, as it gives rise to molecular effectors that increase intracellular-free calcium, a parameter that may play a major role both in cell killing and in the induction of heat shock proteins (hsp).

Hyperthermia-induced changes in the cytoplasmic matrix are important in the cellular response to heat. The matrix comprises a system of interlocking filaments that connect the extracellular matrix to the nuclear matrix. Components include both extracellular macromolecules and cytoplasmatic systems, which include microfilaments, intermediate filaments, and microtubules. Intermediate filaments are particularly sensitive to heat, with the filament lattice collapsing into a perinuclear zone after HT. A possibly connected change observed in heated cells is an increased adherence of cellular proteins to the cytoskeleton, particularly to the intermediate filament–nuclear matrix system. This change appears to correlate well with alterations in cell survival.

The behavior and synthesis of proteins are central to cellular responses to HT. A primary effect of heat is a change in the folding of proteins, a process that leads to denaturation and aggregation of proteins. HT also alters the pattern of protein synthesis. The expression of the majority of cell proteins is inhibited, while a number of families of heat shock genes are induced. These effects are regulated by changes in the transcription, translation, and messenger RNA processing. The resulting heat shock proteins are homeostatic in nature and may be important mediators of thermotolerance, protecting the cell from further heat damage. These proteins possess a high capacity to bind to the hydrophobic domains of other proteins in addition to processing adenosine triphosphatase (ATPase) activity. Heat shock proteins bind to hydrophobic sites on aggregates of denaturated proteins with high affinity, resulting in removal of the bound hsp-unit from the aggregate. The hsp molecule then removes itself from the protein in a step that involves ATP hydrolysis. The "rescued" protein is then able to refold and recover its function or, if damaged, be recognized by components of the cellular protein degradation apparatus, which is induced by heat. The hsp/degradation system may rescue cells from the deleterious effects of protein denaturation and aggregation (PLEHAM 1986). It is commonly believed, but still debated, that these heat shock proteins either protect against subsequent heat stress or enhance the ability of cells to recover from the toxic effects of heat (CARPER et al. 1987).

There is still a lack of understanding of how the many changes induced by heat lead to the ultimate cellular effects. Initial changes, such as protein denaturation or radical generation, may induce a multistep cascade response. The cascade response, depending on the magnitude of the time–temperature stimulus, might lead to the induction of heat resistance with a mild stimulus or to cell killing with an intense stimulus. Alterations in intracellular Ca^{2+} could function as a signal for thermotolerance induction and could activate enzymes such as phospholipases, proteases, and endonucleases that are involved in cell death.

Hyperthermia also modifies the effects of ionizing radiation and a number of chemotherapeutic agents. The extent of interaction varies with the time interval between treatments and the temperature achieved. In general, maximum cytotoxicity is observed when the treatments are given simultaneously. The effect decays to an additive or independent interaction over periods of minutes to hours between the treatments. The mechanisms of sensitization of radiation and chemotherapeutic agents by heat are not well understood. HT inhibits the repair of DNA damage induced by ionizing radiation and increases the frequency of chromosomal aberrations (Dewey et al. 1980). The most heat-sensitive cells are in mitosis and in late S phase, whereas the most heat-resistant cells are those in early G_1 phase. Less is known about heat–drug interactions and the mechanisms of enhancement. Heat may enhance or inhibit drug transport and increase membrane permeability. It may increase the rate of reaction between the drug and its target molecules, inhibit the repair of drug-induced lesions, or induce a combination of these effects (Dahl 1986). Current studies do not indicate that the sensitizing effects of heat on ionizing radiation or cytotoxic drugs are intrinsically greater in cancer cells than in normal cells.

Cellular response to HT can be significantly enhanced under microenvironmental or metabolic conditions that have a neutral or protective effect relative to the effects of radiation and some chemotherapeutic agents. These conditions include hypoxia, acidity, and reduced cell (and tissue) energy status (Dewey et al. 1980). Hypoxic, acidic, and energy-deprived conditions occur naturally in tumors secondary to the high rates of aerobic and anaerobic glycolysis, which is an acid-producing and inefficient pathway for ATP production. Tumor hypoxia further enhances the glycolytic pathway. HT would therefore be expected to be selectively toxic to intratumoral regions of solid tumors that are resistant to radiation.

14.2.3 Effects of Hyperthermia on Normal and Tumor Tissues

Based on the data from in vivo studies there is a discrepancy between the magnitude of killing of tumor cells by HT in vivo and in vitro. It has been reported that greater cell killing occurs in tumors in vivo than in vitro with the use of the same heat parameters. Additional direct killing of tumor cells by heat is too small to account for the frequent cure of tumors by HT. On the other hand, it has emerged from in vivo studies that malignant tumors are more heat-sensitive than normal tissues. This differential effect does not appear to be due to an inherent differential heat sensitivity of tumor cells compared to normal cells. This response to HT is related to differences in anatomic and physiologic properties of normal tissues versus tumors. These differences include microcirculation and changes in environmental factors such as pH, O_2, and nutrients. All of the aforementioned factors are known to greatly influence the thermosensitivity of cells to HT. Nutritional status, pH, and O_2 concentration are dependent on the functional integrity of the vasculature. The tissue temperature during heating is directly related to the efficacy of the heat dissipation by blood perfusion (DEWEY et al. 1980).

The microcirculation of normal tissues is characterized by well-organized, predictable networks of capillaries. The capillary structure consists of endothelium, basement membrane, and pericytes, surrounded by an adventitia. Although there is a difference in organization and blood flow rates in different tissues, there is a uniform physiologic intracapillary blood flow at a steady state. Upon heating to 43°–45 °C there is an increase in blood flow rate, expansion of functional vascular volume by dilation, and alteration in vascular permeability, allowing heat conduction and diminishing heat toxicity (Table 14.1). After termination of heating, changes in microcirculation and permeability return to normal levels within 2 h. It should be mentioned that the magnitude of these changes may vary considerably in different tissues and they are dependent upon the degree of initial heating (EMAMI and SONG 1984).

The neovascularization of malignant tissues is characterized by formation of buds, sprouts, and lacuna-like sinusoids. The tumor capillaries are devoid of an external coat of basement membrane, with the single layer of endothelial cells occasionally being lined by cords of tumor cells. This capillary network, which is formed by random fusion of sprouts, is tortuous, with redundant bending, elongation, and dilation. The blood flow through such a coarse network is intermittent and slow owing to inadequate drainage of sinusoids, easily leading to thrombosis. The relative vascular volume, vascular density, and blood flow decrease as the tumor grows. Moreover, the continuous growth of tumor mass within a limited space exerts progressively increasing pressure on capillaries, particularly on those located in the inner part of the tumor, causing capillary collapse and deterioration of blood flow in the central areas of growing tumors.

Hyperthermia at modest temperatures (40°–41 °C) causes either no effect or a slight increase in blood flow. At the higher therapeutic temperatures (43°–45 °C) commonly used for clinical HT, there is a temperature-dependent reduction of blood flow, exerting a significant detrimental effect preferentially on the microvasculature and blood flow in tumor. Irreversible damage by rupture

Table 14.1. Vascular changes caused by hyperthermia at 43 °C for 1 h in rat extremities (from EMAMI and SONG 1980)

	Blood flow (ml/min 100 g)	Vascular volume (ml/g)	Vascular permeability (mg/g h)
SKIN			
Control	7.82 ± 0.76	0.0165 ± 0.0014	0.0438 ± 0.0040
Heated	29.13 ± 3.39	0.0483 ± 0.0056	0.1559 ± 0.0274
MUSCLE			
Control	4.97 ± 0.55	0.0187 ± 0.0012	0.0022 ± 0.016
Heated	14.61 ± 1.75	0.0297 ± 0.0024	0.0549 ± 0.0073

and destruction of capillaries is due to deformability of red blood cells and changes in platelets, white blood cells, and endothelial structure and finally leads to thrombosis. Changes in vascular permeability lead to pronounced interstitial edema and cellular infiltrates, accounting partially for retardation of blood flow in the heated tumors (Fig. 14.1).

The differential reduced heat dissipation and consequent heat accumulation in malignant tissues compared to normal tissues leads directly to relatively higher cellular heat toxicity and necrosis in tumor tissues. On the other hand, inefficient drainage resulting from heat-induced vascular damage and activation of the anaerobic glycolytic pathway with increased production of metabolites such as lactic acid and β-hydroxybutyric acid creates a hypoxic and acidotic microenvironment in these tissues. The relatively acidotic condition of tumor tissue compared to normal tissues not only enhances lethal responses to HT but also inhibits the repair of thermal damage and the development of thermotolerance (Figs. 14.2, 14.3) (VAUPEL and KALLINOWSKI 1987; EMAMI and SONG 1984).

The rationale for the combined use of HT with radiotherapy has been, in addition to the already mentioned thermal enhancement of cellular radiosensitivity, HT preferential cytotoxicity toward hypoxic cells and cells in S phase, which are relatively radioresistant. The increases in blood flow caused by low HT temperatures in some types of tumor may lead to an increase in oxygenation of tumors and, thus, an increase in the response of the tumors to subsequent

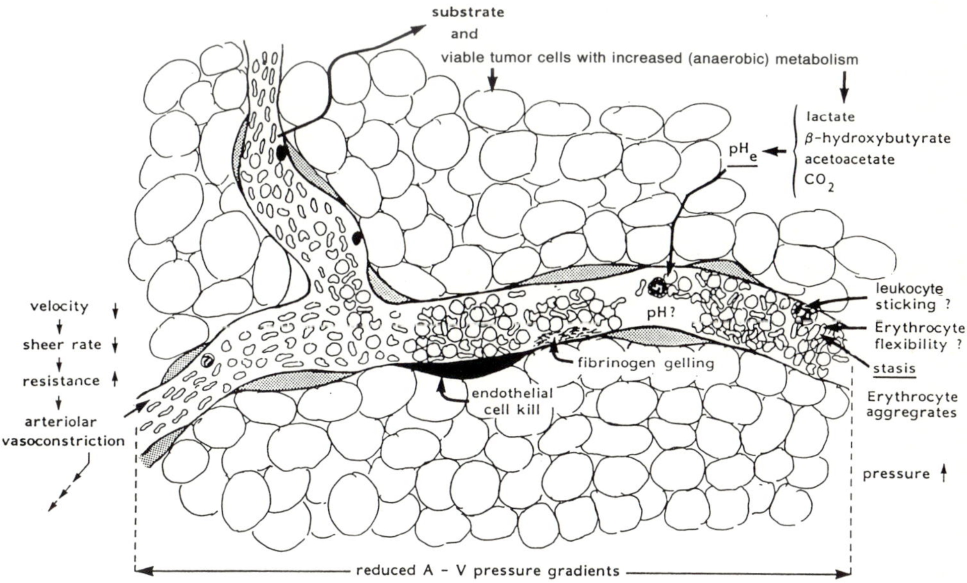

Fig. 14.1. Schematic representation of some of the reported changes in tumor physiology and microcirculation during a hyperthermic treatment. (From REINHOLD 1988)

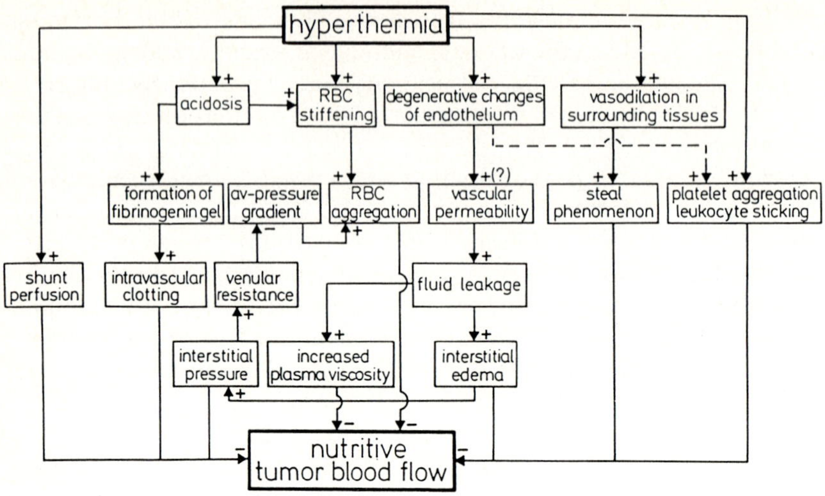

Fig. 14.2. Possible mechanisms involved in HT-induced breakdown of blood flow in malignant tumors. (From VAUPEL and KALLINOWSKI 1987)

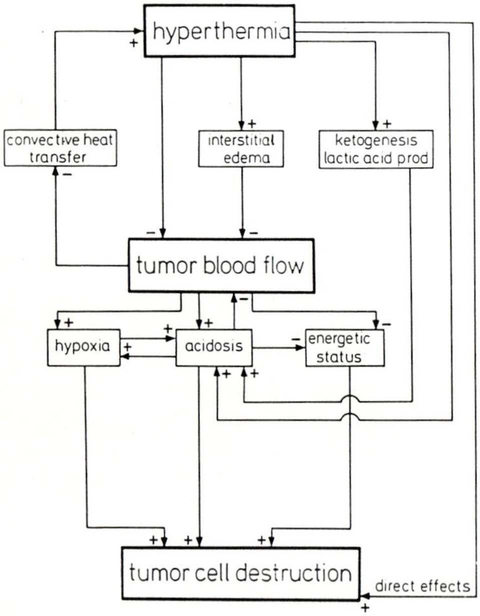

Fig. 14.3. Diagram showing the principles of heat-induced tumor cell destruction in vivo. (From VAUPEL and KALLINOWSKI 1987)

radiation. Unfortunately, heat may also increase the oxygen supply in normal tissues, which would increase their radiosensitivity, too. These facts should imply that the therapeutic gain may be greater if radiotherapy is applied prior to HT rather than vice versa. The differential response of tumor vasculature and normal tissue vasculature to HT should also be taken into account in the combined use of HT and chemotherapy. Inefficient delivery of drug to tumor due to vascular occlusion or stasis and an increase in drug concentration in normal tissues as a result of the increased blood flow and vascular permeability caused by HT may entail greater damage in normal tissues than in tumors. However, there is an intriguing possibility that heat-induced hypoxia in tumors could be exploited to enhance the effect of drugs which are specifically cytotoxic to hypoxic cells. Induction of hypoxia in tumor by HT would increase the fraction of tumor cells vulnerable to the drugs, leading to a greater destruction of tumor. On the other hand, heating at relatively low temperatures may increase the uptake of drugs in some tumors by virtue of an increase in blood flow. Both mechanisms would further potentiate the drug's cytotoxicity at subsequent heating (Song 1984).

14.2.4 Principles of Thermotolerance

In clinical practice HT is given in multiple fractions, analogous to the use of conventional treatment such as radiotherapy. Knowledge of the biologic response to repeated heat treatments is essential for the planning of clinical treatments. A major consideration is the development of thermotolerance. This phenomenon can be seen in vitro as well as during in vivo testing.

Living cells, including normal as well as tumour cells, can increase their thermal resistance during or after an appropriate heat treatment. Two types of thermotolerance were initially described in cells in vitro. One type is induced by prolonged heating at temperatures below 42.5 °C, the cells becoming more resistant to heat after 3–4 h of HT. The second type develops after short exposures to hyperthermic temperatures (41°–46 °C) if the cells are returned to normal physiologic temperatures. The cells then become increasingly resistant to subsequent heat treatment, the maximum effect being observed after a few hours. Both types of thermotolerance have been observed in tissues in vivo. In general, thermotolerance increases to a maximum during the first few hours after the priming heat treatment and then decays with a normal thermal sensitivity being regained within 1–2 weeks. For a given tissue, the degree of thermotolerance is greater and is expressed later following the more severe priming treatment. Moreover, the in vivo development of thermotolerance depends on the temperature as well as on the duration of heating. Although it is difficult to generalize conclusions concerning capacity to develop thermotolerance from tissue to tissue, there is a general relationship between the heating time and temperature required for its induction for a given tissue.

The extent to which thermotolerance in tissues is due to a decrease in intrinsic cellular thermal sensitivty or is secondary to vascular changes which modify the cellular environment is not clear. The similarities between thermotolerance in tissues in vivo and cells in vitro indicate that it is a cellular phenomenon. Recent studies have implicated an important role of the abovementioned heat shock proteins which are synthesized after a thermal insult. In vivo, however, changes in vascular perfusion may alter the cellular response. In some situations heat-induced increases in blood flow may augment heat loss and nutrient supply, thus making later treatments less effective. In other situations vascular damage could reduce heat loss so that subsequent local heating would cause a greater increase in temperature and lead to nutrient deficiency with a consequent reduction in pH. These factors would make cells more sensitive to subsequent heating and the reduced pH would inhibit the further development of thermotolerance.

Based on these data, knowledge of the development of thermotolerance is of major importance in considering fractionation of HT. Thermotolerance can develop during a single session of HT and reduce its efficacy. On the other hand, thermotolerance can be built up during a fractionated regimen if the intervals between fractions are not long enough to allow the complete development of tolerance. Clinically, superficial tissues may become resistant to temperature elevations after the first thermal exposure, due to intrinsic thermotolerance, vasodilation, and interstitial edema. This selective thermotolerance of superficial tissues may be used to enhance the relative cytotoxicity of deeper tissues at sequential treatments (VAUPEL and KALLINOWSKI 1987).

These concepts are important in multiple fractions of prostate HT. Duration of treatments, thermal dose, and intervals between sessions are important parameters in the development of thermotolerance. Hypothetically, sequential therapy, especially in transurethral application, can benefit from the relative thermotolerance of superficial periurethral tissues to heat more efficiently deeper adenoma tissue. This method increases therapeutic efficacy and lowers local toxicity of HT.

14.2.5 Clinical Relevance of Experimental Hyperthermia Data

As mentioned above, most of our knowledge about heat effects stems from laboratory work performed in cell lines of murine or other mammalian origin. Further experience has been gained with animal tumors treated after transplantation or, more seldom, at the site of their origin. It seems likely that the physical and biologic phenomena in these experiments will also be found in human tissues and tumours. In developing clinical approaches, one has to be aware of a huge number of complex interactions between the patient, the tumor, the heat, and combined modalities such as irradiation and drugs. Therapeutic outcomes are influenced by inter- and intraindividual tumor heterogeneity together with HT variables, such as heating rate and dose, duration, timing and fractionation of treatments, thermotolerance, and finally application techniques. These multiple variables have to be taken into account in discussing prostate HT.

14.3 Biologic Effects of Hyperthermia on Prostatic Tissue

14.3.1 Introduction

Reported data on effects of HT on prostatic cells and tissues are very scarce. In interpreting data, we face various, already mentioned methodologic problems. Experimental results of in vitro studies in prostatic cell cultures cannot simply be extrapolated to animal or human tissues. Moreover, the morphometric characteristics of animal prostates differ from those of human prostates.

No data exist on whether the hyperplastic tissue of BPH reacts to HT in the same way as normal tissue or, instead, like malignant tumor. The differential heat sensitivity of malignant and normal cells is well known. Temperatures of 43 °C cause a greater degree of damage to malignant tissue than to normal tissues, where no lasting damage occurs. The effects of local heating depend on a dose–time relationship. These effects on malignant tissues are difficult to demonstrate if the temperature does not reach 43 °C. Until proven otherwise, we have to hypothesize that BPH has a response to HT which is similar to that of malignant tissues. This would allow for extrapolation of the data on heat response of malignant tumors to heat response of BPH.

The minimum temperature at which histologic lesions in prostatic tissues are obtained is around 43 °C. The thermal isoeffect dose, however, is dependent upon intrinsic prostatic factors and technical variables. The size, morphology, and shape of the prostate, local blood flow conditions, and epithelial–stromal ratio are important determinants in tissue reaction to heat. The method of application (TUHT/TRHT/TURF/TUMT), applied temperature and penetration depth, duration and number of sessions, fractionation, and thermotolerance are important technical variables which influence treatment efficacy. All these variables have to be kept in mind in discussing HT effects on the prostate.

We shall first present HT effects on various cell lines in culture and also HT effects on animal tissues. This review will allow us to understand and interpret better the biologic effects seen in humans. After describing the normal anatomy and histology of human and animal prostates, we shall systematically discuss HT effects and heat sensitivity of the separate constituents of prostatic hyperplasia. Subsequently, histologic changes after clinical HT in benign and malignant human prostates will be described. These changes will be evaluated and compared among the different HT modalities. Other biologic effects will also be considered, such as biochemical and immunologic changes occurring as a result of prostatic HT. Finally, possible mechanisms of HT action on the prostate will be discussed.

14.3.2 Effects of Hyperthermia on Prostatic Carcinoma In Vitro and In Vivo

To date, there have been no studies to evaluate the effect of HT on normal and BPH prostatic tissues in vitro. Recently, however, there have been some in vitro studies evaluating the effectiveness of heat on human prostatic tumor cells in culture and identifying parameters which may enhance the cytotoxic effectiveness of HT treatments.

KAVER et al. (1989, 1991a) reported on the effects of heat and radiation on human prostatic tumor cells in culture. The purpose of their first study was to evaluate in vitro the effect of HT on various human CaP cell lines and related sublines under exposure time and temperature conditions mimicking parameters which may be applied in a clinical setting using temperatures > 43 °C. Cell suspensions of different established tumor lines (PC-3, DU-145, 1-LN, and 125-1L) were exposed to heat at 43 °C for 1 h. The effect of this HT on cell growth was assessed by evaluating rates of colony formation and measuring cell growth rates. Statistically significant inhibitory responses were seen in these parameters, with some differential cytotoxic effect between various cell lines due to variable thermal sensitivity. Critical parameters in achieving maximum cell killing rate were applied temperature and exposure time (KAVER et al. 1989).

In the subsequent experiments, the same investigators studied the effects of radiation combined with heat on tumor cell lines (PC-3, DU-145, and 1-LN) evaluating the same parameters. Cells were exposed to different radiation doses up to 200 cGy followed by heat treatment at 43 °C for 1 h. Heat treatment significantly enhanced the radiation response of all the cell lines studied. The combined effect of radiation and heat produced greater cytotoxicity than predicted from the additive effects of the two individual treatment modalities alone (Fig. 14.4) (KAVER et al. 1991a).

These in vitro findings were confirmed in vivo in animal tumor models. KAVER et al. (1991b) investigated the effect of radiation and/or HT on human

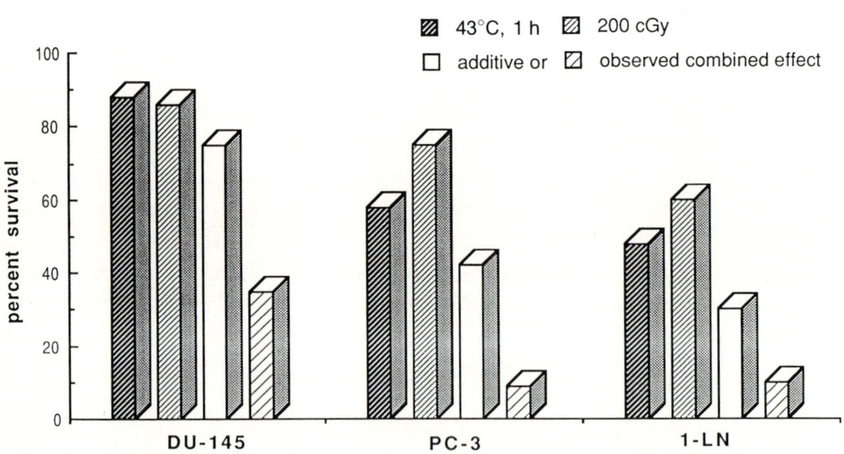

Fig. 14.4. Effects on survival of three human prostate tumor cell lines (DU-145, PC-3, and 1-LN) in cultures after irradiation (200 cGy) or hyperthermia (43 °C for 1 h) or combined treatment. The observed effect of the combined treatment was compared to the calculated additive effects. (From KAVER et al. 1991a)

CaP xenograft in athymic nude mice. A human CaP subline (1-LN-PC-3-1A) was inoculated subcutaneously in the thigh of male athymic nude mice. When tumors reached the appropriate size, they were treated with either radiation (RT) up to 750 cGy in one session or HT by water bath immersion of the leg at 43 °C ± 0.2 °C for 45 min, or an HT-RT combination. In the combined treatment, HT was delivered immediately after radiation exposure. Comparison of the time required to reach twice the tumor volume observed at the time of treatment was used to define therapeutic impact on tumor growth. The tumor doubling time in the combined treatment group was substantially increased over the doubling time obtained for HT alone and radiation alone, suggesting an additive effect of the combined treatment modality (Fig. 14.5). These data were in agreement with those obtained by GOTTLIEB et al. (1988), who used microwave-induced HT and radiation in the Dunning rat prostate tumor model.

TUCKER et al. (1991) reported a substantial decrease in tumor volume in the Dunning prostate tumor model after interstitial HT of 46.5 °C for 2 h. Two HT treatments were administered 48 h apart. These investigators questioned the importance of sequencing of HT treatments in this animal model. More importantly, however, histologic analysis of the tumors demonstrated that the HT caused cell necrosis. Other documented changes were an increased amount of focal solid tumor morphology and an increased amount of stroma. This analysis was performed 27 days after the final treatment. One would, however, expect necrosis to be more evident 1 week after the final treatment. Such necrosis would gradually be absorbed and the normal cell characteristics of the tumor replaced by increased stroma and solid areas of tumor cells (TUCKER et al. 1991).

In conclusion, these in vitro and in vivo observations have indicated therapeutic efficacy of HT as a monotherapy or in combination with radiotherapy. The adjuvant effect of HT on radiation therapy, as well as the importance of several treatment variables such as the applied temperature, exposure time, and

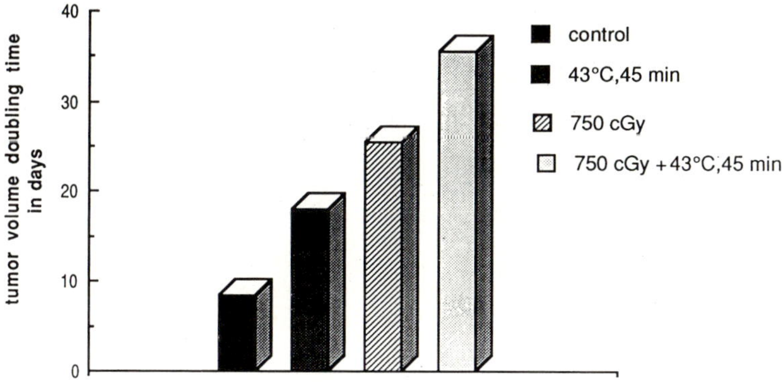

Fig. 14.5. Tumor volume doubling time for human prostatic carcinoma sublines inoculated in the thigh of male athymic nude mice after radiation (750 cGy), hyperthermia (43 °C for 45 min), or combined treatment. (From KAVER et al. 1991b)

fractionation, has been well demonstrated. These data may serve as an important basis for applying heat treatment in BPH patients or as adjunctive treatment for CaP. However, this remains to be elucidated by further well-designed in vivo studies and well-controlled prospective clinical trials with long-term follow-up.

14.3.3 Normal Anatomy and Histology of the Human Prostate

Knowledge of the anatomy and histology of the normal and hyperplastic gland is necessary to understand and interpret observed HT effects in each of these constituents. The relative amounts and location of stromal and epithelial prostatic elements, together with possible differential heat sensitivities, may explain the varying clinical results obtained with different methods of HT application.

The human prostate is a composite organ made up of several glandular and nonglandular components that are tightly fused together within a common capsule. The nonglandular tissues of the prostate include the preprostatic sphincter, striated sphincter, anterior fibromuscular stroma, and prostatic capsule. They are concentrated anteromedially and are responsible for the anterior convexity of the organ. The contour of the glandular prostate approximates a disc with lateral wings that fold anteriorly to encircle the nonglandular tissue. There are four distinct glandular regions (peripheral zone, central zone, transition zone, and periurethral gland region). McNEAL (1988) extensively described this concept of zonal anatomy (Fig. 14.6).

The urethra is considered to be the key anatomic reference structure. The *prostatic urethra* is divided into proximal and distal segments. The proximal

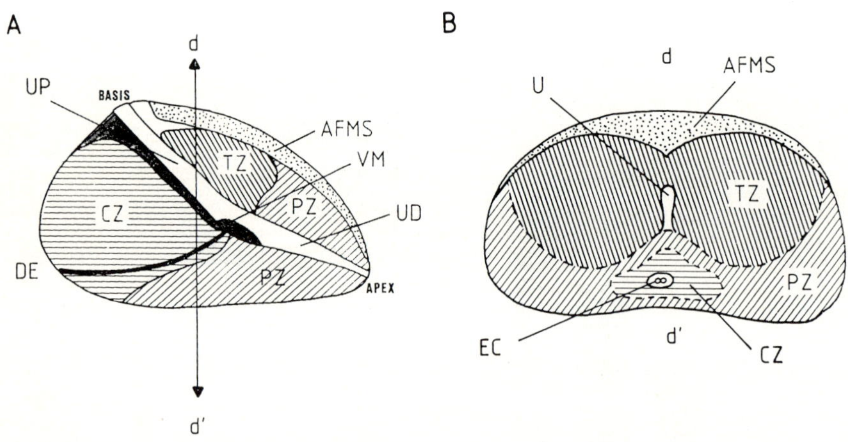

Fig. 14.6A, B. Schematic presentation of prostate zonal anatomy along **A** the sagittal and **B** the coronal prostatic axis. *AFMS*, anterior fibromuscular stroma; *CZ* central zone; *DE*, ejaculatory duct; *EC*, ejaculatory complex; *PZ*, peripheral zone; *TZ* transition zone; *U* urethra; *UD*, Distal urethra; *UP*, proximal urethra; *VM*, verumontanum; *d*, superior part; *d'*, inferior part

urethral wall consists of longitudinal smooth muscle fibers into which the periurethral glands are embedded. The *preprostatic sphincter* surrounds the proximal portion of the urethra from the bladder neck to the top of the verumontanum. The preprostatic sphincter fibers are circular and merge anteriorly with the *anterior fibromuscular stroma*, which comprises the anterior third of the prostate. The *distal smooth sphincter* is located around the distal portion of the urethra, extending from the verumontanum to the apex, where it is in continuity with the external striated sphincter. The *central zone* is a cone-shaped structure consisting of large glands with papillary epithelium surrounded by dense stroma. The ducts of the central zone glands open into the urethra at the verumontanum on either site of the ejaculatory ducts. The *peripheral zone* surrounds the central zone at the posterior, lateral, and inferior aspects. Its glands, which are small and spherical, are composed of smooth epithelial and loose stromal tissue. The ducts drain into the distal urethra on either side of the verumontanum and the crista urethralis. The *transition zone*, which represents only 5% of glandular tissue, consists of two small paraurethral lobes located at the midlevel. Transition zone glands are identical to peripheral zone glands but are less numerous and surrounded by denser stromal tissue. The ducts of this glands arborize and open at the verumontanum just above the ejaculatory duct openings. The *periurethral gland region* is only a fraction of the size of the transition zone. It consists of tiny ducts and abortive acinar systems scattered along the proximal urethra. These glands lie within the longitudinal periurethral smooth muscle stroma. In addition to this zonal anatomy, other anatomic features of the *prostatic capsule* have been identified. The glandular tissue is surrounded by a layer of circularly arranged smooth muscle fibers, which are in continuity with the stromal fibers of the gland. This layer represents the prostatic capsule, which has an average thickness of 0.5 mm.

McNeal (1969) stated that the sites of origin of BPH are in the periurethral glandular area, at the posterior section of the proximal urethra, and in the transition zone, where the transition glands are embedded in the preprostatic sphincter. Nodular enlargement of the periurethral glands and transition zone become, respectively, the "median and lateral lobes" of BPH. Sclerosis of the bladder neck or median bar was not categorized as a prostatic disease but rather as a bladder neck disease. Morphometric analysis of BPH prostate specimens demonstrated the importance of the stromal-to-epithelial ratio in the development of fibromuscular or glandular hyperplasia. McNeal (1969) described the fibromuscular zone distinctly separate from the glandular zone. The transition zone was characterized as having the highest ratio of stromal to epithelial tissues. The second highest ratio was found in the peripheral zone. In the central zone, this ratio was smaller, despite the dense stromal bands of smooth muscles that extended between the large glandular lobules. According to McNeal (1969), 70% of cancers arise in the glandular structures of the peripheral zone, 25% in the transition zone, which may be enlarged by BPH, and 5% in the central zone.

Summarizing, the human prostate is composed of various amounts of glandular tissue embedded in stromal tissue, consisting of smooth muscle and fibrous tissues. These elements are surrounded by a capsule which is surrounded by the major preprostatic venous plexus of Santorini. The ratio of stromal to epithelial elements is dependent upon the zonal region. Since different prostatic tissues may show different heat sensitivities, treatment efficacy can differ depending upon the hyperthermia technique. Important for TUHT is the small amount of glandular tissue and relatively high concentration of stromal elements in the immediate periurethral prostate. The central, deeper-seated target tissues of applications for deep heat penetration (TURF or TUMT) are mainly composed of glandular elements. The main target tissues of TRHT are the glands of the peripheral zone and to a lesser degree of the transition zone. Moreover, the preprostatic venous plexus has major heat-conductive properties, influencing heat absorption during TRHT.

14.3.4 Normal Histology and Anatomy of Animal Prostate

The canine model is considered to be the best prostate model to study histologic and functional changes in the gland following administration of treatment modalities such as hyperthermia and laser therapy. However, it is important to realize that there are major differences between human and canine prostates. Findings from animal studies can only be extrapolated to human disease with appropriate reservations.

Canine prostatic hyperplasia arises diffusely throughout all areas of the prostate, and tissue closer to the urethra may often be less involved than the subcapsular tissue. There are no nodules in canine hyperplasia, unlike in human BPH, in which this enlargement is most often limited to the periurethral tissues and constituted of nodular formations.

Moreover, prostatic hyperplasia in the dog appears to consist purely of proliferation of epithelial cells, whereas the human situation is characterized by both glandular and stromal hyperplasia. The prostate accommodates the increased epithelial cell population by enlargement of existing ducts and acini by displacement of the crowded epithelium into tufts and papillations which partially fill gland lumina (Fig. 14.7). Stereologic analysis has confirmed the visual impression of a primary epithelial hyperplasia without stromal involvement (McNEAL 1990).

Finally, the prostate of dogs has a thinner capsule than that in humans. Dog prostates do not develop a median lobe. This difference in capsule thickness can alter heat penetration patterns and its pathologic effects, especially in transrectal applications of HT.

To summarize, the canine model can be used to study the thermophysical and pathologic effects of HT in prostatic target tissues and surrounding tissues such as the rectum. In view of the above-mentioned interspecies differences, one has to be cautious about extrapolating these data indiscriminately to the human situation.

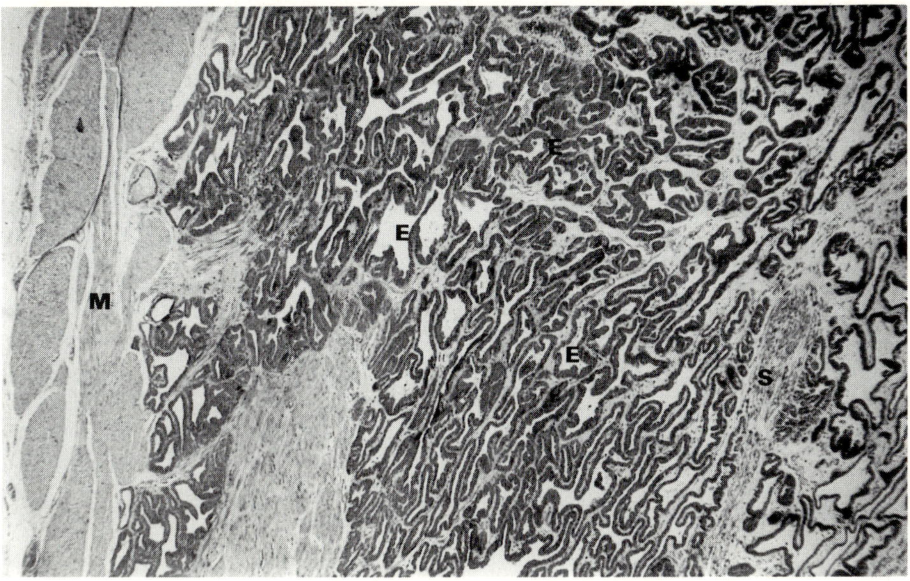

Fig. 14.7. Normal histology of prostatic hyperplastic tissues of the dog. The hyperplasia consists purely of proliferation of epithelial cells (*E*) with minimal stromal involvement (*S*), surrounded by skeletal muscle fibers (*M*). The increased epithelial cell mass is ordered in tufts and papillations that partially fill the gland lumina

14.3.5 Effects of Hyperthermia on Stromal and Epithelial Tissues

There are no published data on the intrinsic heat sensitivity or susceptibility of the different components of the prostatic stromal and epithelial portions such as fibrous, muscular, vascular, and glandular elements. Therefore, we have to rely on general and specific pathologic changes of these elements in other organs and extrapolate the findings to prostatic tissues.

The histopathologic changes following local HT to different *normal* tissues have been only sparsely described, the data deriving mainly from experimental studies in mammals (FAJARDO 1984). Descriptions of pathology are available principally for skin, mesenchymal tissues (skeletal muscle and adipose tissue), liver, small intestine, brain, kidney, and cartilage. Of interest are the lesions previously reported in normal mesenchymal tissues of swine. The early lesions consisted of edema, focal hemorrhage, necrosis, and granulocytic infiltrates, the latter two being more important in muscular tissues (MARTINEZ et al. 1983; MESHORER et al. 1983). The described lesions probably resulted from vascular damage, one of the manifestations of which was increased endothelial permeability. This permeability initially allowed for extravasation of serum, and at a later stage with increasing endothelial damage, also for extravasation of cellular elements, finally leading to thrombosis. In general, the severity of these acute lesions increased with temperature, but never reached the levels of delayed lesions. The delayed lesions consisted of chronic lymphohistiocytic infiltrates, persistent muscle necrosis with some foci of muscle regeneration, and reparative fibrosis.

Also of particular interest are lesions seen in the small intestine of the mouse, as they were found by HUME et al. (1979) to be composed of glandular and subepithelial vascular and smooth muscle elements. The enteric mucosa appeared to be rather thermosensitive. Following application of higher temperatures, lesions were characterized by necrosis of epithelial cells of both villi and crypts, which cessation of mitotic activity. Necrosis of smooth muscle cells was most likely due to the dynamics of heat transfer in vivo. It is of interest to note that smooth muscle cells were initially preserved in blood vessel walls. A probable explanation for this phenomenon was the cooling effect of blood flow in the lumina of the blood vessels, which protected the vessel wall myocytes from more severe heat damage. This blood flow is enhanced by increased tissue temperature and, although able to cool vessel walls sufficiently, was probably insufficient to protect the smooth muscle fibers in the surrounding tissues (EMAMI and SONG 1983; SONG 1984).

14.3.6 Effects of Hyperthermia on Human Malignant Tumors

Morphologic changes have been described in numerous experimental and human tumors exposed to various types of heat treatment. Unfortunately, most observations have again been sporadic; only a few investigators have focused on this specific subject, and then mostly in experimental systems. Nevertheless, the histopathologic changes in human and animal tumors agree and are so characteristic that they justify a general description.

In studies of different experimental animal tumors, the histopathologic reaction following heat treatment in the temperature range from 40.5 °C to 45 °C has been investigated at different times after treatment. The early histopathologic reaction after HT has shown characteristic morphologic changes in all studied experimental tumors. Hemorrhage and edema occur in tumor during and immediately after treatment. They are probably a consequence of early vascular damage that results in stasis and increased vascular permeability combined with a reduction of the functional vascular volume. Progression of tumor damage is seen. Usually, complete cell destruction with the presence of small, apparently destroyed tumor cells is observed within a few to 24 h after heat treatment. In contrast, the stroma and surrounding normal tissues are not generally primarily affected except for moderate edema and hemorrhage, and the stroma cells persist with an apparently normal morphology. It is a typical finding that the nonmalignant cells (such as fibroblasts and endothelial cells) do not manifest the same massive destructive changes as the tumor cells. Within a few days after treatment, a large number of fibroblasts and macrophages gradually invade the necrotic tumor tissue, replacing it by a fibrous scar within 1 or 2 weeks. The pathologic reaction is most pronounced at the upper end of the 40.5°–45 °C range; at the lower temperatures some tumor cells show the described reaction, but a few only minor, and probably reversible, damage, which may be responsible for tumor recurrence within a few days or weeks.

Whereas the initial histopathologic response to HT has been similar in all tumors investigated, the late histopathologic reaction, with subsequent elimination of the destroyed tumor cells and restoration of the tissue architecture, differs widely. In general, tumors are replaced by an ingrowth of fibroblasts and macrophages, ultimately resulting in the formation of a fibrotic scar. In normal tissues, heat-damaged tissue is either completely restored or a permanent fibroserous scar develops.

Treatment with low temperatures and/or short exposure times which do not yield a curative response generally result in the same over all histologic reaction, except that a few apparently morphologically undamaged cells are occasionally found at the tumor periphery or around larger intact blood vessels. Characteristically, recurrences after application of low temperatures are located at the tumor periphery or around larger intact blood vessels. There is experimental evidence that cells situated in such a normal physiologic environment are biologically more resistant to heat than cells situated under environmental conditions characterized by increased acidity, hypoxia, and nutritional depletion. Probably the most decisive factor for heat sensitivity is that the extracellular acidity and the influence of other environmental conditions act indirectly by changing the milieu into a more acidic state. Such environmental conditions are characteristic of large areas in solid tumors and may explain why tumor cells in general are much more sensitive in vivo than similar cells treated in vitro under normal conditions. Furthermore, tumors in vivo are subjected to secondary heat-induced changes in the vascularization, which again may alter the environmental conditions (Overgaard 1983).

14.3.7 Effects of Hyperthermia on Animal Prostatic Tissues

The thermal sensitivity and HT-induced pathologic lesions have been studied in rabbit and canine prostates. Magin et al. (1980) treated the prostates of eight dogs with microwaves (60 °C for 15–22 min) after shielding the rectum and some of the adjacent muscles. At the end of this severe therapy, the prostate was edematous and dark. One week later (four dogs), although the prostate volume was not decreased, there was coagulation necrosis of the entire organ with some foci of neutrophilic infiltrate and/or liquefaction necrosis. Six months later (four dogs) there was no recognizable prostate. The organ had been replaced by a fibrous tissue. Minor lesions were seen in the bladder and the vasa deferentia, but not in the (shielded) rectum (Magin et al. 1980).

Yerushalmi et al. (1982) evaluated normal tissue response to localized deep microwave HT in the prostate and rectal tissues of 59 rabbits. Localized 2450-MHz microwave HT at 43 °C was delivered by means of a coaxial probe in the rectal cavity. This HT was given for 30 min once or twice at an interval of

2 days, without surface cooling. Temperature measurements were performed by placing interstitial thermocouples in the prostate and in rectal mucosa. The 59 rabbits thus treated were examined histologically at multiple times from 1 day to 3 months after exposure. Except in an insignificant number of cases, the authors found no evidence of internal and organ injury up to 3 months after hyperthermic treatment of the prostate. Only minimal changes were present in the rectum, consisting in focal karyopyknosis, inflammatory infiltrates, and edema. These changes were seen in one control and two treated animals. The observed damage in the control animal can be attributed mainly to the mechanical pressure produced in this animal with a smaller than normal rectal cavity. In the treated animal, pressure injury could be enhanced by the addition of heating. More important, however, was the absence of prostatic lesions in all of the treated and examined animals. The short HT sessions and low temperature may have been responsible for this phenomenon.

LEIB et al. (1986) demonstrated definite prostatic and urethral lesions, applying higher temperatures and longer treatment sessions. The investigators applied localized microwave HT to the prostate of dogs, using a transrectal water-cooled skirt-type antenna, operating at 915 MHz. The prostate of 20 male dogs was heated repeatedly under general anesthesia, at temperatures between 40 °C and 47 °C, using treatment times varying from 15 min to 10 h. Histopathologic examination of the prostate invariably showed a mononuclear inflammatory infiltration and edema in the interstitium and polymorphonuclear infiltration in the glandular elements of the prostate. These tissue changes appeared to be time and temperature dependent and correlated well with the applied temperature and the number of HT fractionations. Repeated and prolonged heating at low temperatures (40 °C) did not produce any appreciable histologic lesions, whereas severe necrosis was seen following treatment at 44.5 °C for 1.5 h. Heating at 42.5 °C during multiple sessions of 1.5 h has been found to induce definite histologic evidence of local tissue damage without major toxicity to the surrounding tissues (LEIB et al. 1986).

SERVADIO et al. (1990) applied the same HT with some minor treatment modifications. HT sessions were given for different lengths of time ranging from 90 min to 5 h. Prostate temperatures were monitored by specially constructed copper–constantan thermocouples and ranged between 42.5 °C and 44.5 °C. Grossly, prostate specimens from all dogs showed the same pattern of mononuclear inflammatory infiltrates in the interstitium and polymorphonuclear infiltrates in the glandular elements as already described by LEIB et al. (1986). Rectal lesions consisted of localized venous and lymphatic congestion with consequent submucosal edema; they were believed to be caused by the indwelling applicator in the rectal cavity. Once again, histologic lesions were time and temperature dependent, with the optimal temperature range and time being ca. 42.5 °C for several hours. An important outcome of this study was possible enhancement of cellular immune reactivity as expressed by the high levels of peripheral blood monocytosis found following HT. The authors postulated that this reaction was possibly due to enhanced expression of antigens on the surface of heat-affected cells. On the other hand, values of creatinine phosphokinase (CPK) and serum glutamic oxaloacetic transaminase (SGOT) were found to be irreversibly elevated in those animals which were later found to have definite histopathologic evidence of localized necrosis. These SGOT and CPK levels were perhaps indicators of the degree of cellular damage caused by HT and could allow for treatment monitoring (SERVADIO et al. 1990).

We have recently performed preclinical testing with HT (45 °C for 60 min, one session) in dogs, using a combined transurethral and transrectal approach (DEBICKI et al. 1992). Macroscopic examination showed a distinct area of necrosis between the two target areas of both applicators. At light microscopy, areas of interstitial edema were seen. The glands were dilated and surrounded by interstitial edema. The lumina of the glands were sludged with cellular necrotic material (Fig. 14.8). Some areas showed pronounced focal glandular necrosis with complete destruction of glandular structures and interglandular stroma. The epithelial cells of the glands showed signs of cellular necrosis such as hyperchromatic and pyknotic nuclei (unpublished data).

The pathologic changes observed in animals correlate well with previously reported HT effects. Inflammatory infiltrates are common findings. The presence of more extensive lesions or necrosis, however, is related to treatment temperature and number of HT sessions. Pathologic changes in human prostatic tissue will most likely be influenced by the same treatment variables.

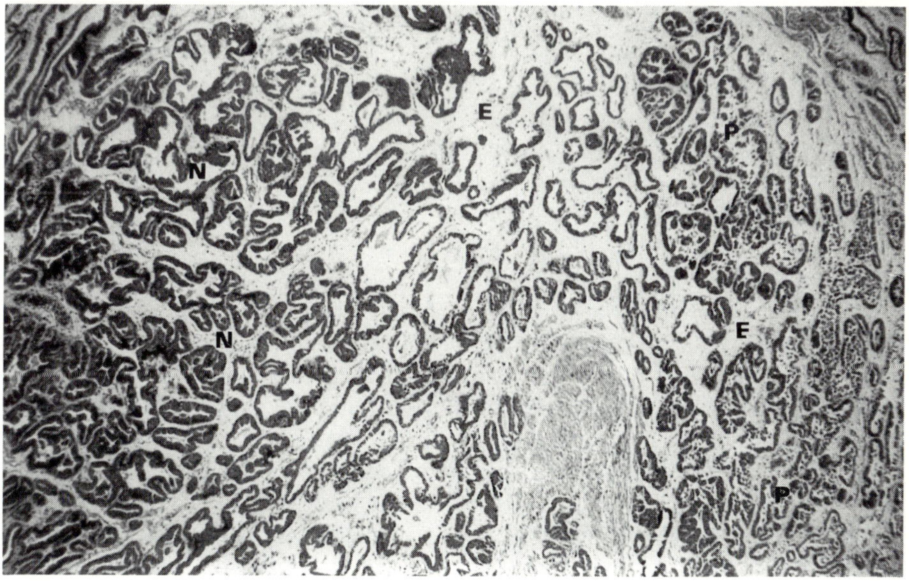

Fig. 14.8. Hyperthermia-induced lesions in the dog's prostate. Early changes after one session of combined TUHT-TRHT (45 °C, 1 h). The normal epithelial structures (*N*) are next to the HT-induced interstitial edema (*E*) and structural changes in glandular epithelium (*P*). The latter consist in dilation of the glands with intraluminal sludging

14.3.8 Hyperthermia Effects in BPH

14.3.8.1 Histologic Lesions in BPH After Transurethral Hyperthermia

The effects of TUHT on benign prostatic tissues were first reported by our group (LAUWERYNS et al. 1991). Histologic lesions were evaluated in adenomectomy specimens of patients who had received TUHT. The first group consisted of patients in acute retention who had failed previous TUHT. All patients received ten TUHT sessions of 60 min at temperatures about 45 °C, Prostates were removed at different intervals (1 week or 4 weeks) to evaluate late lesions in different stages after HT. Early lesions were evaluated in patients who received one TUHT session of 1 h at 45 °C, 24 or 48 h before adenomectomy.

Macroscopically, lesions were seen in the immediate vicinity of the prostatic urethra, particularly in its distal two-thirds, without affecting the bladder neck or external sphincter. These symmetrical, periurethral lesions were cup shaped and consisted of dark and hemorrhagically infiltrated parenchyma. The lesions extended approximately 6 mm radially from the urethra and 4–5 cm longitudinally, and corresponded well with the heating profile of the helical microwave antenna, as determined in phantoms (ASTRAHAN et al. 1991).

Acute changes, 24–48 h after HT, consisted of periurethral edema and parenchymal hemorrhages; the edema extended farther radially from the urethra than did the interstitial hemorrhages. The immediately adjacent smooth muscle fibers showed early coagulation necrosis. The vessel walls and their smooth muscles, however, were normal. In the immediate periurethral area, occasional early venular thrombosis and dense lymphocytic infiltrates were seen. Initially, no changes in periurethral prostatic ducts were seen (Fig. 14.9).

Microscopic examination of the macroscopically observed dark areas revealed the presence of complete hemorrhagic necrosis of the prostatic parenchyma, including the glands and ducts. There was thrombotic obliteration of blood vessels with necrosis of their walls; these changes were less severe deeper in the parenchyma. They consisted of coagulation necrosis, which was limited to the smooth muscle fibers, or fibrinoid necrosis of the blood vessel walls without thrombotic obliteration of their lumina. A sharp transition was present between the abnormal (fibrinoid necrosis) and normal walls of the vessels (Fig. 14.10).

Clear evidence of a varying degree of organization by ingrowing granulation tissue was seen. In the earliest stage this process was restricted to a band-like area which extended along the border of the periurethral hemorrhagic necrotic zone. Progressively, the entire necrotic zone was infiltrated by ingrowing granulation tissue. Edematous loose connective tissue was noted containing the same mononuclear cells and leukocytes as well as hemosiderin-laden macrophages and occasional collagen fiber deposits. In this stage of organization, early attempts at reepithelialization of the urethra were present (Fig. 14.11). In a later phase after 4 weeks, lesions were generally more organized and advanced, although all phases of organization of granulation tissue could be

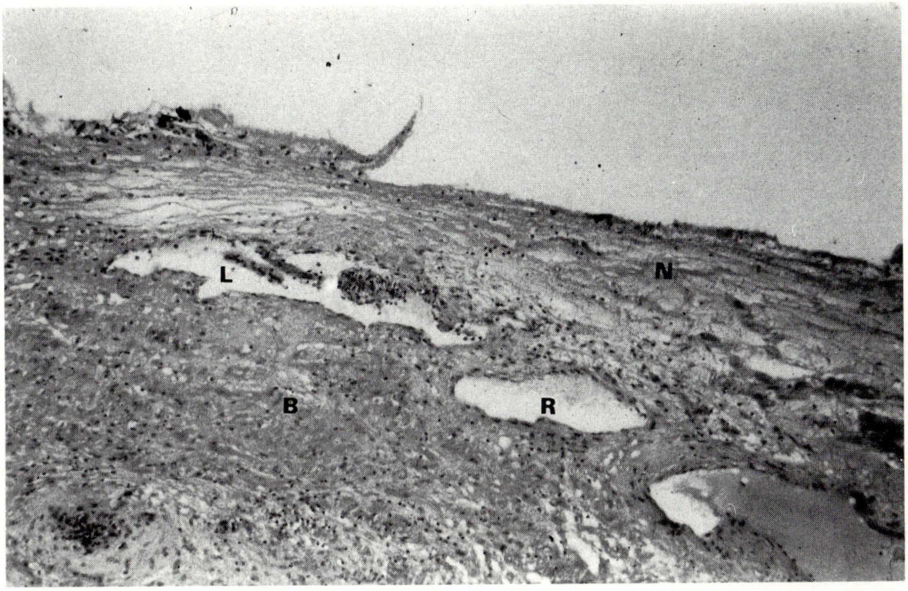

Fig. 14.9. Early lesions after one session of TUHT in human prostates. The urothelium is eroded. The corium shows bleeding and edema (*B*). The latter extends between normal underlying smooth muscle bundles. The upper submucosal corium is nearly necrotic (*N*). Some superficial venules demonstrate partial thrombosis (*L*). The other venules appear normal (*R*). Sparse lymphocytic infiltrates are present

seen (Fig. 14.12). In this organized tissue, several round and oval units were seen. These units had a central core of cell-poor and organized fibrous tissue (Fig. 14.13). Likewise, occasional ghost vessels with hyalinized walls and obliterated lumina with loose connective tissue were observed. They probably represented the final stages of organization of thrombosed and necrotic blood vessels (Fig. 14.14).

Grossly, the same lesions were seen after TURF. Macroscopically, these lesions extended 5–10 mm radially from the urethra. Histologic examination revealed areas of focal glandular necrosis around a preserved urethra. Microscopically, these necrotic areas had a ghost-like outline containing eosinophilic material. The glands had undergone malpighian metaplasia but were well preserved. The necrotic glands were further surrounded by inflammatory infiltrates consisting principally of lymphocytes. The severity and distribution of these histologic changes depended upon the applied temperature, the fractionation scheme, and the heating characteristics of the applicator (van den Bossche et al. 1991).

Heat-induced pathologic changes in the prostate were evaluated at various intervals after TUMT with interstitial temperatures $> 45\,^{\circ}\mathrm{C}$. Serial radial sections of the gland showed preservation of urethral mucosa and periurethral tissue within a distance of 2–4 mm from the urethral lumen. Beyond, necrosis of

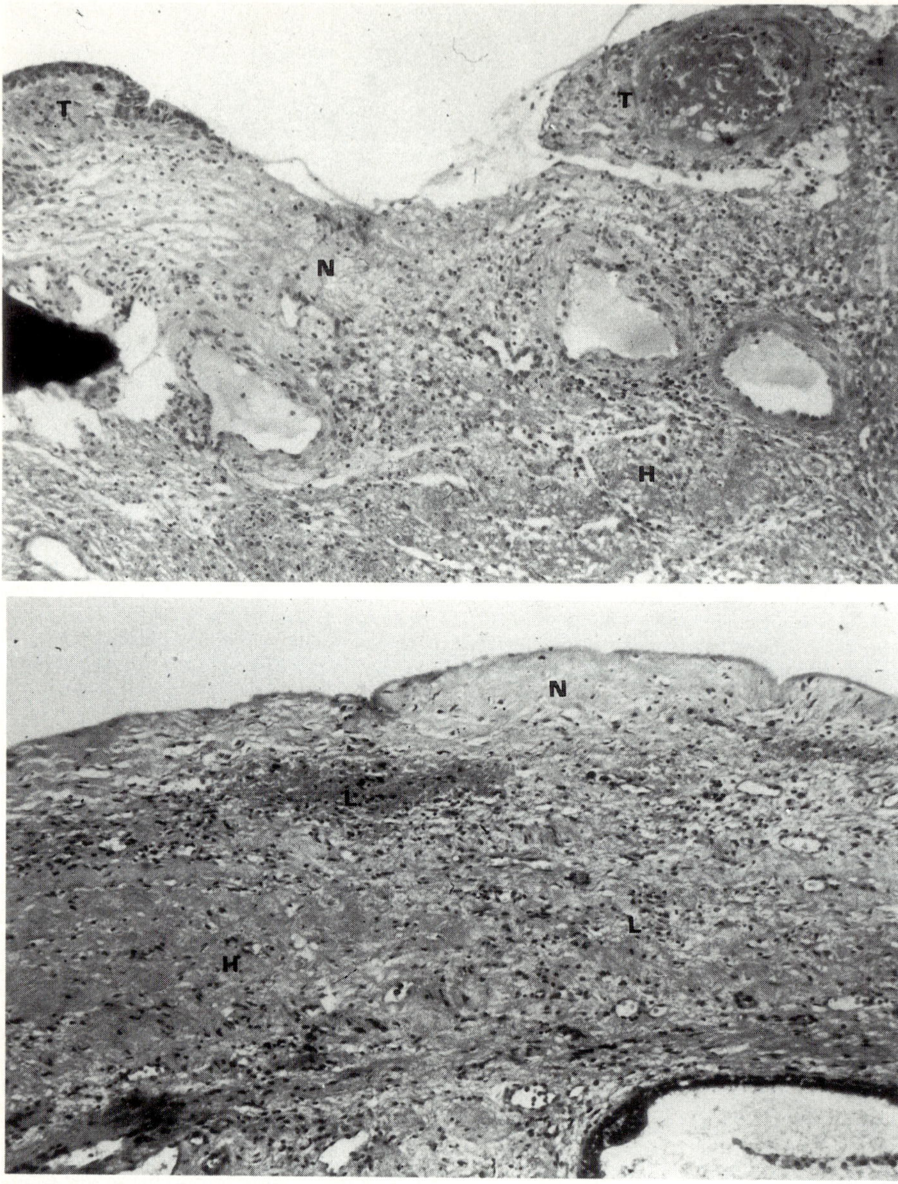

a

b

Fig. 14.10a,b. Early lesions after ten sessions of TUHT in human prostates. **a** After ten sessions, blood vessels are completely thrombosed (*T*), and there is marked interstitial hemorrhage (*H*). The superficial urethral area shows further necrosis (*N*) with completely eroded urothelium. **b** Necrotic (*N*) and hemorrhagic (*H*) areas are infiltrated by lymphocytes (*L*) and hemosiderin-laden macrophages, clearing up the hemorrhagic areas

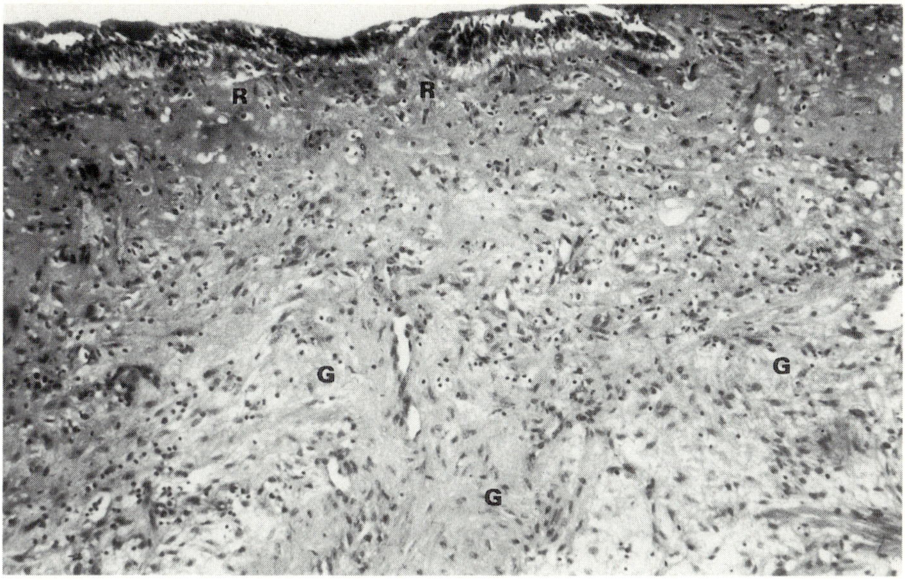

Fig. 14.11. Early organization phase after TUHT in human prostate. At 26 days after TUHT, an early organization phase is demonstrated. Ingrowing granulation tissue (*G*) is invading the periurethral parenchyma, replacing the interstitial edema and necrotic tissues. At the same time, a process of urethral reepithelialization is observed (*R*)

adenomatous tissue was observed up to a depth of 15 mm from the urethra and was roughly symmetrical in both lobes. At 2 months the necrotic tissue had been replaced by a homogeneous fibrotic tissue. Microscopic examination of the treated area after 1 week showed an intense edematous reaction and destruction of stromal and glandular cells. A mild inflammatory reaction with lymphocytes and mononucleated cells was observed. Capillaries had been destroyed, while vessels with a larger diameter were preserved, probably protected by an efficient blood flow. The transition between the treated and nontreated area was sharp (1–2 mm in width), suggesting that the cell toxicity threshold is sharp as well. At the cellular level, smooth muscle cells were found to be more sensitive to heat than acinar cells. After 2 months the treated area was replaced by a retractile fibrosis comparable to the ischemic fibrosis observed after infarction (DEVONEC et al. 1991).

14.3.8.2 Histologic Lesions in BPH After Transrectal Hyperthermia

Histologic evaluations of BPH tissue after TRHT have not been performed extensively. Changes in prostatic tissue on light microscopy or morphometric analysis have been reported by some authors. However, their data have generally been controversial.

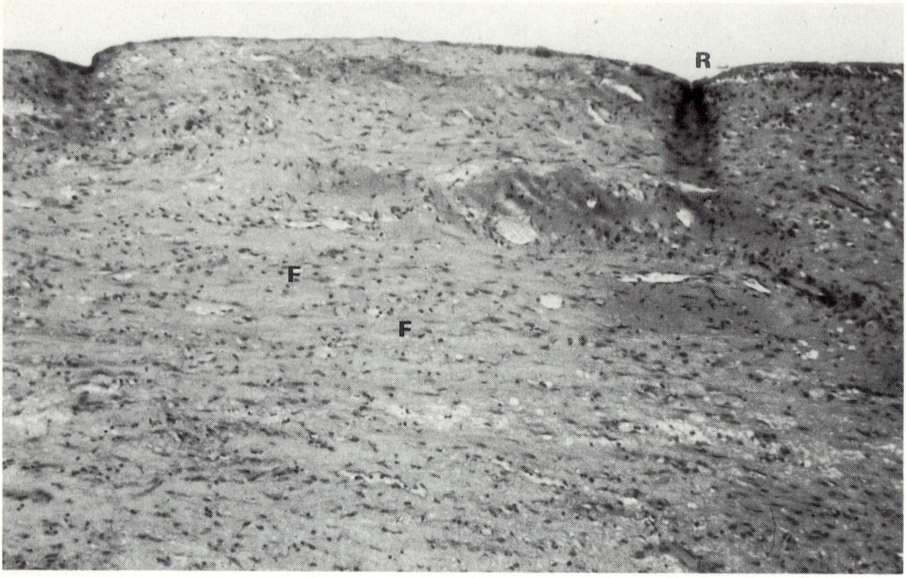

Fig. 14.12. Late organization phase after TUHT in human prostate. In a later stage, end-stage periurethral fibrosis (*F*) with reepithelialization is demonstrated (*R*). The well-layered fibrotic reorganization contrasts with normal periurethral corium structure and previous hyperthermia-induced lesions

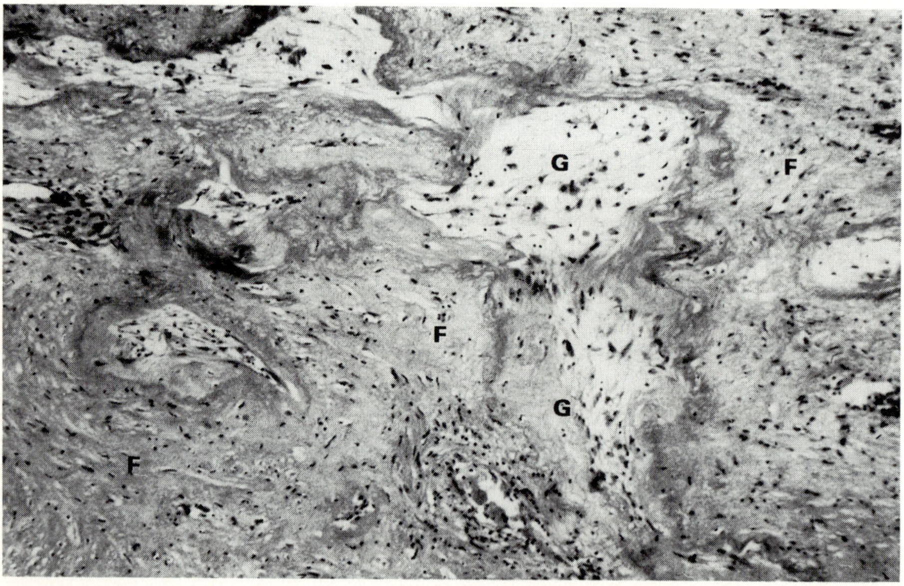

Fig. 14.13. Fibrotic reorganization of periurethral tissue after TUHT. In some areas, end-stage periurethral fibrosis (*F*) is characterized by strands of fibrotic tissues, infiltrated by fibroblasts and macrophages, and the presence of ghost vessels (*G*)

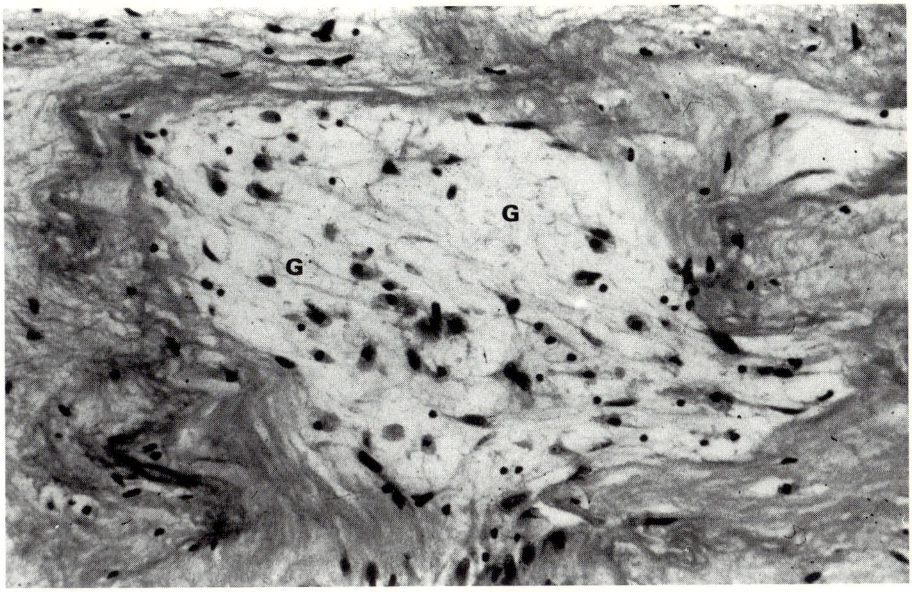

Fig. 14.14. Details of ghost vessels in end-stage periurethral fibrotic tissue after TUHT. Occasional ghost vessels (*G*) with hyalinized walls and obliterated lumina with loose connective tissue are observed. They represent the final stages of organization of thrombosed and necrotic blood vessels

MONTORSI et al. (1992) performed extensive morphologic studies with light microscopy on heated prostates and nonheated controls after surgical treatment. This group showed mild chronic inflammatory infiltrates throughout the gland. Inflammatory infiltrates often presented with a pseudofollicular appearance which was particularly evident in the interstitium around the periurethral glands. The glandular epithelium did not show any morphologic changes induced by TRHT. Morphometric analysis of the prostates surgically removed after TRHT did not show any significant changes in the area of the glandular epithelium and stromal tissue in heated and nonheated specimens. In contrast, morphometric analysis did reveal an HT-induced increase in the number of capillary-like vessels, which was statistically significant. These vessels had thin walls and a tortuous course, suggestive of a neovascularization process.

SIEGEL et al. (1991) recently evaluated morphometrically changes in the volume of different prostatic components after TRHT (ten 1-h sessions at 42° ± 1.5°C). The volumes of glandular, fibrous, muscular, and vascular components were evaluated in patients who failed to respond to HT treatment and underwent adenomectomy or TURP at various intervals after the last TRHT session. These data were compared with a matched BPH control group. The glandular and vascular elements appeared to play no part in this phenomenon. There were no intergroup differences in the volume fraction of these components. Conversely, the nonglandular tissue of the prostate appeared to be heat sensitive. Included in this component are the preprostatic sphincter, the anterior fibromuscular stroma and the prostatic capsule, the nerves, and the blood vessels. A significant reduction in the volume of fibrous tissue was found in the study group compared with the control group, as was a significant increase in the volume occupied by muscle cells. Given the random selection of patients to the HT group, the investigators postulated that at the onset of the study the various tissue components which were evaluated occupied the same volume fractions in all patients. Therefore, the differences observed after treatment would represent the effect of HT. On the other hand, since one cannot anticipate an increase in muscular elements in response to treatment, it is possible that patients become responders or nonresponders to HT on the basis of BPH morphology. According to this theory, higher response rates would be expected in fibromuscular hyperplasia, depending upon the relative fraction of the fibrous and muscular components. Perhaps the most favorable BPH histology from the HT point of view consists of glands with a high proportion of fibrous elements. Lower response rates could be found in glandular hyperplasia (SIEGEL et al. 1991).

These data on gross morphometric histologic analysis, however, seem to contradict the reports of the same authors on immunohistochemical changes in the prostate following TRHT (SIEGEL et al. 1992). The authors performed morphometric analysis on biopsies of prostatic tissue before and after TRHT in an attempt to determine which components within the stromal (fibromuscular) fraction may respond to heat. Three cytoskeletal proteins have been shown to represent reliable discrimination markers between smooth muscle cells and fibroblasts. α-Smooth muscle actin (α-SM) and desmin (DES) express the phenotypic features of smooth muscle cells whereas vimentin (VIM) expresses the phenotypic features of fibroblasts. A significant increase ($P < 0.04$) was seen in VIM levels, while there were less pronounced increases in α-SM and DES. The investigators concluded that this VIM increase represented the growth and hyperplasia of fibroblasts stimulated most probably by heat. These data conflict with the observation of a decrease in the relative volume fraction of fibrous tissues in these authors' previous report (SIEGEL et al. 1991). Further studies are needed to explain this discrepancy in the reported data. Nonetheless, this morphometric analysis represents an attractive method for the evaluation of morphologic changes in prostates after HT.

14.3.8.3 Histologic Lesions in Human Prostatic Carcinoma After TRHT

STROHMAIER et al. (1991) investigated the effects of heat on prostatic cancer. Twenty patients with untreated CaP underwent local HT, each receiving four sessions of 60 min at temperatures of 43 °C. Pathology of pretreatment punch biopsies was compared to posttreatment specimens, obtained by radical prostatectomy ($n = 8$) and punch biopsy or TURP ($n = 12$). Histologic effects were generally in all patients. The prostatic stroma showed distinct edema and diffuse lymphoplasmacellular infiltration throughout the whole gland, suggesting interstitial inflammation. Bleeding into the interstitium and hyperemic capillary blood vessels could be found. Damaged blood vessels showed a swelling of the wall. In the center of the prostatic glands macrophages laden with hemosiderin were observed as a sign of previous bleeding. In some patients, groups of necrotic glands were seen. Definite signs of tumor cell necrosis however, could not be observed in any of the patients. Only slight vacuolation of the cytoplasm of some tumor cells was observed, which was also seen before HT. The authors concluded that previously described volume decrease in prostatic cancer cannot be explained by histologically proven tumor cell destruction (Strohmaier et al. 1991).

14.4 Biochemical and Immunologic Changes in Patients After Hyperthermia

Histologic changes in prostatic tissues after HT are an indicator of HT-induced effects. However, the presence of specific histologic lesions cannot be considered as proof of therapeutic efficacy. Changes in prostate specific antigen (PSA) may be a biochemical sign of HT-induced cellular damage. However, there have been conflicting reports on PSA changes with different HT applications. Immunologic changes after HT can suggest a stimulation of cell-mediated immunity and explain therapeutic response in CaP patients, but reported results are again controversial. A systematic review of these two items will be presented.

14.4.1 Changes in Prostate Specific Antigen After Hyperthermia

Prostate specific antigen is a kallikrein-like, serine protease that is produced exclusively by the epithelial cells lining the acini and ducts of the prostate. After immunoperoxidase staining techniques, none of the other cellular components of the prostate, including the stromal and vascular elements, stain for PSA. PSA is further secreted into the lumina of the prostatic ducts and is present in the seminal plasma at rather high concentrations. This protein has also been detected in the epithelial cells of BPH tissue and primary and metastatic CaP tissue. Serum PSA is a highly organ-specific marker but has a low sensitivity since it is produced by normal, hyperplastic, and cancerous tissues. Furthermore, PSA can be elevated after prostatitis, acute retention, infarction, transrectal and transurethral manipulations, and prostate biopsies. This serum marker, however, is actually the most accurate marker for monitoring residual tumor activity after surgery, radiation, or hormonotherapy.

Serum PSA elevations occur by leakage of PSA out of epithelial cells due to hyperplastic increase in the epithelial mass, trauma, or structural changes due to inflammation, necrosis, or malignancy. This phenomenon in the latter situations is most likely due to locally high PSA concentrations produced by cellular damage or proliferation and/or disorganization of the basal cell layer. It is possible that a disruption of the epithelial basement membrane allows the low-molecular-weight PSA molecule to diffuse more easily from the lumina of the acini to the lumen of the adjacent capillary or lymphatic (OESTERLING 1991). PSA could be a marker of HT-induced changes and/or necrosis in periurethral and adenomatous tissues, as suggested by the various pathology reports. Furthermore, PSA could allow monitoring of HT application and assessment of treatment efficacy.

The reported results on PSA changes in BPH patients are conflicting and dependent upon the applied HT modality and technique. LINDNER et al. (1990) reported no PSA changes during and after five sessions of TRHT at 43 °C. The authors concluded that this treatment apparently has no destructive effects on the epithelial cells. These biochemical data correlated with the histologic absence of cellular necrosis after TRHT (MONTORSI et al. 1992). After TUHT, we noticed no PSA changes after five sessions at 45 °C (unpublished data). This lack of PSA change can be explained by the heating profile of the helical antenna, which only affects the periurethral tissues at a radial distance of $\pm$ 6 mm. This periurethral region is mainly constituted of stromal elements and not of epithelial elements.

A threefold increase in PSA was seen after TURF at 45 °C. Although advocates of this method claim a deeper penetration pattern, histologic lesions were not seen beyond 5–10 mm radially from the urethra (VAN DEN BOSSCHE et al. 1991). These results conflict with the TUHT data, since both techniques show approximately the same degree and distribution of lesions. After one session of TUMT at temperatures between 45 °C and 55 °C, very high PSA levels were seen immediately after treatment, normalizing to the pretreatment levels at a later follow-up. The higher treatment temperatures, together with necrosis in central adenomatous tissues, were a possible explanation for the elevated PSA levels (LADUC et al. 1992).

The role of PSA in monitoring HT application and evaluating treatment efficacy remains to be determined. However, the amount of PSA increase does not correlate well with therapeutic efficacy. The above data clearly indicate that PSA changes are dependent upon the applied method and cannot simply be considered as a general indicator of efficacy for all HT applications.

14.4.2 Immunologic Changes Following Prostatic Hyperthermia

Immunologic changes after HT have been extensively studied in laboratory animals and in patients treated with whole-body HT. Recently, SZMIGIELSKI et al. (1991) studied the reactions of the host immune system to local TRHT (see Chap. 15). The authors evaluated several parameters of cell-mediated immunity such as T-lymphocyte and T-cell subsets, mitogenic responses, and natural killer

(NK) cytotoxic activity in BPH and CaP patients before and after TRHT. The group of CaP patients showed a depressed cell-mediated immunity prior to the administration of TRHT. A transient significant ($P < 0.01$) stimulation of the tested cell-mediated immune parameters and NK cytotoxic activity was noted after TRHT. The peak of this stimulation was noted at 2 months with a subsequent decrease to the pretreatment levels at 6 months. The 15 BPH patients had immune parameters within the normal limits and showed a lesser degree of immune stimulation after TRHT.

We recently evaluated several immunologic parameters in CaP patients after TUHT. These parameters consisted of lymphocyte transformation tests, NK cell activity, mixed lymphocyte cultures, and cellular differentiation of human lymphocytes. In the first analysis of our data, we could not reproduce the data reported by SZMIGIELSKI et al. (1988) nor confirm changes in cell-mediated immunity parameters (unpublished data).

It is apparent that more work should be done to investigate the mechanisms involved in the stimulation of cell-mediated immunity by local HT, especially in the treatment of CaP. Analysis of the role of granulocytic and lymphocytic infiltrations, as seen in several histopathologic studies of prostatic tissues after HT, is mandatory. These infiltrates can indicate inflammatory reactions that might be responsible for triggering the general stimulation of the host's cell-mediated immunity. The importance of applied temperature and degree of tissue-heat interaction cannot be overlooked. We recently started an evaluation of cell-mediated immunity after combined TUHT and TRHT, which assures higher and more homogeneous heating of the prostate. If more pronounced immunologic changes are seen with this method, it is indicative that HT can induce immunologic effects.

14.5 Possible Mechanisms of Action of Hyperthermia in BPH and Prostatic Carcinoma

The working mechanism of action of local HT on benign and malignant prostatic tissues remains unknown. At present, histologic examination of prostates after different HT applications serves only to define pathologic lesions. These lesions, seen on light microscopy, do not necessarily prove therapeutic efficacy. Moreover, the degree and site of these lesions differ not only between transrectal and transurethral modalities, but also between different transurethral applications. Differences in antenna heating profiles, microwave penetration depth, and treatment temperatures may all account for heterogeneous pathologic and biochemical results. Nonetheless, most authors report similar clinical results, suggesting multiple interactions at different levels of the pathophysiology of BPH. Possible mechanisms of action can only be postulated by correlating these new pathologic findings with previous findings and knowledge of general HT effects in other tissues. Finally, these mechanisms and treatment outcomes can be influenced by the complex multifactorial pathogenesis of prostatic diseases, in particular BPH.

14.5.1 Hypothetical Mechanisms of Action of Hyperthermia in BPH Patients

The mechanism of action of local microwave HT in BPH patients is intrinsically related to the pathophysiology of BPH. The mechanism of infravesical obstruction in men is dependent upon a balance of detrusor function and static and/or dynamic low outflow obstructive components.

The static component is related to the obstruction of the bladder outlet resulting from enlargement of the adenoma. The morphology and stromal/epithelial ratio of the enlarged prostate are important pathophysiologic variables. The valve-like action of a median lobe or the sclerotic bladder neck stenosis due to median bar represents a urodynamically severe obstacle which only can be cured by surgery. The histologic composition of the prostatic adenoma seems clearly related to the development of symptomatic BPH. The mean stroma-to-epithelium ratio is significantly higher in symptomatic men than in asymptomatic ones (SHAPIRO et al. 1992).

The dynamic component is related to the tone of the smooth muscles at the bladder neck, prostatic tissue, and capsule, which is mediated by α_1-adrenoreceptors. However, the development of clinical BPH does not appear to be only related to increased adrenergic activation, since inverse relationships have been observed between norepinephrine tissue levels and severity of symptoms (LEPOR et al. 1990).

The exact mechanism of action of local HT on BPH tissues remains unknown. From our pathologic findings, we have formulated a hypothesis to explain the mechanism of TUHT action on the prostatic tissue (Fig. 14.15). Following HT, there is marked parenchymal edema, microhemorrhages, and destruction of myofibrillar proteins leading to superficial myonecrosis. This leads to progressive endothelial damage with increased vessel wall permeability and extravasation of serum and cellular elements. The end lesion results in complete obliteration and thrombosis of superficial vessels. This leads to a reduction in local blood flow and compromised heat conduction, which promotes elevation of local tissue temperatures and secondary necrosis. Multiple HT sessions cause progressive increase in parenchymal injury and help to increase the radial extent of histologic changes. This in turn results in further reduction of blood flow and secondary narrowing and obliteration of deeper blood vessels followed by a reparative process consisting of phagocytosis and granulation with subsequent fibrosis and retraction of the urethra. This fibrosis of periurethral tissues to a depth of 6–8 mm leads to periurethral shrinking, dilates the prostatic urethra, and lowers the static outflow obstruction component of BPH. Especially the progressive increase in the degree of parenchymal injury and the

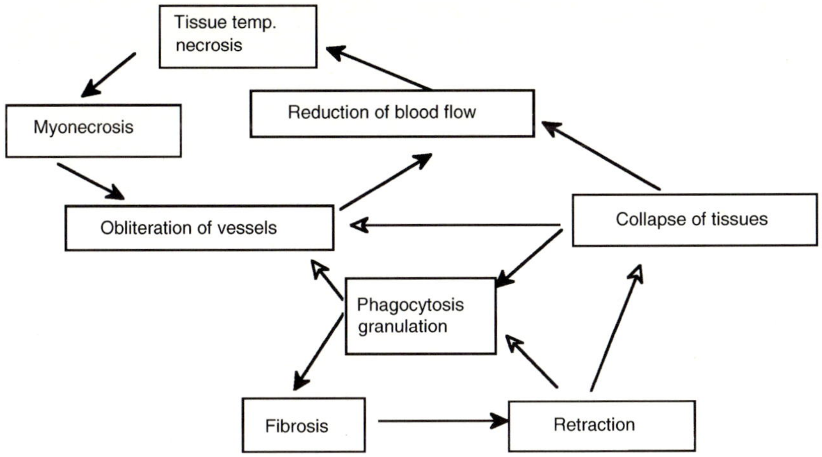

Fig. 14.15. Hypothetical mechanism of action of TUHT in BPH

increase in the depth of HT penetration are important factors which justify the need for repetitive treatment sessions in TUHT applications. The depth of penetration is further related to the heating profiles of the different antennas. The maximum effect of TUHT treatments occurs at between 5 and 10 mm radially from the urethra (Astrahan et al. 1991). This limited penetration can explain the moderate improvements in objective outflow parameters and the possibility of recurrence at long-term follow-up. The posttreatment periurethral fibrosis can be cleared up by dynamic reparative processes. The morphology of the prostate remains another important determinant. Bilobar hyperplasia is characterized by a regular, symmetrical prostatic urethra, assuring optimal tissue-heat interaction by close contact between antenna and target tissues. TUHT is not indicated in patients with median lobe or median bar prostate configurations since only the superior parts of the obstructive tissues are treated, without substantially relieving the mechanical obstruction at the bladder neck (Baert et al. 1991).

The discrepancy between good subjective response and moderate pathologic lesions without necrosis, as seen after TRHT, raises questions as to other possible mechanisms of action. Interaction or modification of α-receptors after local HT can lower dynamic obstructive components. Differential heat sensitivity of the various elements of the prostate adenoma can explain varying treatment outcomes in morphometrically different prostates. Siegel et al. (1991) postulated that fibrous elements in the prostatic stroma are highly heat sensitive. Heat-induced changes in this component which constrict the stromal supporting structure of the entire gland can reduce tissue tone, and hence dynamic obstruction (Lepor et al. 1990). It is possible that differences in the stromal-to-epithelial ratio and relative proportions of stromal fibrous elements of the treated adenomas determine treatment response.

14.5.2 Hypothetical Mechanisms of Action of Hyperthermia in Prostatic Carcinoma Patients

The in vivo mechanism of action of local HT on CaP is questionable. Pathologic examinations did not reveal any significant tumor necrosis or significant tissue changes which can explain shrinkage of CaP mass after local HT (SZMIGIELSKI et al. 1988). The presence of lymphoplasmacellular infiltrates after local HT, however, indicates the existence of inflammatory reactions that might possibly be responsible for triggering the general stimulation of the host's cell-mediated immunity and inducing secondary tumor regression (STROHMAIER et al. 1991). Until further research explains its mechanism of action, HT monotherapy cannot be considered as a treatment for patients with CaP. Hyperthermia may, however, be useful as an adjuvant treatment when it is combined with prostatic irradiation.

14.6 Conclusion

Pathologic effects of HT on various benign and malignant tissues have been well studied in vitro and in vivo. Changes in prostatic tissues, however, have not been well documented. Despite this limited knowledge, we can assume that these tissues show some similar histologic and pathophysiologic response patterns.

Since the introduction of local microwave HT for BPH and CaP, renewed efforts have been made to define biophysical effects and possible mechanisms of action of prostate heating. Fundamental insights into the mechanisms will allow us to optimize HT treatments for prostatic diseases.

The importance of a number of treatment variables on dose–effect relationships and treatment outcome has to be studied. Duration, length, and fractionation of sessions, temperature, and penetration depth all influence the severity of pathologic lesions after local HT. Hence, optimization of technique is expected to improve treatment outcome. The effect of vasodilation in heated tissues is to improve drug diffusion and molecular interactions. The adjuvant role of HT in drug therapy for BPH (5α-reductases inhibitors, α-blockers, etc.) and CaP (antiandrogens, LH-RH analogues, etc.) needs further research. The radiosensitizing effect of HT in combination with several radiotherapeutic options (external beam or interstitial radiotherapy) probably opens new perspectives for the treatment of locally advanced CaP. Further insights into biologic effects are needed to optimize HT as monotherapy or adjuvant therapy for prostatic diseases.

References

Astrahan MA, Ameye F, Oyen R, Willemen P, Baert L, Petrovich Z (1991) Interstitial temperature measurements during transurethral microwave hyperthermia. J Urol 145: 304–308

Baert L, Ameye F, Willemen P, Vandenhove J, Lauweryns J, Astrahan M, Petrovich Z (1990)

Transurethral microwave hyperthermia for benign prostatic hyperplasia: preliminary clinical and pathological results. J Urol 144: 1383–1387

Baert L, Willemen P, Ameye F, Petrovich Z (1991) Treatment response with transurethral microwave hyperthermia in different forms of benign prostatic hyperplasia: a preliminary report. Prostate 18: 315–320

Carper SW, Duffy JJ, Gerner EW (1987) Heat shock proteins in thermotolerance and other cellular processes. Cancer Res 47: 5249–5255

Dahl O (1986) Hyperthermia and drugs. In: Watmough DW, Ross WM (eds) Hyperthermia. Blackie, London, pp 121–153

Debicki P, Astrahan MA, Ameye F, Oyen R, Baert L, Haczewski A, Petrovich Z (1992) Temperature steering in prostate by simultaneous transurethral and transrectal hyperthermia. Urology 40: 300–307

Devonec M, Berger N, Bringeon N, et al. (1991) Short and long term histological effects of transurethral microwave therapy (TUMT) on benign prostatic hypertrophy. J. Urol 145: 363A, abstract 603

Dewey WC, Freeman ML, Raaphorst GP, et al. (1980) Cell biology of hyperthermia and radiation. In: Meyn RE, Withers HR (eds) Radiation biology in cancer research. Raven, New York, pp 589–621

Dickson JA, Calderwood SK (1980) Temperature range and selective sensitivity of tumors to hyperthermia: a critical review. Ann NY Acad Sci 335: 180–205

Emami B, Song CW (1984) Physiological mechanisms in hyperthermia: a review. Int J Radiat Biol Phys 10: 289–295

Fajardo LF (1984) Pathological effects of hyperthermia in normal tissues. Cancer Res (suppl) 44: 4826s–4835s

Gerweck LE (1985) Hyperthermia in cancer therapy: the biological basis and unresolved questions. Cancer Res 45: 3408–3414

Gottlieb CF, Seibert GB, Block NL (1988) Interaction of irradiation and microwave induced hyperthermia in the Dunning R3327G prostatic adenocarcinoma model. Radiology 169: 243–252

Hume SP, Marigolld JC, Field SB (1979) The effects of local hyperthermia on the small intestine of mouse. Br J Radiol 52: 657–662

Kaver I, Ware JL, and Koontz WW (1989) The effect of hyperthermia on human prostatic carcinoma cell lines: evaluation in vitro. J Urol 141: 1025–1027

Kaver I, Ware JL, Wilson JD, Guice JM, Ware JL (1991a) Effect of radiation combined with hyperthermia on human prostatic carcinoma cell lines in culture. Urology 37: 88–92

Kaver I, Koontz WW, Wilson JD, Guice JM, Ware JL (1991b) The effect of radiation therapy and hyperthermia on a human prostatic carcinoma cell line grown in athymic nude mice. J Urol 145: 654–656

Laduc R, Bloem F, Debruyne F (1992) Transurethral microwave therapy (TUMT) in benign prostatic hyperplasia. J Urol 147: 344A, abstract 527

Lauweryns J, Baert L, Vandenhove J, Petrovich Z (1991) Histopathology of prostatic tissue after transurethral hyperthermia. Int J Hyperthermia 7: 221–230

Leib Z, Rothem A, Lev A, Servadio C (1986) Histopathological observations in the canine prostate treated by local microwave hyperthermia. Prostate 8: 93–102

Lepor H, Shapiro E, Bowsher RR, Henry DP (1990) Determination of norepinephrine levels in the adult human prostate. J Urol 144: 1263–1266

Lindner A, Siegel YI, Korczak D (1990) Serum prostate specific antigen levels during hyperthermia treatment of benign prostatic hyperplasia. J Urol 144: 1388–1389

Magin RL, Fridd CW, Bonfiglio TA, Linke CA (1980) Thermal destruction of the canine prostate by high intensity microwaves. J Surg Res 29: 265–275

Martinez A, Meshorer A, Meyer L, Hahn G, Fajardo L, Prionas S (1983) Thermal sensitivity and thermotolerance in normal porcine tissues. Cancer Res 43: 2072–2075

McNeal JE (1969) Origin and development of carcinoma in the prostate Cancer 23: 24–33

McNeal JE (1988) Normal histology of the prostate. Am J Surg Pathol 12: 619–633

McNeal JE (1990) Pathology of benign prostatic hyperplasia. Insight into etiology. Urol Clin North Am 17:477–486

Mendecki J, Friedenthal E, Botstein C, Paglione R, Sterzer F (1980) Microwave applicators for localized hyperthermia treatment of cancer of the prostate. Int J Radiat Oncol Biol Phys 6:1583–1589

Meshorer A, Prionas S, Fajardo L, Meyer J, Hahn G, Martinez A (1983) The effects of hyperthermia on normal mesenchymal tissues. Arch Path ol Lab Med 107:328–339

Montorsi F, Galli L, Guazzoni G, et al. (1992) Transrectal microwave hyperthermia for benign prostatic hyperplasia: long-term clinical, pathological and ultrastructural patterns. J Urol 148:321–325

Oesterling JE (1991) Prostate specific antigen: a critical assessment of the most useful tumor marker for adenocarcinoma of the prostate. J Urol 145:907–923

Oleson JR, Calderwood SK, Coughlin CT, Dewhirst MW, Gerweck LE, Gibbs FA, Kapp DS (1980) Biological and clinical aspects of hyperthermia in cancer therapy. Am J Clin Oncol 11:368–380

Overgaard J (1983) Histopathologic effects of hyperthermia. In: Storm FK (ed) Hyperthermia in cancer therapy. G.K. Hall, Boston, pp 163–185

Pleham HRB (1986) Speculations on the function of the major heat shock proteins. Cell 46:959–961

Reinhold HS (1988) Physiological effects of hyperthermia. Recent Results Cancer Res 107:32–43

Sapozink MD, Boyd SD, Astrahan MA, Korczak D, Lindner A (1990) Transurethral hyperthermia for benign prostatic hyperplasia: preliminary clinical results. J Urol 143:944–950

Servadio C, Leib Z, Lev A (1990) Local hyperthermia to canine prostate. A pilot study. Urology 35:156–163

Shapiro E, Becicj MJ, Hartanto V, Lepor H (1992) The relative proportion of stromal and epithelial hyperplasia is related to the development of symptomatic benign prostatic hyperplasia. J Urol 147:1293–1297

Seigel YI, Zaidel L, Hammel I, et al. (1991) Histopathology of benign prostatic hyperplasia after failure of hyperthermia treatment. Br J Urol 68:383–386

Siegel I, Lidner A, Zaidel L, Hammel I (1992) Immunohistochemical changes in the prostate gland following rectal hyperthermia. J Urol 147:345A, abstract 529

Song CW (1984) Effect of local hyperthermia on blood flow and microenvironment: a review. Cancer Res 44:4721s–4730s

Song CW, Kang MS, Rhee JG, Levitt SH (1980) Effect of hyperthermia on vascular function in normal and neoplastic tissues. Ann NY Acad Sci 335:35–47

Streffer C, van Beuningen D (1987) The biological basis for tumour therapy by hyperthermia and radiation. Recent Results Cancer Res 104:24–70

Strohmaier WL, Bichler KH, Böcking A, Flüchter SH (1991) Histological effects of local microwave hyperthermia in prostatic cancer. Int J Hyperthermia 7:27–33

Szmigielski S, Zielinski J, Stawarz B, et al. (1988) Local microwave hyperthermia in the treatment of advanced prostatic adenocarcinoma. Urol Res 16:1–7

Szmigielski S, Sobczynski J, Sokolska G, Stawarz B, Zielinski H, Petrovich Z (1991) Effects of local prostatic hyperthermia on human NK and T cell function. Int J Hyperthermia 7:869–880

Tucker RD, Loening SA, Landas S, Mardan AH, Zong-Ying R, Lubaroff DM (1991) The in vivo effect of regional hyperthermia on Dunning R3327 prostatic tumor. Prostate 18:321–329

van den Bossche M, Noel JC, Schulman CC (1991) Transurethral hyperthermia for benign prostatic hypertrophy. World J Urol 9:2–6

Vaupel P, Kallinowski F (1987) Physiological effects of hyperthermia. Recent Results Cancer Res 104:71–109

Yerushalmi A, Shpirer A, Hod I, Gottesfeld F, Bass DD (1982) Normal tissue response to localized deep microwave hyperthermia in the rabbit's prostate: a preclinical study. Int J Radiat Oncol Biol Phys 9:77–82

Yerushalmi A, Fishelovitz Y, Singer D, et al. (1985) A. Localized deep microwave hyperthermia in the treatment of poor operative risk patients with benign prostatic hyperplasia. J Urol 133:873–876

15 Cell-Mediated Immune Response in Patients Undergoing Prostatic Hyperthermia

STANISLAW SZMIGIELSKI, BRONISLAW STAWARZ, and ZBIGNIEW PETROVICH

CONTENTS

15.1 Introduction

The use of hyperthermia (HT) treatment regimes for advanced cancer of the prostate (CaP) and symptomatic benign prostatic hyperplasia (BPH) has now led to the accumulation of considerable clinical experience (BICHLER et al. 1992; PERLMUTTER 1992; MEIER et al. 1992), although the mechanisms underlying HT-evoked remissions of prostatic diseases are not known. Most of the HT systems applied at present for the treatment of prostatic disease use various frequencies of microwave (MW) radiation as the source of thermal energy (PERLMUTTER 1992), with 2450 MHz, 915 MHz, and 434 MHz being most frequently utilized. The MW energy of these frequencies is rapidly absorbed in tissues and effective penetration of 434-2450 MHz MWs to tissues surrounding HT antennas is relatively limited (see Chap. 13). A transurethral (TUHT), 630- or 915-MHz MW applicator described by ASTRAHAN et al. (1989), which was

STANISLAW SZMIGIELSKI, MD, PhD, Professor, Center for Radiobiology and Radiation Safety, MMA Postgraduate Medical School, ul. Szaserow, Warsaw, Poland
BRONISLAW STAWARZ, MD, PhD, Professor and Chairman, Department of Urology, MMA Postgraduate Medical School, ul. Szaserow, Warsaw, Poland
ZBIGNIEW PETROVICH, MD, Professor and Chairman, Department of Radiation Oncology, University of Southern California, Kenneth Norris Jr. Cancer Center, 1441 Eastlake Avenue, Los Angeles, CA 90033, USA

Petrovich/Baert (Eds.)
Benign Prostatic Hyperplasia

built of three antennas located in a modified Foley-type catheter, could effectively heat periurethral tissues to a depth of about 0.5–1.0 cm (Chap. 13). When the applicator was installed intraurethrally and the feedback thermoregulation was set at 46 °C, a cylindrical volume approximately 4 cm in length and 0.5 cm outward from the catheter was heated from 47 °C to 42 °C. The temperature gradient was measured as 6 °C/cm of prostatic tissue (ASTRAHAN et al. 1991). Similar temperature gradients were registered during transrectal hyperthermia (TRHT) of the prostate with the use of systems and applicators at 2450 MHz (MAGIN et al. 1980). In the case of TRHT the exponential decrease in temperature in tissues surrounding the applicator results in the highest temperature being achieved in the rectal mucosa and not in the prostate. The heating conditions can be considerably improved by installation of a cooling system which effectively reduces the temperature of the adjacent rectal wall.

Limited penetration of MW energy into tissues and the resulting sharp temperature gradients registered in the prostate during HT treatments clearly indicate that both TRHT and TUHT allow only for local heating of parts of the prostate located in the proximity of radiating antennas. The parts of the prostate more distant from an applicator remain unaffected. Heating of prostatic tissues exceeding 42 °C results in the appearance of detectable morphologic changes (LEIB et al. 1986) that seem to be related quantitatively and qualitatively to temperature levels and duration of heating (LAUWERYNS et al. 1991; MAGIN et al. 1980; MONTROSI et al. 1992). Six 1.5-h HT treatments of canine prostate at 42.5 °C resulted in diffuse infiltration of the heated area with mononuclear cells and slight edema but without symptoms of irreversible or severe damage of prostatic glandular cells or stroma (LEIB et al. 1986). Increasing temperature to 44.5 °C using the same HT scheme (six 1.5-h sessions) led to considerably more profound histopathologic changes, with the appearance of local necrotic foci, hemorrhages, and inflammatory infiltrations. From experimental studies performed on canine prostate heated with MWs (LEIB et al. 1986) a general relation between conditions of HT treatment (temperature levels, duration of heating, number of sessions) and morphologic injury of prostatic tissues can be established (PERLMUTTER, 1992). Treatment temperatures in the range of 42°–43 °C are considered to be safe and lack the ability to damage normal tissues permanently, while temperatures exceeding 45 °C will result in local necrosis with an intensity approximately related to the thermal load (temperature level × duration of heating). In the range of 42°–45 °C only slight morphologic changes in the stroma and glandular cells of the prostate can be found, while diffuse infiltration with mononuclear cells (macrophages and lymphocytes) predominates (LEIB et al. 1986). This histologic evidence of mononuclear cell infiltrates can be found in a substantial part of the prostate following administration of intracavitary HT.

Histopathologic examination of HT-treated patients was performed mostly in those who suffered from symptomatic BPH and failed to respond to this therapy. Some of the patients who failed HT subsequently underwent surgical resection of the prostate (LAUWERYNS et al. 1991; MONTROSI et al. 1992). Five or ten 60-min TRHT sessions with an intraprostatic temperature of 42.5 °C did not cause irreversible damage to the glandular epithelium or to the stroma, but mild inflammatory infiltrates were seen throughout the gland (MONTROSI et al. 1992). Evidence of inflammation in prostatic tissues heated to 42°–45 °C was also clearly visible in histologic examinations of glands resected surgically after failure of TUHT treatments (DUMANSKI et al. 1994; LAUWERYNS et al. 1991). Diffuse and localized infiltrations of mononuclear cells were found at a distance of 1–2 cm from the surface of the TU applicator (the urethral temperature was 45 °C) and were accompanied by other typical signs of inflammation (edema and hyperemia) (DUMANSKI et al. 1994).

15.2 Immunologic Considerations

Histologic evidence of inflammation in considerable parts of the prostate heated with TR or TU applicators suggests that a reaction may be triggered from the immune system, particularly in view of the fact that most of the HT treatment protocols include repeated heating sessions. Surprisingly, present knowledge concerning immune reactions to local heating of tissues, both normal and neoplastic, is limited. Earlier studies revealed that local HT of experimental tumors stimulated cell-mediated immune reactions and enhanced immunogenicity of HT-suppressed cancer cells. Until recently, however, no systematic studies have been undertaken on this subject. A review of the literature revealed that most of the investigations on the effects of HT on the immune system were devoted either to whole-body hyperthermia or to in vitro studies of immunocompetent cells exposed to elevated temperatures. Whole-body HT at core body temperatures of 38.5°–40 °C caused only minimal effects on the immune responses of normal mice after 2–4 h exposure to radiant heat (GREELEY et al. 1992). Under these conditions whole-day HT did not influence the absolute number of blood lymphocytes, although the proportion of lymphocyte subjects was temporarily changed, with an immediate increase in splenic CD^{4+} (helper) cells. This was followed within 18 h by an overall decrease in Lyt 2^+ and Thy 1.2^+ cells and an increase in the percentage of mature T lymphocytes in the thymus (GREELEY et al. 1992). More intensive whole-body HT (core body temperature 40°–41.5 °C) induced in mice by exposure in MW chambers (SZMIGIELSKI et al. 1984) or by conventional heating stimulated cell-mediated immunity in normal mice with a transient increase in lymphocytosis. There was also enhanced reactivity of blood lymphocytes to mitogens [phytohemagglutinin (PHA) and concanavalin A (Con A)] and stimulation of cytotoxicity. The above signs of immune stimulation were demonstrated after a single 2-h exposure to MW HT. Similar responses from the immune system were observed in mice treated with daily 2-h HT sessions for 4 days. Prolonged exposure to daily HT sessions (e.g., for 7–11 days), however, gradually diminished the intensity of immune stimulation and finally led to signs of suppression of lymphocyte function (SZMIGIELSKI et al. 1984). Whole-body HT can be induced in experimental animals and in patients at significantly lower temperatures (not exceeding 41.5°–42 °C) than are used for the local heating of tissues. Therefore, it is expected that morphologic changes and inflammatory reactions appearing in organs heated locally to 42°–47 °C will not be the same as in the case of whole-body HT. The mechanisms responsible for effects of whole-body HT on the immune systems also may be quantitatively different from those operating in local heating of tissues to higher temperatures. Analysis of immune reactions in normal mice exposed to whole-body HT suggested that the observed phenomena may be mediated by an altered distribution of lymphocyte pools in the heated organs (homing of lymphocytes) and by circulating factors rather than by some heat-induced alterations in the cells themselves (GREELEY et al. 1992).

Immunocompetent cells, including macrophages, T-lymphocytes, and natural killer (NK) lymphocytes, are among the cells most sensitive to temperature elevation (YOSHIOKA et al. 1990). In vitro studies revealed a biphasic reaction of lymphocytes to HT, showing stimulation of physiologic functions (e.g., transformation rates in PHA/Con A microcultures, release of cytokines) at 38°–39 °C followed by rapid inhibition of these functions as the temperature was increased to 41°–42 °C (IZUMI et al. 1983). NK cells isolated from murine or rat spleen lost their lytic activity following exposure to 1°–42.5 °C for 30 min, but the activity was partially recovered after reincubation at 37 °C (YANG et al. 1992). Exposure to temperatures exceeding 43 °C inhibited irreversibly the lytic activity of NK cells (GREELEY et al. 1992).

Reaction of the immune system to local HT may result both from thermal injury of immunocompetent cells in the heated tissues and from factors released from the areas where temperatures do not reach the levels inhibiting lymphocyte functions (YOSHIOKA et al. 1990). Hind limbs of normal mice heated locally in hot water after maintaining temperature of muscles at 43 °C for 45 min showed a biphasic reaction of the NK cytotoxic activity. The NK activity was noted to be suppressed 2 days following a single session of local HT and significantly enhanced (by 25%–30%) 7 days following the heat exposure. The authors concluded that this enhancement of NK cytotoxic activity following local HT may play an important role in the antitumour effect of heat therapy. However, they were not able to provide direct evidence to support their hypothesis, particularly in view of the fact that the mice used in the study did not bear tumors (YOSHIOKA et al. 1990). Mice bearing transplanted Lewis lung carcinoma also showed stimulation of cell-mediated cytotoxicity in response to local HT with circulating hot water (ROBINS et al. 1991). Two sessions of local HT applied 6 and 10 days after implantation of cancer cells resulted in inhibition of growth of the primary tumor and lowering of the number of lung metastases, accompanied by enhanced activity of splenic granulocyte-macrophage progenitor cells. The authors concluded that the antimetastatic effect in HT-treated tumor-bearing mice reflected the immune-associated responses, including activation of cytotoxic mechanisms (ROBINS et al. 1991).

15.3 Immune Responses to Local Hyperthermia for Cancer of the Prostate

15.3.1 Preliminary Results

YERUSHALMI et al. (1982) reported preliminary results of the use of TRHT in patients with advanced CaP. This treatment method has been applied in several other clinical studies (SERVADIO et al. 1986, 1987; STROHMAIER et al. 1992; SZMIGIELSKI et al. 1988) with results varying from temporary remission in a considerable percentage of treated patients to no effects at all. TRHT of canine prostate with a water-cooled 915-MHz microwave applicator with prostatic temperatures ranging from 42.5 °C to 44.5 °C and maintained from 9 min to 5 h resulted in localized necrosis in regions close to the rectal wall and in inflammation with diffuse infiltrations of mononuclear cells and polymorphonuclear leukocytes throughout the gland (LEIB et al. 1986; SERVADIO et al. 1990). A differential count of blood leukocytes in these dogs showed significant monocytosis lasting for about 1 week after TRHT. Additionally, serum levels of creatinine phosphokinase (CPK) and serum glutamic oxoaloacetic transaminase (SGOT) rose considerably in animals treated with higher temperatures. This rise in CPK and SGOT was subsequently found to have a definite correlation with histologic evidence of localized necrosis (SERVADIO et al. 1990). The use of TRHT in patients with CaP (42°–43 °C for 60 min) did not cause detectable tumor cell necrosis, but hyperemia, microhemorrhages, and edema of the stroma with diffuse infiltrations of lymphocytes, macrophages, and plasma cells were observed throughout the gland (STROHMAIER et al. 1992). As diffuse interstitial inflammation of the prostatic stroma predominated in patients with CaP treated with TRHT, we concluded that the involution of tumors observed in some treated patients may have resulted from the immune responses evoked both by the inflammation itself and by the heat-suppressed, but not killed cancer cells (SZMIGIELSKI et al. 1987). This hypothesis was subsequently subjected to a phase I clinical trial.

15.3.2 Phase I Clinical Studies

From 1987 through 1989 15 patients with advanced CaP received TRHT at the Department of Clinical Urology, MMA Postgraduate Medical School in Warsaw, Poland (SZMIGIELSKI et al. 1987). All treatments were given using a water-cooled microwave applicator at 434 or 2450 MHz. Local TRHT was given twice a week for a total of six sessions. Each TRHT sessions lasted for 30 min at steady-state temperature controlled on the rectal mucosa at 45 °C. In all these patients studies of immune reactions were performed before TRHT, upon the completion of six TRHT sessions, and at 1, 2, 4, and 6 months following this therapy. Monitoring of T and NK cell functions comprised assessment of subsets of peripheral blood lymphocytes. They were identified by an indirect immunofluorescence staining technique using CD3 (pan-T), CD4 (T-helper-inducer) and CD8 (T-suppressor-cytotoxic) mouse monoclonal anti-bodies. The mitogenic response of isolated peripheral blood mononuclear cells (PBMCs) to PHA and Con A in 72-h microcultures and NK cytotoxic activity of PBMCs against a ^{51}Cr-labeled target K-526 erythroleukemic cell line were also studied (SZMIGIELSKI et al. 1991).

This clinical study was repeated in 1990 using another group of 15 patients with advanced CaP (SOBCZYNSKI et al. 1994). TRHT of these patients and monitoring of the NK and T lymphocyte function were performed using methods identical to those used in the first study (SZMIGIELSKI et al. 1988, 1991). Additionally, the function of the granulocyte system was investigated before TRHT, upon the completion of six TRHT sessions, and at 1, 2, and 4 months following this therapy. For assessment of the granulocyte system, granulocytosis, percentage or polymorphonuclear leukocytes reducing Nitro-BT, the size of blood and bone marrow reserve pools of mature granulocytes (released after administration of epinephrine or hydrocortisone), and serum levels of muramidase (lysozyme) were investigated. (SOBCZYNSKI et al. 1993). In the first study of 15 CaP patients, eight responded to TRHT with remissions (three complete and five partial) lasting from several months to more than 5 years (STAWARZ et al. 1993). In the second study, six patients had remissions of their tumors (two complete and four partial), making a total of 14 remissions in 30 patients treated with TRHT (Table 15.1). Of the 30 patients suffering from advanced CaP, 24 had symptoms of suppression of T and/or NK cells functions, including a lower CD^{4+}/CD^{8+} ratio (20 patients), decreased transformation rates of PBMCs by PHA and Con A (18 patients), and weaker NK cytotoxic activity (16 patients). Mean values of the group and dispersion of the results when compared to identical immune tests performed in 30 healthy male volunteers of the same age showed that all parameters were significantly lower ($P < 0.01$) in patients suffering from advanced CaP (SZMIGIELSKI et al. 1991). Depressed cell-mediated immunity in patients with genitourinary cancers had previously been reported by other investigators (CATALONA et al. 1974; MANDEVILLE et al. 1982; ZEMBALA et al. 1977). These studies suggested a relationship between the intensity of immunosuppression, stage of disease, and prognosis for

Table 15.1. Treatment response to TRHT in patients with advanced prostatic carcinoma

Study	No.	Complete response	%	Partial response	%	No response	%
I	15	3	20	5	33	7	47
II	15	2	13	4	27	9	60
Total	30	5	17	9	30	16	53

survival (IZUMI et al. 1983). In patients treated for CaP with cytoreductive techniques (radio- and hormonotherapy) NK-mediated cytotoxic activity has been shown to be inversely related to tumor mass and spread of neoplastic cells (KASTELAN et al. 1992; LAHAT et al. 1989; WHITE et al. 1982). No such correlation was found with tumor grade and NK-mediated cytotoxic activity (KASTELAN et al. 1992; TARLE et al. 1993). In our group of 30 CaP patients treated with TRHT, a wide range of NK cytotoxic activity was noted: 16 (53%) showed lower activity than the healthy males from the control group, while the remaining 14 (47%) was located in the middle (11) and upper (3) ranges of the control group (SOBCZYNSKI et al. 1994; SZMIGIELSKI et al. 1991).

Analysis of immunologic data in our two phase I studies revealed considerable stimulation of granulocyte and lymphocyte function, detectable within 1–2 months after completion of the six sessions of TRHT (Tables 15.2, 15.3).

All 15 investigated patients in the second study showed significant stimulation of the granulocyte system at the completion of six TRHT sessions and 1 month after completion of therapy (Table 15.2). The number of granulocytes in peripheral blood rose from about 5000 cells/mm^3 before TRHT to about 6500 cell/mm^3 at the completion of therapy ($P < 0.05$) (SOBCZYNSKI et al. 1994). This was accompanied by an increase in the percentage of Nitro-BT-reducing blood granulocytes from 5.46 to 8.36 ($P < 0.01$) and in the serum level of muramidase (lysozyme) from 6.32 to 9.68 mg/l ($P < 0.01$). Additionally, the phagocytic index of granulocytes rose from 212 before TRHT to 268 ($P < 0.05$) after completion of the therapy, and the bone marrow reserve pool of granulocytes released after administration of hydrocortisone was significantly larger (increment of granulocytosis of 78.3% before TRHT and 112.1% after

Table 15.2. Stimulation of the granulocyte system in the 15 patients treated with TRHT in the authors' second study

	Responders ($n = 6$)				Nonresponders ($n = 9$)			
	After THRT	1 mo.	2 mo.	4 mo.	After TRHT	1 mo.	2 mo.	4 mo.
Granulocytosis (increment > 30%)	4	5	2	0	6	8	5	3
Nitro-BT reduction (> 10% granulocytes)	3	4	1	1	5	8	4	3
Phagocytic index (score > 240)	3	6	2	1	5	7	1	2
Serum muramidase (> 10 mg/l)	3	6	3	2	4	7	3	2
Bone marrow reserve pool (increment > 120%)	1	4	3	2	1	6	5	3

Table 15.3. Stimulation of the lymphocyte system in the 30 patients treated with TRHT in the authors' two studies

	Responders ($n = 14$)				Nonresponders ($n = 16$)			
	After THRT	1 mo.	2 mo.	4 mo.	After TRHT	1 mo.	2 mo.	4 mo.
T Lymphocytes (CD^{3+}) (> 150% pretreatment)	2	3	8	4	1	2	4	2
T helper cells (CD^{4+}) (> 200% pretreatment)	1	4	9	6	1	3	4	2
CD^{4+}/CD^{8+} ratio (increment > 1.50)	0	3	8	5	1	4	5	3
Transformation in vitro (2x pretreatment transformation rate)	0	4	6	3	0	2	3	2
NK cytotoxicity (– 130% pretreatment)	2	7	13	6	2	3	6	3

completion of the therapy, $P < 0.05$) (SOBCZYNSKI et al. 1994). All the above tests of granulocyte function were still significantly higher 1 months after completion of TRHT therapy but had returned to the pretreatment values at 2 or 4 months posttherapy. On the basis of these results, the authors concluded that TRHT of the prostate evoked fast stimulation of the granulocyte (and probably also macrophage) systems. This was probably in response to diffuse inflammation of the prostatic stroma. Stimulation of phagocytic cell systems appeared early during TRHT therapy and was clearly demonstrable after completion of the six treatment sessions. Analysis of appearance of granulocyte stimulation in TRHT-treated CaP patients failed to show any differences between patients who responded to HT therapy with remissions and those who failed the treatment (nonresponders) (Table 15.2). All patients in both subgroups (responders and nonresponders) showed similar symptoms and duration of stimulation of the granulocyte system after TRHT, the highest test values being found upon the completion of TRHT.

NK and T cell functions have also been found to be stimulated in CaP patients treated with TRHT (SZMIGIELSKI et al. 1991), but the kinetics of stimulation of these cell systems were different from those reported for granulocytes (Table 15.3). Mean values of all investigated parameters (subset of T lymphocytes, T helper/T suppressor ratio, transformation rates in vitro, NK cytotoxic activity) were significantly different from the pretreatment values (at $P < 0.01$). The peak effect of the stimulation was noted 2 months after TRHT, with a subsequent decrease. The administration of TRHT resulted in an increase in the number of CD^{3+} (pan-T) lymphocytes, an increase in the CD^{4+}/CD^{8+} ratio, and an enhancement of mitogenic response of BMNCs to PHA and Con A with a tendency toward greater expression of stimulation of cell-mediated immune reaction in the initially immune-depressed CaP patients (SOBCZYNSKI et al. 1994; SZMIGIELSKI et al. 1991). However, analysis of expression of the stimulation of cell-mediated immune reactions in relation to clinical response to TRHT (responders vs nonresponders) (Table 15.3) did not show a correlation between the degree of stimulation of T lymphocytes and the appearance of remission of the primary tumors after hyperthermia. In contrast to T lymphocyte function, NK-mediated cytotoxicity of BMNCs did show a correlation with clinical results of TRHT in the investigated groups of CaP patients (Table 15.3). In spite of the considerable individual variations in NK activity in patients before TRHT and the higher number of cases with lowered NK activity among nonresponders to TRHT (11 of 16 nonresponders had lowered NK activity, compared to 5 of 14 responders, $\chi^2 = 3.27$, $P < 0.05$), the patients who responded to TRHT with significant enhancement of NK activity (when compared to the individual pretreatment values) more frequently had tumor remission (responders) than did patients with unchanged NK activity following treatment (Table 15.3). Of the 30 CaP patients treated with TRHT, 19 (63%) responded with significant enhancement of NK activity at 1–2 months after therapy (when compared with individual pretreatment values). The 19 cases with enhancement of NK activity were mostly distributed in the group of patients with treatment response (13 of 14 responders); only six patients in the group of nonresponders (16 patients) showed enhancement of NK activity ($\chi^2 = 9.85$, $P < 0.01$). This confirmed recent findings that the assessment of NK activity of BMNCs may be considered a useful test in advanced CaP for predicting the individual reaction of the patient to applied therapy (TARLE et al. 1993).

Clinical studies on local HT of the prostate clearly indicated that TRHT allows heating of prostatic tissues to 42°–43 °C. These temperatures were too low for direct thermal killing of normal or neoplastic cells. However, thermal damage to glandular cells and stroma under these conditions produced a wide range of typical morphologic signs of diffuse inflammation, including massive infiltration of the heated tissues with polymorphonuclear granulocytes, macrophages, and lymphocytes. It is reasonable to assume that in the case of prostatic carcinoma the macrophages and lymphocytes infiltrating neoplastic tissue may become activated by heat-suppressed cancer cells or their products. Experimental evidence exists that heat-damaged neoplastic cells show enhanced immunogenicity and may trigger activation of macrophages.

Application of TRHT in patients with advanced CaP twice a week for a total of six 30-min sessions evoked stimulation of both granulocyte and T/NK lymphocyte systems; however, the kinetics and probably the mechanisms of the stimulation were different. Stimulation of granulocyte function, measured with a battery of tests indicating both activation of the cells (phagocytosis, reduction of Nitro-BT) and kinetics/turnover of granulopoiesis (serum muramidase levels, size of reserve pools of granulocytes), appeared immediately after completion of the TRHT and lasted only for the first month after therapy. The character of the reaction of the granulocyte system after TRHT was typical for the reaction of this system to acute inflammation. In view of the available data, the stimulation of phagocytic cell systems in TRHT-treated patients should be considered as a defensive response to thermal damage (diffuse inflammation) of the prostatic tissues. Lack of signs of granulocyte stimulation 2 and 4 months after TRHT of the prostate may suggest that the inflammation evoked by repeated sessions of HT is a transient event and does not lead to development of chronic inflammation of the prostate.

Stimulation of T lymphocyte function (increased number of T lymphocytes, including an increase in T helper/inducer cells, elevation of the T helper/T suppressor lymphocyte ratio, and a higher mitogenic response of cultured lymphocytes) appeared in TRHT-treated CaP patients much later than the reaction of the granulocyte system and reached a maximum 2 months after HT therapy. Initially, most of the patients with advanced CaP (19 of the 30 under study) had suppression of T lymphocyte function documented in lowered values on one or more of the tested parameters. Therefore, stimulation of the system after TRHT may arise either from a direct response to heat damage of the prostatic tissues or from a complicated chain of events related to interactions between heat-suppressed cancer cells, macrophages, and T lymphocytes. Analysis of individual reactions of the T lymphocyte system in CaP patients who responded to TRHT with measurable improvement (responders) and in those without remissions (nonresponders) revealed that signs of stimulation of T lymphocytes occurred in both subgroups (Table 15.3). There was, however, no significant correlation with the clinical results of HT therapy. More conclusive results were obtained in the analysis of NK-mediated cytotoxic activity of BMNCS in CaP patients treated with TRHT. Before therapy most of the investigated patients (16 of the 30 treated) showed lowered NK cytotoxicity; a significant posttreatment increase in the activity was found more frequently in patients who responded to HT with remissions ($P < 0.01$). This finding may be of clinical relevance and of importance for the long-term prognostic impact of TRHT in CaP patients. This confirmed a recent report indicating NK cytotoxicity to be a useful supplementary test for evaluation of patients with advanced CaP (TARLE et al. 1993). However, as in the case of T lymphocyte reactions, enhancement of NK cytotoxicity following TRHT in patients with CaP did not allow us to conclude whether this phenomenon may be considered (a) a direct response to heat damage of prostatic tissue or (b) secondary to inhibition of growth of cancer cells and effects of HT on neoplastic cells. In order to evaluate these phenomena, a study of immune reactions to TRHT in patients with benign prostatic hyperplasia (BPH) was undertaken simultaneously with the above-described investigations of reactions to TRHT in patients with CaP.

15.4 Immune Responses to Local Hyperthermia for BPH

For local HT of patients with BPH two methods of heating are being applied which include TRHT or TUHT (PERLMUTTER 1992). There is considerable evidence to suggest that TUHT is more effective than TRHT in the treatment of BPH (Baert et al. 1991; Perlmutter 1992; Stawarz et al. 1991). In the reported studies, about 70%–80% of patients responded to repeated (five to ten) sessions of TUHT with a major improvement of subjective symptoms and objective urine flow parameters, while benefits from TRHT were noted in only about 40% of treated patients. The response rates, however, were different in patients with enlargement of the median lobe of the prostate. These patients were relatively resistant to TUHT (Baert et al. 1991), while TRHT allowed for easier heating of the median lobe and, therefore, enhanced the chance of improvement. Long-term effects of both TUHT and TRHT in BPH patients, the duration of this improvement, the number of sessions required to obtain an improvement, and the optimal temperature of HT are not yet known (Perlmutter 1992). Both TRHT and TUHT, however, have been considered safe treatment modalities in patients with symptomatic BPH. Some investigators have advised that HT be repeated in BPH patients who respond to the first treatment course with an improvement but later again develop symptoms of urinary outflow obstruction (Bichler et al. 1992).

Histopathologic studies of the prostate after TUHT in dogs and in patients with BPH revealed that thermal damage of prostatic tissue corresponded with the thermal profile of the radiating antenna (Dumanski et al. 1994; Lauweryns et al. 1991). Under typical conditions of TUHT (temperature at the urethral surface maintained at 45 °C, duration of HT sessions 45–60 min) a 2- to 3-mm zone of necrosis around the applicator and considerable thermal damage to prostatic tissue 5–6 mm from the heating antenna were found. The size and intensity of necrotic lesions in tissue surrounding the applicator depended on the applied temperature and duration of exposure to this temperature (Dumanski et al. 1994). Healing of necrotic lesions occurred by ingrowing granulation tissue with its organization and, finally, fibrosis (Lauweryns et al. 1991). Layers of the tissue surrounding the necrotic zones showed a histologic picture similar to that observed after TRHT. There was vascular wall damage, edema and hyperemia of the stroma, focal parenchymal hemorrhages, and diffuse infiltrations of phagocytic cells (polymorphonuclears, macrophages) and lymphocytes.

Diffuse inflammation of a relatively large part of the prostate with accompanying local necrotic foci suggested the possibility of a generalized reaction of the immune system, particularly since TUHT was applied in multiple sessions that enhanced the intensity of thermal damage to the prostate.

In our first study, conducted from 1987 through 1989, 15 patients with moderate to severe urinary outflow obstruction due to BPH were treated with TRHT given twice a week for a total of six sessions (Szmigielski et al. 1991). TRHT was administered identically as in the group of patients with CaP. This allowed us to compare the results of immune tests in both the BPH and CaP groups and in the simultaneously investigated (but not heated) healthy males, used as the control group. Studies of immune reactions (T lymphocytes and T cells subsets, mitogenic response of PBMCs to PHA and Con A,

NK cytotoxic activity) were performed in the BPH patients using the same methods and time intervals (before TRHT, upon the completion of six TRHT sessions, and at 1, 2, and 4 months following therapy) as for the TRHT-treated CaP patients. Unlike in the CaP group, in the 15 BPH patients the measured immune parameters were all within normal limits before TRHT and there were no cases of suppressions of NK or T cell function. Analysis of immune parameters after TRHT revealed only a slight change in NK and T lymphocyte function (SZMIGIELSKI et al. 1991). The only significant change in this group appeared to be an increased number of T lymphocytes (CD^{3+} cells) in peripheral blood 2 months after TRHT. The other subset of blood lymphocytes, the CD^{4+}/CD^{8+} ratio, mitogenic response to PHA and Con A, and NK cytotoxicity did not show a significant difference when compared to the pretreatment values.

The above study was repeated using another group of 15 patients with symptomatic BPH treated with TRHT (SOBCZYNSKI et al. 1994). This investigation included a total of 45 patients treated with HT. Of these 45 patients, 15 suffered from advanced CaP and were treated with TRHT. The remaining 30 patients had BPH and were randomly assigned to two groups of 15 patients each. One group was treated with TRHT and the other with TUHT. Studies of T and NK cell function and in addition assessment of the granulocyte system (see methods listed in Sect 15.3) were performed in all patients before and after HT therapy. Results obtained in CaP patients revealed signs of stimulation of the granulocyte system immediately after completion of TRHT and 1 month thereafter. In BPH patients treated with TRHT, all tests of the granulocyte system were additionally performed 1 and 2 weeks after HT therapy to follow the kinetics of the stimulation during the first month

Table 15.4. Stimulation of the granulocyte system in the 30 BPH patients treated with TRHT and TUHT

	THRT ($n = 15$)				THUT ($n = 15$)			
	After THRT	1 week	1 mo.	2 mo.	After TUHT	1 week	1 mo.	2 mo.
Granulocytosis (increment > 130%)	10	12	12	4	8	10	11	2
Nitro-BT reduction (> 10% granulocytes)	7	11	9	2	5	8	8	3
Phagocytic index (score > 240)	5	8	7	3	4	6	9	3
Serum muramidase (> 10 mg/l)	9	10	13	4	7	9	9	2
Bone marrow reserve pool (increment > 120%)	6	8	10	2	4	7	9	3

Table 15.5. Stimulation of the lymphocyte system in the 30 BPH patients treated with TRHT and TUHT

	TRHT ($n = 15$)				TUHT ($n = 15$)			
	After THRT	1 mo.	2 mo.	4 mo.	After TUHT	1 mo.	2 mo.	4 mo.
T lymphocytes (CD^{3+}) (> 150% pretreatment)	0	1	1	1	1	0	1	1
T helper cells (CD^{4+}) (200% pretreatment)	0	0	1	0	0	0	0	0
CD^{4+}/CD^{8+} ratio (increment < 1.50)	0	0	0	0	0	0	0	0
Transformation in vitro (– 2x pretreatment transformation rate)	1	1	2	1	0	1	2	1
NK cytotoxicity (– 130% pretreatment)	0	2	3	1	1	3	3	1

after therapy. Both TUHT and TRHT resulted in stimulation of all tested parameters of the granulocyte system during the first month after completion of therapy (Table 15.4). A comparison of pre- and posttreatment results showed in a significant increase in two or three of the four tested parameters of granulocyte function in a majority of patients (75%–85%) (Table 15.4). The kinetics and intensity of stimulation of the phagocytic cell system did not differ between patients treated with TRHT or TUHT. NK and T cell function was only slightly stimulated in a few BPH patients treated with TRHT or TUHT without any typical response that may be related to the applied therapy (Table 15.5). In contrast to the 15 CaP patients, treatment of BPH with TRHT or TUHT influenced NK cytotoxicity in only 4 of the 30 patients, who showed increased cytotoxic activity of PBMCs at 2 months after therapy, when compared to the individual pretreatment values (Table 15.5).

15.5 Conclusion

The available data indicated that HT of the prostate, either with a TR applicator or with the use of a TU antenna, evoked a nonspecific but long-lasting (about 1 month) stimulation of the phagocytic cell system. This was thought to represent a response to thermally induced localized necrosis and diffuse inflammation of prostatic tissues located around the heating part of the applicator. Following HT of the prostate without neoplastic infiltrations (normal prostate in dogs, enlarged prostate in BPH patients), the above-mentioned stimulation of the granulocyte system disappeared after a few weeks without further consequences and no repeatable response from the T and NK lymphocyte systems could be detected. Patients with advanced CaP initially quite frequently showed various signs of suppression of T and/or NK lymphocyte functions, but responded to TRHT with identical stimulation of the granulocyte system during the first month after therapy. This, however, was followed by stimulation of cell-mediated immune reactions, which were more pronounced in CaP patients who responded clinically to TRHT with remissions of the primary tumor. The mechanism underlying stimulation by TRHT of cell-mediated immunity in patients with advanced CaP remains unclear and needs further investigation. The HT-induced inflammatory reaction and enhanced immunogenicity of heat suppressed cancer cells activating tumor-infiltrating macrophages seem to play the basic role.

Acknowledgements. This work was partly supported by research grant No. 4-4018/91/02 from the Committee for Scientific Research (KBN) in Warsaw, Poland.

References

Astrahan M, Sapoznik MD, Cohen D, et al. (1989) Microwave applicator for transurethral hyperthermia of benign prostatic hyperplasia. Int J Hyperthermia 5:283–296

Astrahan M, Imanaka K, Jozsef G, et al. (1991) Heating characteristics of helical microwave applicator for transurethral hyperthermia of benign prostatic hyperplasia. Int J Hyperthermia 7:141–156

Baert L, Willemen P, Ameye F, Petrovich Z (1991) Treatment response with transurethral microwave hyperthermia in different forms of benign prostatic hyperplasia: a preliminary report. Prostate 18:315–320

Bichler KH, Strohmaier WL, Wilbert DM (1992) Hyperthermia of the prostate. State of the art. PMI, Frankfurt

Catalona WJ, Chritien PB, Trahan EE (1974) Abnormalities of cell-mediated immunocompetence in genitourinary cancer. J Urol 111:229–232

Dumanski Z, Stawarz B, Zielinski H, Szmigielski S (1994) Histologic and ultrastructural changes of the prostate following transrectal and transurethral hyperthermia with 434 MHz or 2450 MHz microwave applicators. Urol Res (in print)

Greeley EH, Helfrich BA, Feuerman LL, et al. (1992) Radiant heat-induced hyperthermia in mice: in vivo effects on the immune system. Int J Hyperthermia 8:209–220

Herr HW (1980) Suppressor cell in immunodepressed bladder and prostate cancer patients. J Urol 123:635–639

Izumi A, Koga S, Maeta M (1983) Effects of in vitro hyperthermia on murine and human lymphocytes. Cancer 51:2061–2065

Kastelan M, Kraljic I, Tarle M (1992) NK cell activity in treated cancer prostate patients as a sensitive probe for circulating tumor cells: hormone regulatory effects in vivo. Prostate 21:111–119

Lahat N, Alexander N, Levin DR, Moskovitz B (1989) The relationship between clinical stage, natural killer activity and related immunological parameters in adenocarcinoma of the prostate. Cancer Immunol Immunother 28:208–215

Lauweryns J, Baert L, Vandenhove J, Petrovich Z (1991) Histopathology of prostatic tissue after transurethral hyperthermia. Int J Hyperthermia 7:221–230

Leib Z, Rathem A, Lev A, Servadio C (1986) Histopathological observations in the canine prostate treated by local microwave hyperthermia. Prostate 8 : 93–102

Magin RL, Fridd CW, Bonfiglio TA (1980) Thermal destruction of the canine prostate by high intensity microwaves. J Surg Res 29 : 265–275

Mandeville R, Lamoureux G, Legault-Poisson S, Poisson R (1982) Biological markers and breast cancer. A multiparametric study. II. Depressed immune competence. Cancer 50 : 1280–1288

Meier AHP, Weil EHJ, Van Waalwijk ESC, Verhaegh GTCM, Janknegt RA (1992) Transurethral radiofrequency heating or thermotherapy for benign prostatic hypertrophy: a prospective trial on 65 consecutive cases. Eur Urol 22 : 39–43

Montrosi F, Galli L, Guazzoni G, et al. (1992) Transrectal microwave hyperthermia for benign prostatic hyperplasia: long-term clinical, pathological and ultrastructural patterns. J Urol 148 : 321–325

Perlmutter AP (1992) Prostatic heat treatments. Semin Urol 10 : 169–179

Robins HI, Jonsson GG, Jacobson EL, et al. (1991) effect of hyperthermia in vitro and in vivo on adenine and pyridine nucleotide pools in human peripheral lymphocytes. Cancer 67 : 2096–2102

Servadio C, Leib Z, Lev A (1986) Further observations on the use of local hyperthermia for the treatment of diseases of the prostate. Eur 12 : 38–40

Servadio C, Leib Z, Lev A (1987) Diseases of the prostate heated by local microwave hyperthermia. Urology 30 : 97–99

Servadio C, Leib Z, Lev A (1990) Local hyperthermia to canine prostate. A pilot study. Urology 35 : 156–164

Sobczynski J, Szmigielski S, Stawarz B, Zielinski H, Ogrodnik J (1994) Reaction of granulocyte system and changes in lymphocyte function in patients treated with microwave hyperthermia for prostate cancer and benign prostatic hyperplasia. Eur Urol (in print)

Stawarz B, Szmigielski S, Ogrodnik J, Petrovich Z (1991) A comparison of transurethral and transrectal microwave hyperthermia in poor surgical risk BPH patients. J Urol 146 : 353–357

Stawarz B, Zielinski H, Szmigielski S, et al. (1993) Transrectal hyperthermia as a palliative treatment for advanced adenocarcinoma of the prostate and a study of cell mediated immunity. Urology 41 : 548–553

Strohmaier WL, Bichler KH, Fluchter SH, Wilbert DM (1992) Local microwave hyperthermia of benign prostatic hyperplasia. J Urol 144 : 913–917

Szmigielski S, Zaboklicki S, Gil J, Jeljaszewicz J, Pulverer G (1984) Inhibition of Lewis lung carcinoma in mice by local microwave hyperthermia combined with immunomodulating *Propionibacterium granulosum KP-45*. Cancer Immunol Immunother 16 : 151–159

Szmigielski S, Jeljaszewicz J, Pulverer G (1987) Thermoimmunotherapy of advanced neoplasms. A concept and preliminary results. Biomed Pharmacother 18 : 132–141

Szmigielski S, Stawarz B, Zielinski H, Gil J, Sobczynski J, Sokolska G, Jeljaszewicz J, Pulverer G (1988) Local microwave hyperthermia in the treatment of advanced prostatic adenocarcinoma. Urol Res 16 : 1–7

Szmigielski S, Sobczynski J, Sokolska G, Stawarz B, Zielinski H, Petrovich Z (1991) Effects of local prostatic hyperthermia on human NK and T cell function. Int J Hyperthermia 7 : 869–880

Tarle M, Kraljic I, Kastelan M (1993) Comparison between NK cell activity and prostate cancer stage and grade in untreated patients: correlation with tumor markers and hormonal serotest data. Urol Res 21 : 17–21

White D, Jones DB, Cooke T, Kirkham N (1982) Natural killer (NK) activity in peripheral blood lymphocytes of patients with benign and malignant breast disease. Br J Cancer 46 : 611–616

Yang H, Lauzon W, Lemaire I (1992) Effect of hyperthermia on natural killer cells: inhibition of lytic function and microtubule organization. Int J Hyperthermia 8 : 87–97

Yerushalmi A, Servadio C, Leib Z, Fishelovitz Y, Rokovsky E, Stein J (1982) Local hyperthermia for treatment of carcinoma of the prostate. Prostate 6 : 623–630

Yoshioka A, Miyachi Y, Toda K, Imamura S, Hiraoka M, Abe M (1990) Effects of local hyperthermia on natural killer activity in mice. Int J Hyperthermia 6 : 261–267

Zembala M, Mytar B, Popiela T, Asherson GL (1977) Depressed in vitro peripheral blood lymphocyte response to mitogens in cancer patients: the role of suppressor cells. Int J Cancer 19 : 605–613

16 Transrectal Hyperthermia in Benign Prostatic Hyperplasia

KARL HORST BICHLER, W.L. STROHMAIER, and W. MATTAUCH

CONTENTS

16.1 Introduction

Today the treatment of benign prostatic hyperplasia (BPH) comprises the well-known surgical techniques as well as alternative procedures such as pharmacologic treatment, local hyperthermia, stents, balloon dilation, and procedures causing prostatic necrosis (e.g., by using laser or high-intensive focused ultrasound). In the past, the available alternative procedures have had to stand comparison with operative techniques, particularly with transurethral resection of the prostate (TURP) as the gold standard. With an increasing number of therapeutic options available for patients with BPH, the question arises as to whether these options enable us to practice considerably more selective treatment for different stages of BPH (see Chap. 8).

The aforementioned alternative procedures have been developed for various reasons, e.g., the values to which the medical profession is subject have altered considerably and, most importantly, the patients' view of the role of the doctor has changed. Patients do prefer noninvasive procedures to operative interventions. Moreover, there is a need to reduce costs in medicine generally and this impacts on the operative specialties as well. In this context, the problems identified by Roos et al. (1989) with regard to late mortality and incidence of

K. HORST BICHLER, MD, PhD, Professor and Chairman, W.L. STROHMAIER, MD, PhD, and W. MATTAUCH, MD, Department of Urology, Eberhard-Karls-University, Hoppe-Seyler-Straße 3, 72076 Tübingen, Germany

Petrovich/Baert (Eds.)
Benign Prostatic Hyperplasia

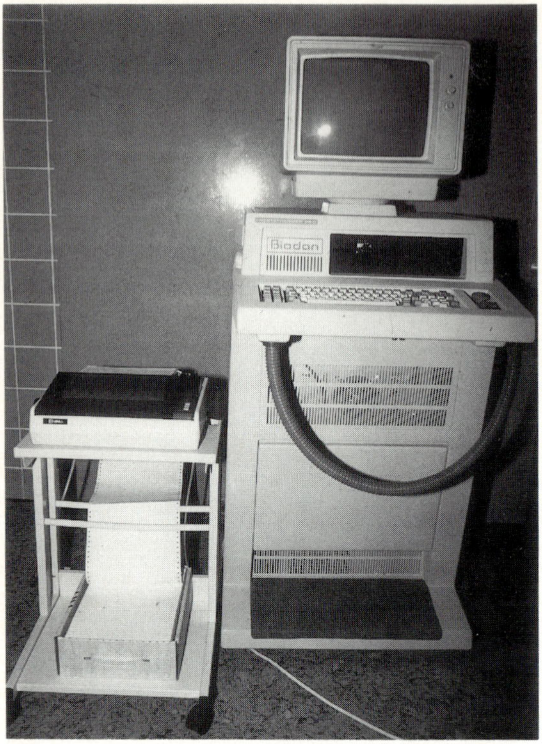

Fig. 16.1. Prostathermer TM System Model 99-D (Biodan Medical System), as used in this study

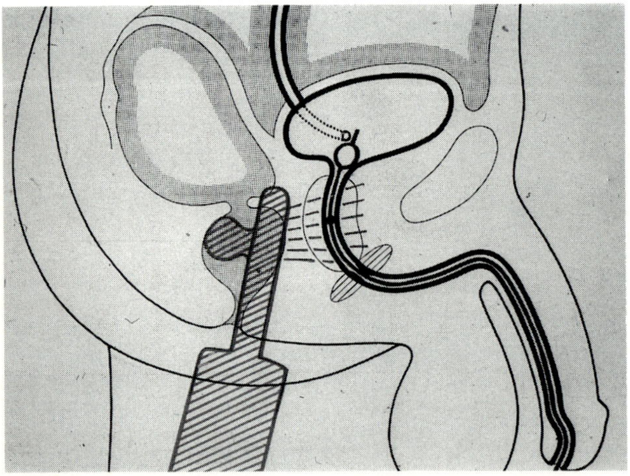

Fig. 16.2. Schematic representation of TRHT. Treatment with the Prostathermer, as used in this study

sequelae with TURP played an important role. In response to the above concerns, the medical equipment industry has designed and produced new, frequently technologically sophisticated instruments which have made possible the application of alternative forms of treatment.

These developments can be illustrated by the example of the application of hyperthermia in BPH. In quick succession, a number of hyperthermia instruments for transrectal and transurethral treatments have been made available. Unfortunately, however, one has to realize that both physicians and patients may sometimes accept these techniques uncritically.

Two procedures are currently available for local hyperthermia in BPH: (a) transrectal and (b) transurethral. The former procedure, the subject of this chapter, is discussed in more detail in Bichler et al. (1992); in both studies our investigations have been conducted with the Prostathermer (Biodan Medical Systems) (Figs. 16.1, 16.2).

16.2 Clinical Study of Transrectal Hyperthermia

16.2.1 Patients and Methods

A total of 32 patients were enrolled in the study, of whom 30 could be evaluated (see below). The patients were divided into two groups. Group 1 comprised 25 patients with prostatism (pollakiuria, nocturia, hesitancy, decreased stream, urgency, terminal dribbling, and sensation of incomplete voiding), while group 2 comprised five patients with urinary retention. The hyperthermia was performed in eight sessions of 60 min each, with two sessions per week; the intraprostatic temperature was 42°–43 °C. Prior to and 4 weeks after completion of treatment we determined the micturition score according to Boyarsky et al. (1977), the volume of the prostate, and residual urine; at the same times we also performed transrectal ultrasonography and uroflowmetry, including the nomogram according to Siroky et al. (1979).

Transrectal hyperthermia (TRHT) was tolerated well by almost all patients and no major complications were observed. Temporary voiding discomfort caused by insertion of a transurethral catheter to measure the temperature was noted in all patients. A bacterial urinary tract infection occurred in one patient. Following appropriate antibiotic treatment, TRHT could be continued. One of the 32 study patients discontinued hyperthermia after a single session because of urethral discomfort due to catheterization. An additional patient did not present for follow-up examination and thus only 30 of the 32 patients who entered the study could be evaluated. The mean thermal equivalent dose applied was 16.025 ± 6.460.

16.2.2 Results

General improvement in voiding following hyperthermia was reported by 15 patients (54%), whereas 13 (46%) noticed no change. A comparison of voiding complaints before and after hyperthermia is shown in Table 16.1.

No significant improvement in symptoms was observed as assessed by the symptom score according to BOYARSKY et al. (1977). Of the five patients with urinary retention, only one could be weaned off the catheter (recovery of voiding, residual urine volume < 50 ml, and a peak flow rate > 15 ml/s). In the remaining patients, no relevant change was observed. The size of the prostate did not decrease significantly. There was also no improvement in the objective voiding parameters such as residual volume, peak flow rate, and voiding time (Fig. 16.3).

16.2.3 Discussion

Our results do not agree with those reported by ZERBIB et al. (1992a, b) who used the same hyperthermia device for the treatment of patients. These investigators

Table 16.1. Subjective parameters

	No. of pts. with score 1–3	No. of pts. improved after hyperthermia
Nocturia	18/23	6/18 (33%)
Daytime frequency	21/23	10/21 (48%)
Hesitancy	20/23	9/20 (45%)
Terminal dribbling	14/23	5/14 (36%)
Urgency	9/23	4/9 (44%)
Weak stream	21/23	10/21 (48%)
Dysuria	3/23	3/3 (100%)
Sensation of incomplete voiding	7/23	2/7 (29%)

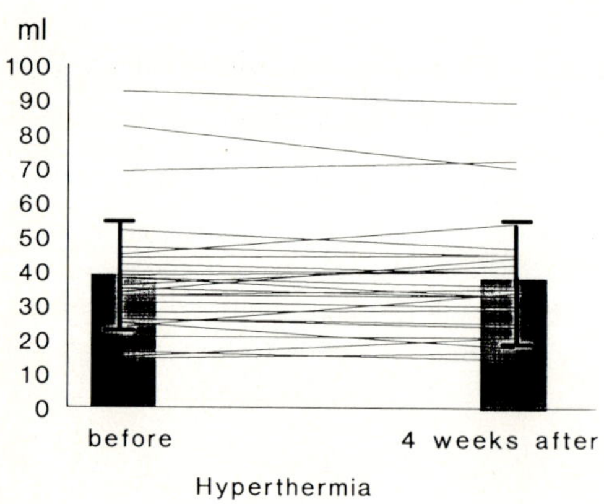

Fig. 16.3a

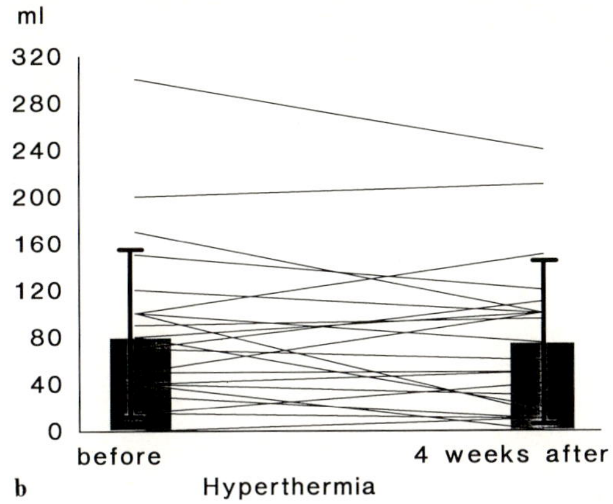

b

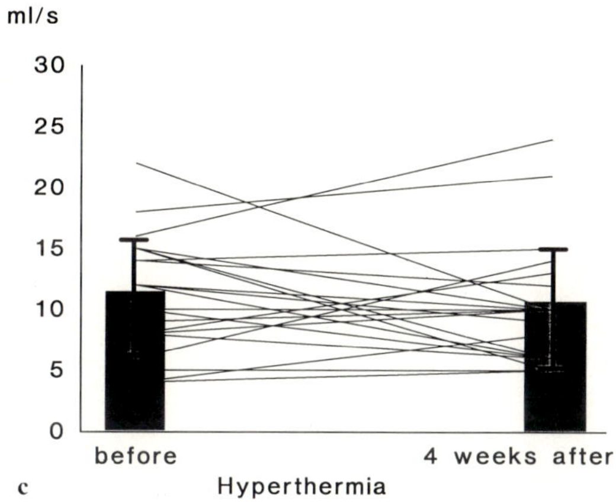

c

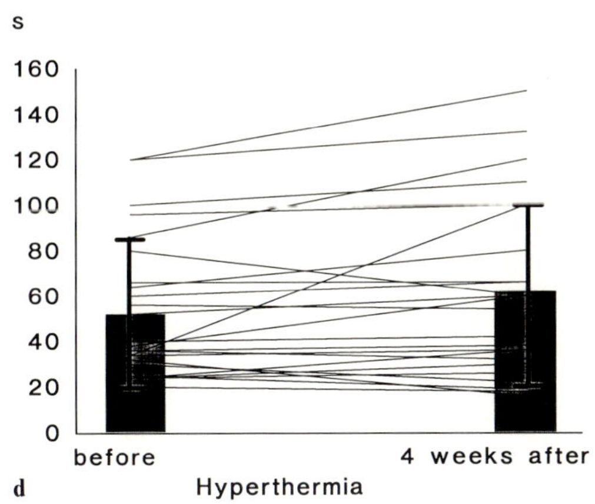

d

Fig. 16.3a-d. Objective parameters before TRHT and 4 weeks following completion of the treatment course

treated a total of 68 patients in a prospective randomized study. Of the 68 patients, 38 (56%) received TRHT, while the remaining 30 (44%) received placebo treatment. An objective response was seen in 50% of the treatment group and in 13% of the placebo group. Subjective improvement was reported

Table 16.2. Survey of the most important clinical studies on hyperthermia of the prostate

Author	No.	Hyperthermia device	Evaluation criteria	Study type	No. of sessions and HT duration	Objective response	Subjective response
Fabricius (1993, personal communication)	51	Primus Transrectal	Max. flow Residual urine Prostate size	Randomized and placebo	10 × 80 min	TRHT 20% Placebo 20%	TRHT 57% Placebo 32%
Zerbib et al. (1992)	68	Biodan Transrectal	Max. flow Residual urine	Randomized and placebo	6 × 60 min	TRHT 50% Placebo 13%	TRHT 60% Placebo 50%
van Erps and Denis (1992)	144	Primus Transrectal	Max. flow Residual urine	Single arm	10 × 60 min	24%	61%
Strohmeier et al. (1992)	30	Biodan Transrectal	Max. flow Residual urine Prostate size	Single arm	6 × 60 min	10%	50%
Van Den Bossche and Schulman (1992)	50	(Thermex II) Transurethral	Max. flow Residual urine Nocturia	Single arm	1 × 3 h	45%	70%
Baert et al. (1992)	74	BSD 300 Transurethral	Max. flow Residual urine	Single arm	5–10 × 60 min	33%	60%
Nissenkorn (1992)	37	(Thermex II) Transurethral	Max. flow Residual urine	Single arm	6 × 60 min	56%	56%
Devonec et al. (1992)	170	Prostatron Transurethral	Max. flow Residual urine	Single arm	1 × 120 min	60%	

by 60% of the treatment group and 50% of the placebo group. Objective response criteria included peak flow rate and residual urine. In another clinical study, the same investigators demonstrated that a majority of patients who had a treatment response maintained this response for 13 months or longer (ZERBIB et al. 1992b).

Another TRHT device manufactured by Technomatics Medical (Antwerp, Belgium) was used by VAN ERPS and DENIS (1992). In a study of 144 BPH patients, an objective response was reported in 24% and a subjective response in 61% of the patients. Comparable results were obtained by BERNHARDT et al. (1992) in a similar pilot study of transrectal microwave hyperthermia in patients with BPH.

FABRICIUS (1993, personal communication) reported on a placebo-controlled study with the Primus device. Of the 51 study patients, 26 (51%) received hyperthermia, while 25 (49%) received placebo only. Objective responses were not obtained in the treatment or in the placebo group. A subjective response was reported by 32% of patients in the placebo group. In the treatment group, a subjective amelioration of obstructive symptoms was reported by 57% of patients, while 61% reported an improvement in irritative symptoms. In transurethral systems (Prostatron, Thermex, The Prostate Machine) temperatures ranging from 44 °C to 50 °C were delivered via an applicator in the urethra. Treatment results obtained with these transurethral systems are shown in Table 16.2; the results of these studies were presented at the workshop held in Tübingen in the spring of 1991 (BICHLER et al. 1992).

16.3 Mode of Action of Prostatic Hyperthermia

The most important question when assessing the quality of transrectal and transurethral hyperthermia in BPH is: What is the effect of heat on the prostate?

It is supposed that when applying heat transrectally, shrinkage of the prostate results as a consequence of various processes induced by hyperthermia. An impairment of α-receptors and subsequent dilation of the bladder neck have also been discussed as a possible mode of action of TRHT.

The histologic effects of TRHT on the prostate consists of diffuse lymphocytic and plasma cell infiltrates, hyperemia, edema, and interstitial bleeding (Fig. 16.4). Subsequent resorption of the edema may cause shrinkage of the prostate.

More circumscribed changes caused by heat delivered transurethrally, with expansive necrosis of the periurethral glands, have been described by DEVONEC et al. (1992).

Another question relating to the mechanism of action of hyperthermia in the prostate is the reaction of prostate specific antigen (PSA). It has been postulated that transrectal or transurethral manipulation during hyperthermia may cause an increase in PSA levels (LINDNER et al. 1990). A study conducted in our department showed that eight of ten patients with BPH treated with TRHT showed a transient 10% increase in PSA levels during TRHT. The reason for the

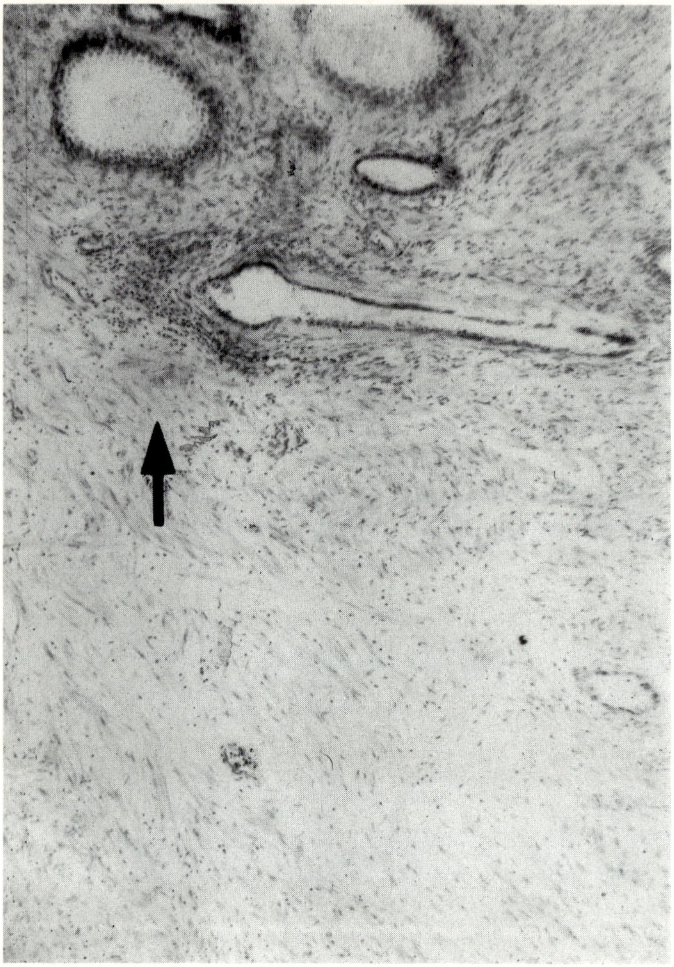

Fig. 16.4. Histologic changes following TRHT. The *arrow* points to lymphoplasmacellular infiltrates. There is also prominent edema of the stroma. H&E × 150

discrepancy in PSA levels between our study and that reported by LINDNER et al. (1990) is not clear. It may well be that it was caused by the use of different assays for PSA determination. However, the increase in PSA during hyperthermia is in accordance with the observations of FABRICIUS (1993, personal communication). Most probably, PSA elevation is caused not only by prostatic manipulations during hyperthermia but also by hyperthermia-induced effects on the epithelial cells.

In evaluating TRHT, it is important to compare treatment outcomes obtained using hyperthermia with those obtained using other treatment modalities. It is also necessary to compare TRHT with transurethral resection.

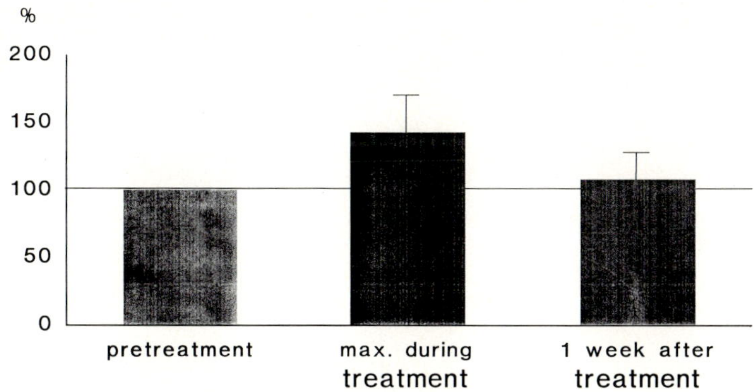

Fig. 16.5. Mean percentage change (± SD) in serum PSA levels obtained before TRHT, during the treatment, and 1 week following completion of the treatment course

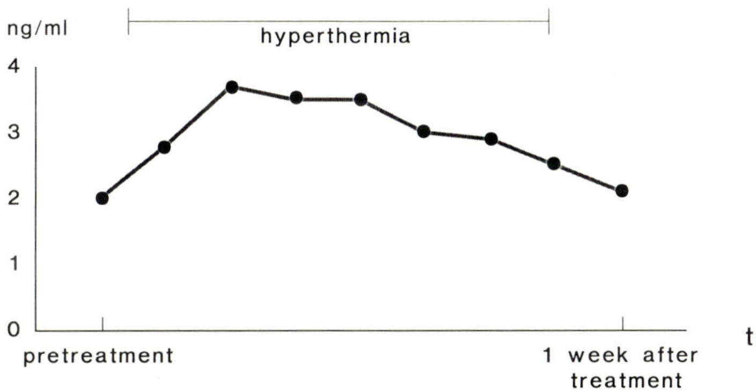

Fig. 16.6. A typical serum PSA profile in a 73-year-old patient treated with TRHT

Table 16.3. TURP: micturition parameters ($\bar{X} \pm SD$)

	Preoperative		Postoperative	
	Peak flow (ml/s)	Residual (ml)	Peak flow (ml/s)	Residual (ml)
ABRAMS et al. (1979) ($n = 152$)	6.9 ± 4.1	106	19.9 7.1	28
Tübingen (1990) ($n = 20$)	11.4 ± 6.3	125 ± 95	25.1 ± 11.8	21 ± 18

Table 16.4. Criteria for the selection of patients to receive local hyperthermia of BPH

Small prostate
No middle lobe
Residual urine 100–200 ml
Younger patients
No urinary tract infection
"Operation anxiety"
High-risk patients
Carcinoma of the prostate
No urinary retention

Investigations by Abrams et al. (1979) and results obtained at our department showed that after TURP, peak flow rates increased from 7 or 11 cc/s to 20 or 25 cc/s, respectively. Residual volume could be reduced from a mean of 106 or 125 cc to 28 or 21 cc, respectively (Table 16.3).

In the process of assessing any kind of treatment for BPH, one needs to be cognizant of the unpredictable natural course of this disease, which is often characterized by spontaneous improvement (see Chap. 3). It is not unusual to observe little change or no change in objective or subjective parameters in BPH patients studied over a long period (several years) (Ball et al. 1981).

It remains to be seen whether an escalating, stepwise therapeutic approach in BPH – beginning with pharmacologic treatment and proceeding through hyperthermia, stent, and balloon dilation to transurethral resection (after a period of varying duration) – will meet our demands, especially in patients unwilling to undergo an operation. On the basis of our results and those obtained with transurethral hyperthermia (42°–47 °C), the indications for hyperthermia in BPH are shown in Table 16.4.

To summarize, it can be said that local hyperthermia (42°–47 °C) is applicable as a palliative treatment. Subjective symptoms in particular are improved considerably following administration of hyperthermia. Moreover, a favorable effect of varying degree is found for uroflow and residual urine. Side-effects are common but of no importance and include dysuria and involuntary bladder spasm.

In our opinion, the trend in the application of local hyperthermia will be towards the refinement of appropriate technological precautionary measures (cooling), permitting more controlled thermocoagulation, localized exclusively to the prostate.

The treatments that are being tested at present are laser, high-intensive focussed ultrasound, and last but not least, thermocoagulation either by way of local hyperthermia application at temperatures ranging around 60 °C or in the form of thermoablation (Technomed) at temperatures of approximately 80 °C. It remains to be seen whether advances in technology in the form of computer-aided machines will render it possible to introduce such methods into clinical practice. The trend in BPH treatment – when making the best use of the various

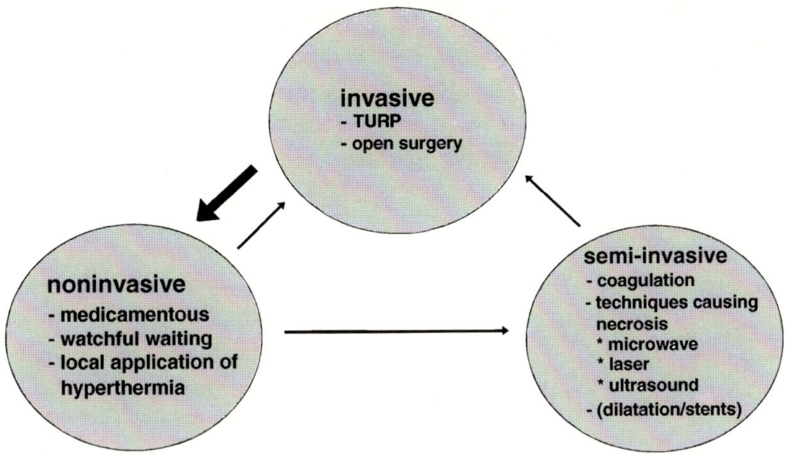

Fig. 16.7. Treatment options in patients with symptomatic BPH

options – might be as illustrated in Fig. 16.7. It seems likely that there will be a continuing shift in urologic practice away from operative methods and towards less invasive treatment techniques. It is not expected, however, that surgical treatment will be totally replaced by the new and less invasive therapeutic modalities.

References

Abrams PH, Farrar DJ, Turner-Warwick RT, et al. (1979) The results of prostatectomy: a symptomatic and urodynamic analysis of 152 patients. J Urol 121 : 640–642

Baert L, Ameye F, Willemen P, Petrovich Z (1992) Transurethral microwave hyperthermia for benign prostatic hyperplasia, the Leuven clinical experience. In: Bichler KH, Strohmaier WL, Wilbert DM (eds) Hyperthermia of the prostate. State of the art. PMI, Franfurt, pp 90–97

Ball AJ, Feneley RCL, Abrams PH (1981) The natural history of untreated prostatism. Br J Urol 53 : 613–616

Bernhardt K, Basting RF, Hammer H (1992) Transrectal hyperthermia – pilot study. In: Bichler KH, Strohmaicr WL, Wilbert DM (eds) Hyperthermia of the prostate. State of the art. PMI, Franfurt, pp 87–89

Bichler KH, Strohmaier WL, Wilbert DM (eds) (1992) Hyperthermia of the prostate. State of the art. PMI, Frankfurt, pp 5–125

Boyarsky S, Jones G, Paulson DF, Prout GR Jr (1977) A new look at bladder neck obstruction by the Food and Drug Administration regulators: guidelines for investigation of benign prostatic hyperplasia. Trans Am Assoc Genitrourin Surg 68 : 29–32

Devonec M, Cathaud N, Dufrieuux-Berger N, et al. (1992) Histology of thermal injury induced by transurethral microwave thermotherapy of benign prostatic hyperplasia In: Bichler KH, Strohmaier WL, Wilbert DM (eds) Hyperthermia of the prostate. State of the art. PMI, Franfurt, pp 98–103

Lindner A, Siegel Y, Korczak D, et al. (1990) Serum prostate specific antigen levels during hyperthermia treatment of benign prostatic hyperplasia. J Urol 144 : 1388–1389

Nissenkorn I (1993) Transurethral hyperthermia for benign prostatic hyperplasia (BPH) using the Thermex II. In: Bichler KH, Strohmaier WL, Wilbert DM (eds) Hyperthermia of the prostate. PMI, Franfurt, pp 104–105

Roos NP, Wennberg JE, Malenka DJ, et al. (1989) Mortality and reoperation after open and transurethral resection of the prostate for benign prostatic hyperplasia. J Med 320:1120–1124

Siroky MB, Olsson CA, Krane KE (1979) The flow rate nomogram. I. Development. J Urol 121:665–668

Strohmaier WL, Fluchter SH, Wilbert DM, Bichler KH (1993) Influence of transrectal hyperthermia on prostate specific antigen in prostatic cancer and benign prostatic hyperplasia. Urol Int 51:28–31

van den Bossche M, Schulman CC (1992) Transurethral hyperthermia for benign prostatic hypertrophy. In: Bichler KH, Strohmaier WL, Wilbert DM (eds) Hyperthermia of the prostate. State of the art. PMI, Franfurt, pp 105–107

Zerbib M, Conquy S, Steg A, et al. (1992a) A prospective randomized study of localized hyperthermia vs. placebo in obstructive benign hypertrophy of the prostate. In: Bichler KH, Strohmaier WL, Wilbert DM (eds) Hyperthermia of the prostate. State of the art. PMI, Franfurt, pp 71–72

Zerbib M, Conquy S, Steg A, et al. (1992b) Long-term follow-up of 40 patients treated by transrectal hyperthermia of obstructive benign prostatic hypertrophy. In: Bichler KH, Strohmaier WL, Wilbert DM (eds) Hyperthermia of the prostate. State of the art. PMI, Franfurt, pp 73–74

17 Transurethral Microwave Thermotherapy

MARIAN DEVONEC, JEAN-PHILIPPE FENDLER, PATRICE JOUBERT, and PAUL PERRIN

CONTENTS

17.1 Introduction

Current therapeutic options for benign prostatic hyperplasia (BPH) include medical management, which has only a limited effect and is essentially palliative and reversible at the end of the treatment (LEPOR 1989), and endoscopic surgery, which clearly has an important effect made permanent by the removal of prostatic tissue and the creation of a cavity within the prostate (LEPOR and RIGAUD 1990; HOLTGREWE et al. 1989). In addition to these two treatment options, there is a possibility of using minimally invasive alternative therapy whose aim is essentially to induce irreversible tissue changes in order to obtain

MARIAN DEVONEC, MD, PhD, JEAN-PHILIPPE FENDLER, MD, PATRICE JOUBERT, MD, and PAUL PERRIN, MD, Professor and Chairman, Department of Urology, Antiquaille Hospital, Claude Bernard University, 69321 Lyon, France

Petrovich/Baert (Eds.)
Benign Prostatic Hyperplasia

therapeutic effectiveness more optimal than that of medical treatment. Treatment outcome of this minimally invasive therapy should be as close as possible to that of transurethral resection of the prostate (TURP), the standard management of BPH, but at a lesser cost in terms of associated morbidity and clinical burden.

17.2 The Difference Between Hyperthermia and Thermotherapy

The application of microwave energy to tissue results in heating and, consequently, the activation of protective mechanisms against heat, i.e., thermoregulation. Only when these mechanisms become saturated beyond thermal threshold is the tissue damaged. Histologic changes resulting from this treatment can be easily observed and are dependent on the physical characteristics of the microwave emission. Microwave thermotherapy of BPH should be distinguished from microwave hyperthermia in that its goal is to cause an irreversible tissue lesion with a favorable outcome in the irritative and obstructive symptoms of BPH. Hyperthermia elevates the temperature of the target tissue to 42°–44 °C (COSSET 1989). Repeated exposures to such temperatures have been shown to affect cancerous tissue and are essentially used in combination with radiation therapy. Hyperthermia treatment of cancer is safe because temperatures of 42°–44 °C do not produce immediate tissue necrosis (see Chaps. 13, 14). Normal or benign tissue treated with transrectal hyperthermia requires much higher temperatures, well above 45 °C, before it undergoes necrosis (SERVADIO et al. 1989; LINDNER et al. 1990a; STROHMAIER et al. 1990; MONTORSI et al. 1992; ZERBIB et al. 1992; VAN DEN BOSSCHE et al. 1991). On the other hand, repeated applications of transurethral hyperthermia produces a well-defined but superficial necrosis of the prostatic urethra (BAERT et al. 1990; SAPOZINK et al. 1990; LAUWERYNS et al. 1991).

Thermotherapy elevates the temperature of the target tissue to between 46° and 60 °C (DEVONEC et al. 1991). At such high temperatures, a single exposure of 1 h has been shown to induce thermocoagulation of benign hypertrophy of the prostate. Thermotherapy is safe if there is constant monitoring of the rectal and urethral temperatures. Above 60 °C, thermoablation of prostatic tissue can be observed with the formation of a cavity inside the prostate gland.

The treatment goals, thermokinetic characteristics, and pathology results of the two techniques are so different that the World Health Organization has drawn a distinction between thermotherapy (intraprostatic temperature between 46° and 60 °C) and hyperthermia (intraprostatic temperature between 42° and 44 °C) (SMITH et al. 1992).

17.2.1 Safety, Pain, and Efficacy Thresholds of Microwave Therapy

Three thresholds have been demonstrated during the use of microwave therapy in the treatment of BPH: a safety threshold, a pain threshold, and an efficacy threshold (DEVONEC et al. 1992a). These three thresholds are close to each other. Homeostasis in man means that the pain threshold lies above 45 °C. Below 45 °C, a 1-h exposure is not harmful to normal cells in that it does not create cell necrosis (see Chap. 14). This is the safety threshold. Well above 45 °C, a 1-h exposure results in tissue necrosis. This is the cellular toxicity, or efficacy threshold. Pain occurs above 45 °C and warns the organism that prolonged exposure (beyond 45 °C) will be harmful to the organism as a whole.

17.2.1.1 Safety Threshold

The abundant vasculature of the rectal wall provides an efficient and natural shield against the heat not only for the rectum itself but also for the contiguous posterior part of the prostate. This explains why the temperature recorded in Denonvilliers' fascia can be up to 18 °C lower than that recorded elsewhere at the same distance from the urethral antenna, but laterally in the adenomatous tissue. The continuous recording of rectal temperature monitors the safety of the procedure.

17.2.1.2 Pain Threshold

Tolerance to microwave treatment is satisfactory, especially rectal tolerance. Urethral temperatures beyond 45 °–47 °C appear to be the limiting factor, whereas within the prostate, a much higher temperature (up to 60 °C) can be recorded and well tolerated. This observation suggests an organ-specific sensitivity to heat and/or a concentration of pain receptors in the prostatic capsule and urethra.

17.2.1.3 Efficacy Threshold

Prostatic tissue destruction requires temperatures well above 45 °C, and preferably beyond 50 °C. Thus pain appears to play a natural homeostatic role, preventing tissue damage due to exposure to higher temperature. The treated area has a distinct margin, indicative of a precise cell toxicity threshold; cytoplasmic enzymes are probably destroyed beyond this threshold, causing cell death.

17.2.2 Principles of Transurethral Microwave Thermotherapy

Microwave heating is the consequence of electromagnetic energy absorption by tissue (DEVONEC et al. 1992c). The principle of radiative heating differs from the principle of cooling, which is based on conductivity from a limited depth

(Fig. 17.1A). The combination of these two modes of energy diffusion, i.e., radiative heating and conductive cooling, results in a temperature curve with a steep ascending slope and a progressive descending slope (Fig. 17.1B). As long as the temperature remains below the cell's toxicity threshold, no histologic effect is observed (Fig. 17.1C). Tissue destruction occurs when the ascending

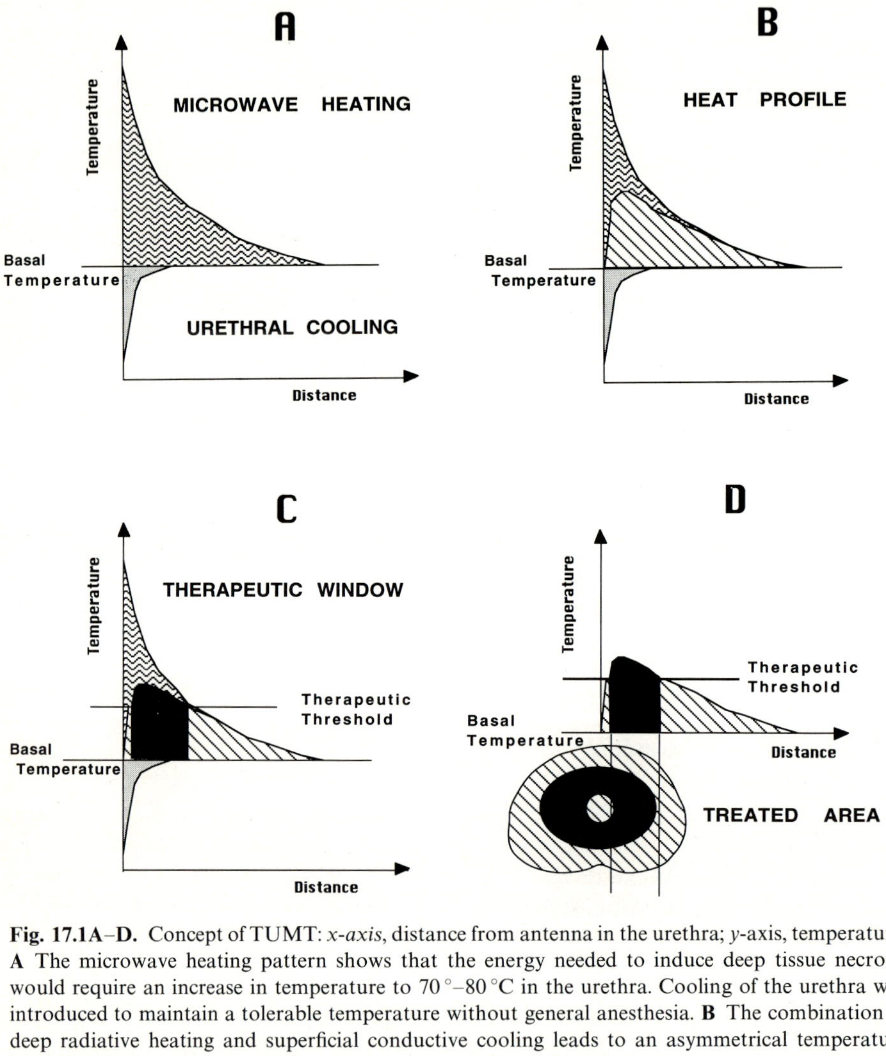

Fig. 17.1A–D. Concept of TUMT: *x-axis*, distance from antenna in the urethra; *y*-axis, temperature. **A** The microwave heating pattern shows that the energy needed to induce deep tissue necrosis would require an increase in temperature to 70°–80°C in the urethra. Cooling of the urethra was introduced to maintain a tolerable temperature without general anesthesia. **B** The combination of deep radiative heating and superficial conductive cooling leads to an asymmetrical temperature profile, with a steep ascending slope and a progressive descending slope. **C** Because of the cell toxicity threshold, periurethral tissue is preserved as long as the temperature is below the therapeutic threshold. Tissue destruction (*area in dark*) is observed as soon as the ascending slope crosses the therapeutic threshold and continues until it is crossed again by the descending slope. **D** Theoretical application of TUMT concept of prostate. The gland is protected centrally and surrounded by a crown of treated prostatic tissue (*area in dark*)

slope of the curve goes beyond this toxicity threshold and is maintained for at least 30 min. Tissue destruction does not occur when the tissue temperature is below 45 °C. Consequently, the integration of a cooling system permits the preservation of the urethra and the periurethral mucosa in the center of the necrotic zone. The cooling allows the urethral temperature to be maintained below the pain threshold.

17.3 Histology of Thermal Injury (46°–60 °C)

The histology of the thermal injury induced in the prostate by transurethral microwave thermotherapy (TUMT) was studied using suprapubic adenomectomy specimens of TUR chips from patients undergoing operation subsequent to TUMT (Devonec et al. 1992a, d).

17.3.1 Evolution of Thermal Injury

The thermal injury evolves with three phases: coagulation necrosis, granulomatous reaction, and fibrous scar.

17.3.1.1 Acute Phase

After adenoma enucleation post thermotherapy, radial sections of the two lobes showed a thermocoagulation lesion with a butterfly shape. Tissue destruction was symmetrical around the urethra.

Transurethral resection of a treated prostate showed a preserved urethra: superficial bites removed chips with a pink mucosa on one side and underlying necrotic tissue; deeper bites removed necrotic tissue.

At this stage, microscopic examination showed coagulation necrosis. In the center of the lesion glandular cells and smooth muscle cells were totally destroyed and were replaced by a reticular pattern with an intense edematous reaction; small vessels (capillaries) were thrombosed, whereas larger vessels were preserved. Interstitial hemorrhage was common. Peripherally, the inner limit of the lesion showed a preserved urethra with a sharp transition from the treated to the nontreated area, as did the outer limit of the lesion.

17.3.1.2 Intermediate Phase

The intermediate phase occurred within the second to third week and was characterized by the appearance of a granulomatous reaction peripherally. The features were: neo-angiogenesis with the appearance of neocapillaries and a mild lymphohistiocytic infiltrate, penetrating into the center of the lesion. Centrally, the edematous reaction diminished and mild collagen deposition was observed. Interestingly, there was no tissue liquefaction and no abscess formation.

17.3.1.3 Late Phase

The late phase (within 1–2 months) was the phase of scar organization. Centrally there was no regeneration of acini or of smooth muscle cells. The treated area was replaced by bands of collagen and fibroblasts. Lymphocytic infiltration was less pronounced.

17.3.2 Important Features of the Thermal Lesion

The healing process of the thermal lesion induced by TUMT in the prostate evolved in a similar fashion to the usual healing process of any coagulation necrosis lesion. However, certain features are worth emphasizing.

17.3.2.1 Sharp Delineation of the Lesion

The lesion had sharp margins, whether it was the inner margin near the urethra or the outer margin near the prostatic capsule. There are two possible explanations for this: a steep temperature gradient between the two sides of the margin during treatment or a well-defined cell toxicity threshold. As for the inner margins, the "elevated temperature gradient proposal" may not hold true since the temperature slope ascends rapidly with a temperature gradient of 5°–15 °C between the two sides, i.e., 5–15 °C over a distance of a few millimeters (Fig. 17.1C). The situation was totally different at the outer margin, where the temperature slope was gentle, with a temperature gradient of only 1° or 2°C on either side of the margin. However, it also had a sharp delineation. The well-defined cell toxicity threshold explanation is favored. Experimental work in dogs as well as in humans suggests that this threshold is well above 45 °C (DEVONEC et al. 1991). This explains why the temperature range (42°–44 °C) of transrectal hyperthermia does not induce histologic changes in terms of tissue necrosis in the human prostate (STROHMAIER et al. 1990; MONTORSI et al. 1992).

17.3.2.2 Absence of Abscess Formation

The second feature is the absence of abscess formation in the thermocoagulation lesion. This is possibly related to the persistence of some blood supply and the absence of tissue liquefaction on microscopic examination. The thermocoagulation lesion has similar features to an infarction lesion, except for the preservation of some blood perfusion. With these temperatures, the thermotherapy injury does not lead to the formation of a cavity but rather to a retractile fibrous scar comparable to that observed after infarction.

17.3.2.3 Histologic Features of Thermal Origin

There are no late stigmata characteristic of thermal origin of the fibrotic scar inside the prostate that distinguish it from a natural prostatic infarction; homogenization of smooth muscle cells, and hemosiderin deposits secondary to interstitial hemorrhage resorption by macrophages and histiocytes are not necessarily of heat origin. However, the symmetrical topography and extent of the lesion on both sides of the urethra, as well as the sharp inner delineation at the level of the periurethral region, are highly suggestive of its thermal origin. The initial brown butterfly-shape lesion observed during the first week is the only typical histologic signature of thermotherapy.

17.3.3 Clinical Implications of the Histologic Features of the Thermal Lesion

17.3.3.1 Treatment Efficacy

Irreversible tissue damage is mandatory for a favorable treatment outcome and probably for lasting efficacy. Periurethral tissue destruction beyond the preserved urethra is potentially involved in the α-blocker type effect rapidly experienced by the patient. Indeed, nerve connections with α-receptors of the preserved mucosa are destroyed. The healing process of the lesion leads to a fibrous scar, possibly with a smaller volume and/or with a decreased urethral tone. Thus both the irritation syndrome and the dynamic and static components of the obstructing syndrome of BPH are affected by thermotherapy (Blute et al. 1992; Carter et al. 1991).

17.3.3.2 Treatment Safety

The absence of prostatic abscess and the sharp limits of the treated area are synonymous with the safety of the other normal structures in the region, such as the rectal wall, striated sphincter, and trigone. Preservation of the urethra is the direct consequence of cooling, which anesthetizes the prostatic urethra, allowing a high power output. Without cooling, pain in the urethra impedes power output. Prolonged (van den Bossche et al. 1991) or repeated (Lauweryns et al.

Table 17.1. Effects of heat on normal or benign prostate

	Temperature (°C)	Technique	Effect
Fever	> 37		
Hyperthermia	42–44	Microwaves	No histologic effect
		Radio-frequency	
Thermotherapy	47–60	Microwaves	Thermocoagulation
	60–100	Microwaves	Thermoablation
		Laser	
		Focused ultrasound	
		Piezo-electricity	

1991) sessions of transurethral hyperthermia induce at most superficial burning of the urethral and periurethral tissue.

In conclusion, the thermotherapy technique allows one to work within a new temperature range and provides a new type of lesion in benign tissue. In its present state, microwave thermotherapy works in the temperature range of 46°–60 °C (Table 17.1), i.e., above the hyperthermia temperature range, at which benign tissue is not affected, and below the temperature level of 60 °C, at which tissue ablation will occur.

17.4 Clinical Results

Well-controlled phase II and phase III clinical trials are being conducted to evaluate thermotherapy in patients complaining of BPH.

17.4.1 Randomization Sham vs TUMT

Four well-controlled studies are presently evaluating the placebo response to TUMT: the multicenter Food and Drug Administration study (USA) (150 patients), the Nijmegen study (Netherlands) (50 patients), the multicenter French study (150 patients), and the London study (England) (40 patients). In their present state, they corroborate the results published from the English trial based on the randomization of 40 patients (OGDEN et al. 1993). At 3 months, the thermotherapy group showed a 70% decrease (from 14.5 to 4.3) in the mean Madsen symptom score (Madsen SS), a 53% increase in peak flow rate (PFR) (8.5 to 13.0 ml/s), and a 92% decrease in postvoiding residual volume (PRV) (147 to 12 ml). No significant change was seen in these mean indices in the sham group. There was no difference in the incidence of transient hematuria between the two groups. However, acute retention occurred in 22% of patients in the

TUMT group. The results show little placebo contribution to the significant subjective and objective improvement that occurs in patients who have received TUMT.

17.4.2 Randomization TUMT vs TURP

Sixty patients with obstructing BPH have been evaluated in a prospective randomized study comparing TUMT with TURP (Pettersson et al. 1993). The 12-month evaluation showed that in the TUMT and TURP groups, the PFR increased from a mean of 7.5 and 7.2 ml/s, respectively, before treatment, to 12.0 and 18.9 ml/s after 6 months. The PRV decreased from 110 to 136 ml, respectively, before treatment, to 63 and 16 ml post-treatment. The Madsen SS dropped from 11.8 and 13.3 to 3.6 and 0.8. The side-effects in the two groups were few but more severe in the TURP group. These results show slightly better outcome in the TURP group, but their complications were more severe than those in the TUMT-treated patients. Most of the patients in the two groups have, so far, been happy with the result of the treatment.

17.4.3 Long-Term Efficacy of TUMT

Transurethral microwave thermotherapy has been evaluated in well-controlled long-term studies. In a multicenter study involving 12 centers (Devonec et al. 1992b), 818 patients were treated with a single 1-h session and were followed up to 18 months. Over this period, the Madsen SS fell from 13.3 to 3.4 (74%), the PFR increased from 8.8 to 12.9 ml/s (47%), and the PRV decreased from 121 to 74 ml (39%). TUMT provided a long-lasting effect over a period of 18 months.

Symptom improvement was observed at 1 month post-treatment, this being sooner than the improvement in urinary flow, which was observed at 3 months.

17.4.4 Success Rate of TUMT

Interpretation of the results after TUMT is dependent on the definition of success (Devonec et al. 1992c). If success corresponds to an increase in the PFR of 50% or above 15 ml/s and/or a fall in the Madsen SS of 50% or below 5, the results of TUMT are, on average, as follows: 70% of patients can be considered successfully treated; 20% of patients are mildly improved, not reaching the aforementioned figures but not requiring any other form of treatment; and 10% of patients are clear failures and need a transurethral resection.

17.4.5 Dose Dependence of TUMT

In order to identify features of the ideal candidate and the ideal treatment, a retrospective analysis was conducted in patients treated at eight centers (BERG et al. 1993). Responders (R) were defined as having a PFR increase of 50% and > 15 ml/s post-treatment, a Madsen SS fall of 50% and < 3, and a PRV decrease of 50% and below 100 ml. Nonresponders (NR) were defined as having a PFR increase < 20% and < 10 ml/s post-treatment, a Madsen SS fall < 50% and > 5, and a PRV decrease < 50% and > 200 ml. The responders (77 patients) showed a mean PFR increase of 91%, a Madsen SS fall of 71%, and a PRV decrease of 57%. The NR group (62 patients) showed a PFR increase of 14%, a Madsen SS fall of 16%, and a PRV increase of 25%. Before treatment, no significant differences in patient profile were found between the two groups. However, significant differences in treatment profile were found between them (R vs NR, respectively). The total energy delivered to the prostate was 120 kJ vs 90 kJ, and the total time with a urethral temperature greater than the rectal temperature was 31 vs 24 min. The PSA increase 1 week after treatment was 1300% vs 150%. The results show that currently there is no ideal patient profile, since before treatment, no significant differences were found between the two groups. However, the outcome of treatment is dose dependent and is probably linked to the prostate histology and blood supply specific to each individual.

17.5 Thermoregulation During TUMT

Transurethral microwave thermotherapy in 340 BPH patients treated at our center showed the important role played by the two thermoregulatory processes during the procedure (DEVONEC et al. 1993b). The first one was artificial and automatically driven by the machine (the power output and cooling rate were adjusted to the urethral and rectal temperature safety thresholds). The second one was natural thermoregulation. The latter is species-organ, zone-cell specific. The variability has been demonstrated by interstitial thermometry and histologic study. The human prostate is more resistant to heat than the dog prostate of a comparable volume treated with the same thermal dose. The prostate of a young patient requires a higher thermal dose than that of an old patient with the same prostate volume in order to achieve a comparable intraprostatic temperature, probably due to a more viable blood supply. The transition zone is more sensitive to heat than the peripheral zone, as demonstrated by recorded temperatures of 60 °C and 42 °C, respectively, at the same distance from the antenna. Acinar cells seem to be more resistant to heat than smooth muscle cells when exposed to the same temperature level, as demonstrated by microscopic examination at the periphery of the treated area. Increases in thermal dose can be safely achieved only by accurate management of both the natural and the artificial thermoregulatory processes.

17.6 From Microwave Thermocoagulation to Microwave Thermoablation

The results demonstrating the dose dependence of TUMT led us to increase the temperature in order to improve its efficacy, especially for those patients with clinical evidence of obstruction. Increasing the intraprostatic temperature to greater than 60 °C induces thermoablation of prostatic tissue. At this temperature, tissue blood supply is totally suppressed, whereas the lower temperature (below 60 °C) of the conventional protocol allows partial preservation of the blood supply in the coagulated tissue .

Forty patients were treated with this experimental protocol and 50% had a cavity in their prostate at 3 months (Devonec et al. 1993c). The cavity was cone or cylinder shaped, with its base at the bladder neck and its apex at the verumontanum. No cavity was observed in the remaining 50% of patients, probably because of the relatively low thermal dose received, limited by frequent rectal alarms. No major complications were recorded but morbidity (i.e., acute urinary retention, nonbacterial prostatitis) was higher than that of the conventional protocol (intraprostatic temperature below 60 °C).

In conclusion, the results obtained with TUMT demonstrated the dose dependency of the response based on thermometry and histologic data as well as on the clinical outcome of patients. In its present state, TUMT allows for the treatment of irritation as well as that of obstruction related to BPH, using the same device but with a different treatment protocol according to the patient's profile. In any case, treatment is delivered during a single 1-h session and without the need for neuroleptanalgesia even in the prostate thermoablation protocol for obstructed patients.

17.7 Comparison of Thermotherapy with Other Techniques

Comparison of the results with other techniques using heat produced by nonionizing radiation are hard to make, be it according to the principle of microwave hyperthermia (Servadio et al. 1989; Lindner et al. 1990a; Stawarz et al. 1991) or of diathermia, an earlier technique (Bordier 1928) using "a mixture" of radiofrequencies (van den Bossche et al. 1991). Indeed, any comparison will lead one to compare therapies with different aims, using different technologies, and achieving a different thermal effect (tissue maintained below 45 °C), without any histologic proof (Lauweryns et al. 1991) comparable to that demonstrated by other groups using thermotherapy (Devonec et al. 1992a), nor with any biologic modification of the PSA level (Lindner et al. 1990b).

The future belongs to the technique that offers greater efficacy with regard to objective parameters while maintaining the treatment conditions close to those presently used in thermotherapy, i.e., a single session of short duration, without general anesthesia. It is likely that this improvement will be provided by increasing the thermal dose. The advantage of thermotherapy over hyperthermia, using transrectal or transurethral microwave heating; is that thermotherapy is evolving: the thermal dose can be augmented while maintaining the same conditions, namely the absence of pain and the safety of neighboring organs.

Other techniques aiming at tissue thermoablation, such as the TULIP system (ROTH and ARETZ 1991), focused piezoelectricity using the external route (VALLANCIEN et al. 1991), or focused ultrasound using the endorectal route (FOSTER et al. 1991; CHAPELON et al. 1991), are at the stage of early clinical trials in man, as is microwave thermoablation. Their safety relies on the precision of the permanent echographic localization used to target the therapeutic vector, whereas the safety of microwave thermotherapy relies simply on suprapubic ultrasound confirmation of the correct positioning of the microwave catheter balloon during treatment. The best technique will be the one that provides the best compromise between three parameters: safety for the patient, efficacy, and ease of use.

References

Baert L, Ameye F, Willemen P, et al. (1990) Transurethral microwave hyperthermia of benign prostatic hyperplasia: preliminary clinical and pathological results. J Urol 144:1383–1387

Berg C, Choi N, Colombeau P, et al. (1993) Responders versus nonresponders to thermotherapy in BPH: a multicenter retrospective analysis of patient treatment profiles. J Urol 149:251A

Blute ML, Tomera KM, Hellerstein DK, et al. (1992) Transurethral microwave thermotherapy for prostatism: early Mayo Foundation experience. Mayo Clin Proc 67:417–421

Bordier H (1928) Application de la diathermie en Urologie. In: Bordier H (ed) Diathermie et Diathermotherapie. Bailliere, Paris, pp 359–371

Carter C, Patel A, Reddy P, Royer P, Ramsay JWA (1991) Single session transurethral microwave thermotherapy for the treatment of benign prostatic obstruction. J Endourol 5:137–144

Chapelon JY, Margonari J, Bouvier R, et al. (1991) Ablation tissulaire par ultrasons focalises (ATUF). Proges en Urologie 1:231–244

Cosset JM (1989) Interstitial hyperthermia. In: Gautherie M (ed) Interstitial, endocavitary and perfusional hyperthermia. Springer, Berlin Heidelberg New York, pp 1–37

Devonec M, Berger N, Perrin P (1991) Transurethral microwave heating of the prostate: from hyperthermia to thermotherapy. J Endourol 5:129–135

Devonec M, Berger N, Cathaud M, et al. (1992a) Historical development of transurethral microwave thermotherapy (TUMT): short and long term results in benign prostatic hyperplasia. In: Fitzpatrick JM (ed) Non-surgical treatment of BPH. Churchill-Livingstone, New York, pp 187–206

Devonec M, Tomera K, Perrin P (1992b) Transurethral microwave thermotherapy (TUMT) in benign prostatic hyperplasia. In: Puppo P (ed) Urology. Monduzzi, Bologna, pp 239–244

Devonec M, Tomera K, Perrin P (1992c) Transurethral microwave thermotherapy. In: Stamey TA (ed) Monographs in urology. Montverole, Florida, Medical Directions Publishing 13:77–95

Devonec M, Cathaud M, Dutrieux-Berger N, et al. (1992d) Histology of thermal injury induced by transurethral microwave thermotherapy of benign prostatic hyperplasia. In: Bichler KH, Strohmaier WL, Wilbert DM (eds) Hyperthermia of the prostate. State of the art. Verlagsgruppe, Frankfurt, pp 98–103

Devonec M, Ogden C, Perrin P, St Clair Carter S (1993a) The clinical response to transurethral microwave thermotherapy is thermal-dose dependent. Eur Urol 1993, 23:267–274

Devonec M, Berger N. Fendler JP, et al. (1993b) Thermoregulation during transurethral microwave thermotherpay: experimental and clinical fundamentals. Eur Urol 1993, 23:63–67

Devonec M, Fendler JP, Jouver P, et al. (1993c) Thermotherapy in benign prostatic hypertrophy: an update of clinical results and latest development. J Endourol (in press)

Foster RS, Bihrle R, Sanghvi NT, et al. (1991) Noninvasive ultrasound produced volume lesion in prostate. J Urol 145:396A

Holtgrewe HLM, Mebust WK, Dowd JB, et al. (1989) Transurethral prostatectomy: practice aspects of the dominant operation in American urology. J Urol 141:248–253

Lauweryns J, Baert L, Vandenhove J, Petrovich Z (1991) Histopathology of prostatic tissue after transurethral hyperthermia. Int J Hyperthermia 7:221–230

Lepor H (1989) Nonoperative management of benign prostatic hyperplasia. J Urol 141:1283–1289

Lepor H, Rigaud G (1990) The efficacy of transurethral resection of the prostate in men with moderate symptoms of prostatism. J Urol 143:533–537

Lindner A, Braf Z, Lev A, et al. (1990a) Local hyperthermia of the prostate gland for the treatment of benign prostatic hypertrophy and urinary retention. Br J Urol 65:201–203

Lindner A, Siegel YI, Korczak D (1990b) Serum prostate specific antigen levels during hyperthermia treatment of benign prostatic hyperplasia. J Urol 144:1388–1389

Montorsi F, Galli L, Guazzoni G, et al. (1992) Transrectal microwave hyperthermia for benign prostatic hyperplasia: long term clinical, pathological and ultrastructural patterns. J Urol 148:321–325

Ogden CW, Reddy P, Johnson H, Ramsay JW, St. Clair Carter S (1993) Sham versus transurethral microwave thermotherapy in patients with symptoms of benign prostatic bladder outflow obstruction. Lancet 341:15–17

Pettersson S, Dahistrand C, Fall M, Geirsson G (1993) Transurethral microwave thermotherapy versus transurethral resection for benign prostatic hyperplasia: preliminary results of a randomized study. Eur Urol 23:292–298

Roth RA, Aretz HT (1991) Transurethral ultrasound guided laser-induced prostatectomy (TULIP procedure): a canine prostate feasibility study. J Urol 146:1128–1135

Sapozink MD, Boyd SD, Astrahan MA, Jozsef G, Petrovich Z (1990) Transurethral hyperthermia for benign prostatic hyperplasia: preliminary clinical results. J Urol 143:944–950

Servadio C, Lindner A, Lev A, et al. (1989) Further observations on the prostate gland for the treatment of benign prostatic hypertrophy and urinary retention. Br J Urol 65:204–208

Smith P, Chaussy C, Conort P, et al. (1992) Report of the committee on other nonmedical treatment. In: Cockett ATK, Aso Y, Chatelain C, Denix L, Griffith K, Khoury S, Murphy G (eds) The international consultation on benign prostatic hyperplasia by World Health Organization. Churchill-Livingstone, New York, pp 187–206

Stawarz B, Szmigielski S, Ogrodnik J, Astrahan M, Petrovich Z (1991) A comparison of transurethral and transrectal microwave hyperthermia in poor surgical risk benign prostatic hyperplasia patients. J Urol 146:353–357

Strohmaier WL, Bichler KH, Fluchter SH, Wilbert DM (1990) Local microwave hyperthermia of benign prostatic hyperplasia. J Urol 144:913–917

Vallancien G, Chopin D, Davilla D, et al. (1991) Focal extracorporeal pyrotherapy: preliminary experimental results. Prog Urol 1:84–88

van den Bossche M, Noel JC, Schulman CC (1991) Transurethral hyperthermia for benign prostatic hypertrophy, World J Urol 9:2–6

Zerbib M, Steg A, Conquy S, et al. (1992) Localized hyperthermia versus the sham procedure in obstructive benign hyperplasia of the prostate: a prospective randomized study. J Urol 147:1048–1052

18 Treatment Results with Transurethral Hyperthermia in Patients with Benign Prostatic Hyperplasia

LUC BAERT, FILIP AMEYE, and ZBIGNIEW PETROVICH

CONTENTS

18.1 Introduction

Surgery is the modality of choice in the treatment of patients with moderate to severe symptoms and signs of benign prostatic hyperplasia (BPH) (GRAVERSON et al. 1989). Patients with these signs and symptoms who are poor surgical risks [American Society of Anesthesiologists (ASA) group ≥ 3] have limited treatment options (New Classification of Physical Status 1963). Transrectal microwave hyperthermia (TRHT) has been in use as a treatment for poor surgical risk BPH patients since 1980. Major improvement was reported in more than 70% of patients, with no treatment complications of importance being seen (YERUSHALMI et al. 1985; LINDNER et al. 1990). Other investigators, however, could not reproduce these excellent treatment results (STROHMAIER et al. 1990; STAWARZ et al. 1991). In a report by STROHMAIER et al. (1990), no convincing

LUC BAERT, MD, PhD, Professor and Chairman, Department of Urology, St. Pieter's Hospital, Catholic University of Leuven, Brusselsestraat 69, 3000 Leuven, Belgium and Clinical Professor of Urology and Radiation Oncology, University of Southern California School of Medicine, Los Angeles, CA 90033, USA
FILIP AMEYE, MD, Department of Urology, St. Pieter's Hospital, Catholic University of Leuven, Brusselsestraat 69, 3000 Leuven, Belgium
ZBIGNIEW PETROVICH, MD, Professor and Chairman, Department of Radiation Oncology, University of Southern California, Kenneth Norris Jr. Cancer Center, 1441 Eastlake Avenue, Los Angeles, CA 90033, USA

Petrovich/Baert (Eds.)
Benign Prostatic Hyperplasia

evidence of therapeutic activity was noted in 32 patients treated with TRHT (see Chap. 19).

Since 1985, transurethral microwave hyperthermia (TUHT) has been under investigation for poor surgical risk patients (Astrahan et al. 1989; Sapozink et al. 1990). Two phase I studies have demonstrated therapeutic effectiveness of TUHT, with subjective and objective improvement being noted in more than 70% of patients (Sapozink et al. 1990; Baert et al. 1990). Histologic changes have been reported in periurethral prostate. Their intensity and extent correlated well with the applied treatment temperatures (Lauweryns et al. 1991).

18.2 Patients and Methods

From April 1989 to July 1990, 104 BPH patients were treated with TUHT at the Department of Urology, Catholic University of Leuven in Leuven, Belgium in cooperation with the University of Southern California School of Medicine (USC). The age of the patients ranged from 52 to 95 years, with a mean age of 71 years. Criteria for admission to TUHT studies included: mean peak flow rate < 15 cc/s, postvoiding residual volume (PRV) > 100 cc, or urinary retention. Subjective complaints were assessed using the Food and Drug Administration (FDA) recommended symptom score scale (Boyarsky et al. 1977).

All patients had a detailed general and urologic history and physical examination. Laboratory studies included: general, cytologic, and bacteriologic urinalysis, complete blood count, serum prostate specific antigen (PSA), prostatic acid phosphatase (PAP), blood urea nitrogen, and serum creatinine. Prostatic volume and PRV were measured utilizing transrectal ultrasonography. Flexible cystoscopy was performed to evaluate prostatic and bladder neck anatomy. Radiographic studies were obtained on an as-needed basis. Prostatic needle biopsy was performed only in patients in whom, based on clinical laboratory studies, the presence of adenocarcinoma of the prostate was suspected. ASA class was determined in poor operative risk patients during routine preoperative counseling by the responsible anesthesiologist.

Of the 104 patients treated, 74 (71%) had moderate to severe symptoms and signs of urinary outflow obstruction. The remaining 30 (29%) patients presented with urinary retention. The majority (59%) of patients had bilobar hyperplasia, while 12% had trilobar and 31% had median lobe or median bar enlargement (Table 18.1). Prostate volume ranged from 20 to 150 cc (mean 49 cc). The mean peak flow rate of the 74 patients who were not in retention was 9 cc/s and the mean average flow rate was 5.1 cc/s. Mean PRV was 147 cc. The mean score on the FDA scale was 13.5.

The majority (62%) of treated patients, including all 30 patients presenting with retention, had ASA class ≥ 3. The remaining 40 (38%) patients refused the recommended surgical procedure and were treated with TUHT.

Table 18.1. Distribution of patients by clinical presentation and prostatic morphology

Clinical presentation	Bilobar	%	Trilobar	%	Median Lobe	%	Median bar	%	Total	%
Urinary retention	23	77	0	0	4	13	3	10	30	29
Moderate to severe outflow obstruction	38	51	12	16	14	19	10	14	74	71
Total	61	59	12	12	18	17	13	12	104	100

18.3 Hyperthermia Technique

All 104 patients were treated with TUHT at 915 MHz, using a BSD 50 or BSD 300 apparatus of BSD Medical Corporation (Salt Lake City, Utah, USA). Transurethral applicators consisted of a modified 14-French urologic catheter. This catheter contained a helical antenna and a channel for thermometry. The helical antenna was positioned for TUHT in the prostatic urethra. Its location was verified with transrectal ultrasonography. Hyperthermia was given once per week for 60 min at a steady state in 74 patients without retention. The 30 retention patients were treated twice a week.

The temperature was controlled on the urethral surface at 45 °C ± 1 °C. Continuous temperature monitoring was required throughout each treatment. Additionally, temperature mapping along the prostatic urethra was obtained ≥ 3 times during each treatment session. The temperatures during the mapping procedure were measured at 5-mm intervals. Details on the treatment technique, instrumentation, and temperature monitoring have been published (Astrahan et al. 1989, 1991; Baert et al. 1990; Sapozink et al. 1990).

All TUHT treatments were administered on an outpatient basis without sedation or anesthesia. The 30 patients who presented with retention received a mean of 8.9 TUHT sessions, while the other 74 patients had a mean of 5.2 sessions per patient.

Regular follow-up visits were scheduled at 1, 3, and 6 months after the completion of TUHT. At each follow-up visit, interval general and urologic histories were obtained. Prostatic volume and PRV were measured with transrectal ultrasonography. Peak and average flow rates were obtained. Posttreatment flexible cystoscopy was performed in the first ten patients. Because of the absence of significant changes, its routine use was discontinued. All patients had their symptoms assessed and compared with the pretreatment values utilizing the FDA recommended symptom score scale. Due to an almost universal patient refusal to report for follow-up studies beyond 6 months, their use in otherwise stable patients could not be continued. Follow-up ranged from 6 to 24 months with a mean of 12 months.

Objective treatment response was considered good if an improvement in a measured parameter was $> 50\%$, and fair if it was $\leq 50 \geq 30\%$. An improvement of $< 30\%$ was considered treatment failure. Subjective response was scored as follows: an improvement of > 10 points was considered an excellent response, $> 5 \leq 10$ points was a good response, $\geq 3 \leq 5$ was a fair response, and < 3 points was a treatment failure.

18.4 Results

In the 30 patients who presented with urinary retention, 17 (57%) resumed normal voiding at the end of TUHT. It is of interest to note that of the 23 retention patients who had bilobar or trilobar hyperplasia, 17 (74%) resumed normal voiding. This was in contrast to the seven median lobe or median bar patients, who did not respond to the treatment. The 17 patients who had a treatment response had a mean post-treatment PRV of 80 cc, a mean average flow rate of 6.3 cc/s, and a mean peak flow rate of 11.4 cc/s. Their mean FDA symptom score was 6.0. Of these 17 patients who had a response, 14 were catheter-free at 1 year. Worsening of symptoms was noted in one patient at 6 months post-treatment. He was successfully managed with α-blockers. The remaining two patients died of intercurrent disease before 1 year, maintaining spontaneous voiding until death.

Objective treatment response was seen in 70% of the 74 non-retention patients. There was a significant ($P < 0.002$) decrease in PRV (Fig. 18.1). An increase in the mean average flow rate was measured, ($P = 0.23$) and an increase in the mean peak flow rate was recorded from 9 to 12 cc/s ($P < 0.0026$)

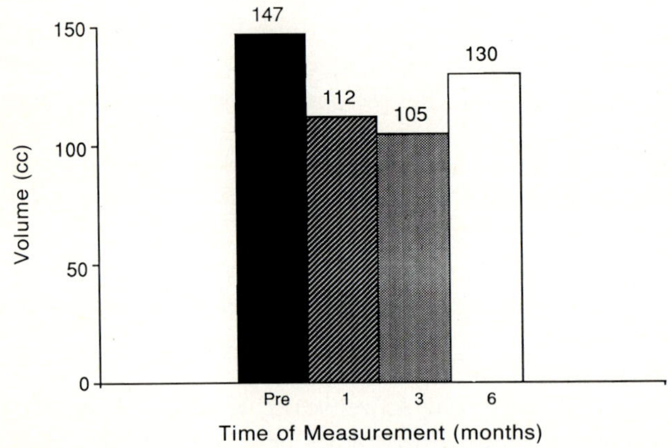

Fig. 18.1. Mean PRV for the 74 nonretention patients before TUHT and at 1-, 3-, and 6-month follow-up visits

(Fig. 18.2). In the 50 patients with bilobar or trilobar hyperplasia, a decrease in the mean PRV was noted from 134.5 cc to 119 cc at 6 months post-treatment (NS at $P = 0.25$) (Fig. 18.3). In the same group of 50 patients, an increase in the mean average flow rate was recorded from a mean of 5.5 cc/s to a mean of 7 cc/s ($P < 0.086$) (Fig. 18.4). There was no change in the mean average flow rate in the 14 median lobe (6.5 cc/s vs 6.4 cc/s) or in the ten median bar patients (4.3 cc/s vs 4.8 cc/s) ($P = 0.822$). The mean peak flow rate increased in the 50 bilobar and trilobar patients. This increase was from 9.8 cc/s before the treatment to 13.6 cc/s at 6 months post-treatment ($P = 0.056$) (Fig. 18.4). In the 14 median lobe patients, the mean peak flow rate increased from 10.4 cc/s to 13.3 cc/s

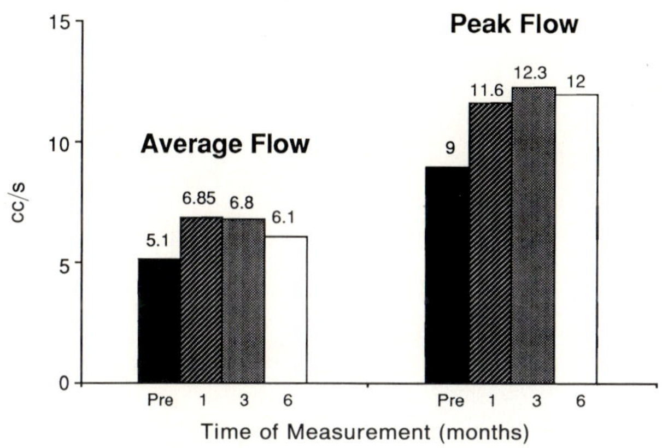

Fig. 18.2. A comparison of mean average and mean peak flow rates before and after treatment for the 74 nonretention patients

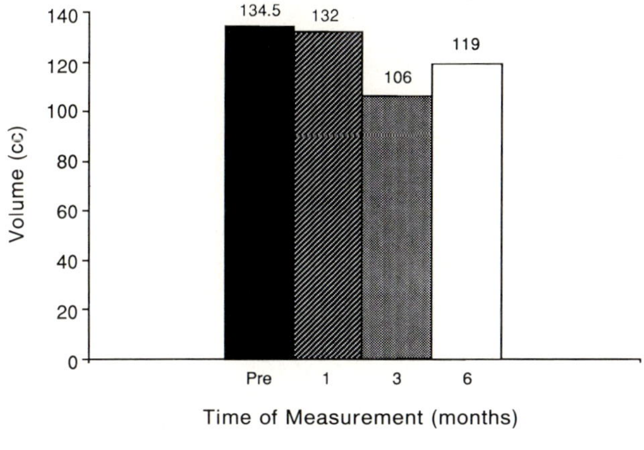

Fig. 18.3. Changes in mean PRV in the 50 bilobar and trilobar hyperplasia patients

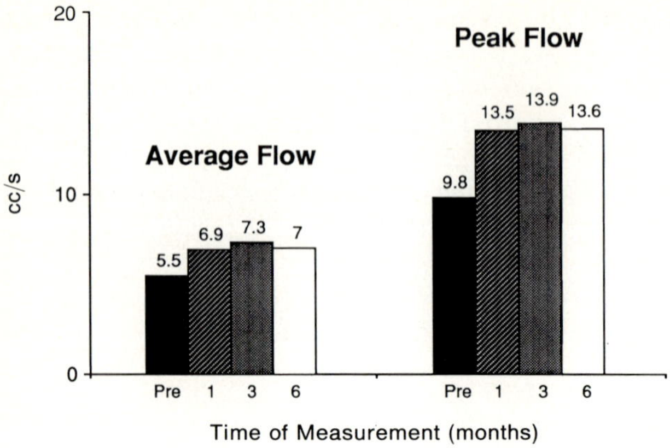

Fig. 18.4. A comparison of mean average and mean peak flow rates before and after treatment in the 50 bilobar and trilobar hyperplasia patients

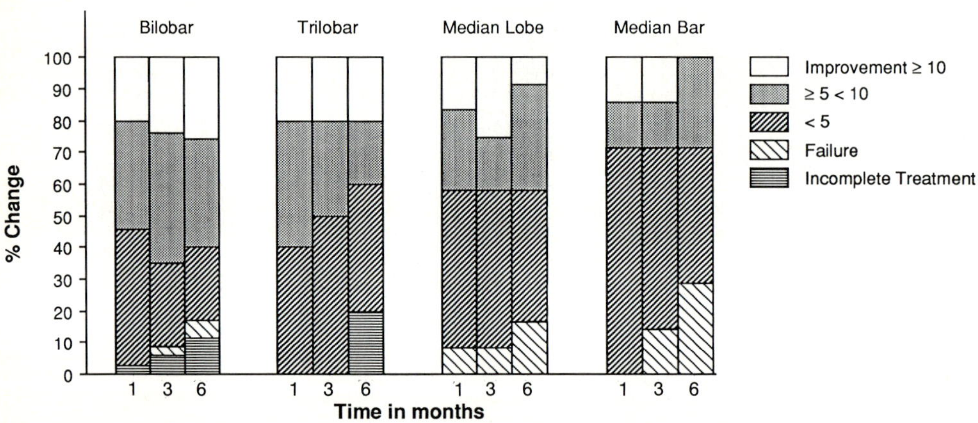

Fig. 18.5. Post-treatment mean FDA symptom score changes for the 74 nonretention patients. In each morphologic group, mean score changes were measured at 1, 3, and 6 months post-TUHT

($P = 0.372$). In the ten median bar patients, this increase was from 8.7 cc/s to 10 cc/s ($P = 0.190$).

An excellent, good, or fair subjective improvement was seen in 75% of the 74 non-retention patients. Of the 38 bilobar hyperplasia patients, 60% showed an excellent or good improvement (> 5 points on the FDA symptom score scale) at 6 months post-treatment (Fig. 18.5). The same degree of improvement was seen in 40% of the 12 trilobar patients, 41% of the 14 median lobe patients, and 29% of the ten median bar patients (Fig. 18.5). The failure rate ranged from a low of 4% for the 50 bilobar and trilobar hyperplasia patients to a high of 30% for the ten median lobe patients (Fig. 18.5).

A decrease in the overall mean symptom score for the 74 nonretention patients was from a mean of 13.5 points to a mean of 8.5 points at 6 months post-therapy (Fig 18.6). There was also a decrease in the mean scores for nocturia and obstructive and irritative symptoms. The decrease in the mean score was greater for the obstructive as compared to the irritative symptom

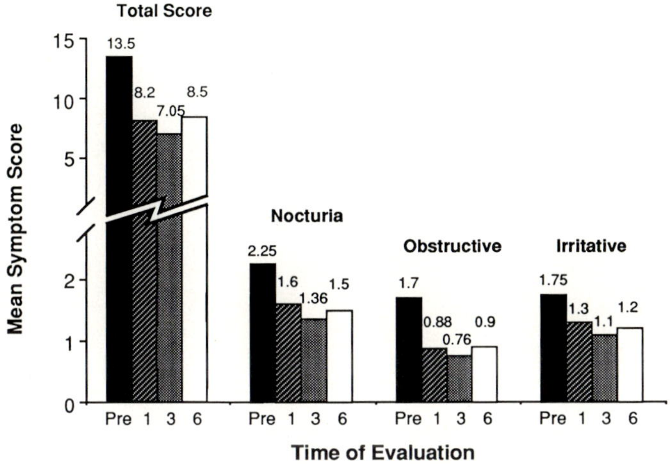

Fig. 18.6. Comparison of mean pre- and post-treatment total FDA symptom scores for the 74 non-retention patients. Changes in mean symptom scores for nocturia, and for obstructive and irritative mean symptom scores

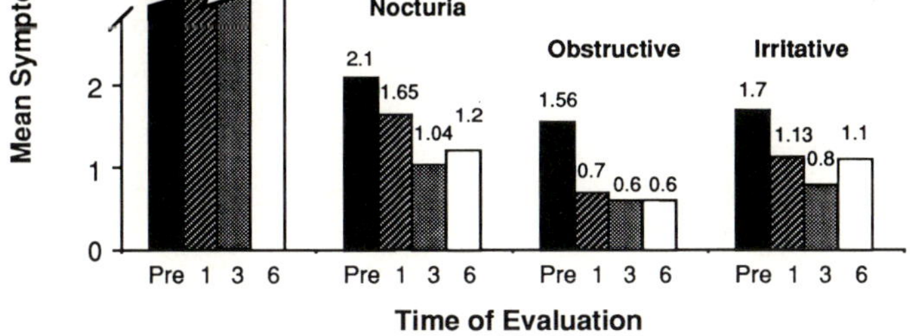

Fig. 18.7. Comparison of mean pre- and post-treatment FDA symptom scores for the 50 patients with bilobar and trilobar hyperplasia. Changes in mean symptom scores for nocturia and for obstructive and irritative mean symptom scores

score (Fig. 18.6). The 38 bilobar hyperplasia patients showed a decrease in the mean symptom score from 13 to 6.5 points while the score was reduced from a mean of 14 to a mean of 6.5 points for the 12 trilobar hyperplasia patients (Fig. 18.7). As expected, there was a corresponding decrease in the mean post-treatment score for obstructive and irritative symptoms. This decrease was again greater for the obstructive than for the irritative symptoms. A lesser reduction in the mean symptom score was seen in the median lobe and median bar patients, i.e., from 13 to 12 and from 14 to 9 points, respectively.

Of the 13 (12.5%) patients who failed TUHT, 11 were salvaged with transurethral resection or an open prostatectomy. The remaining two patients had ASA class 4 and had only a permanent suprapubic catheter placement. It is of interest to note that all of the surgically treated patients showed distinct periurethral histologic changes thought to be induced by TUHT (LAUWERYNS et al. 1991; BAERT et al. 1990).

18.5 Treatment Complications

Bladder spasms were reported in 619 (95%) of the 652 TUHT treatments given to the 104 patients. They were manifested by an urge to void and mild suprapubic discomfort. At the conclusion of 587 (90%) TUHT treatments following the removal of a hyperthermia applicator, minor urethral bleeding was noted. Typically, it was seen as a few to several drops of blood at the meatus. This bleeding did not persist in 97% of sessions. Following 20 (3%) treatments mild hematuria was reported for up to 36 h and following four (0.6%) treatments it lasted for up to 5 days. In no case did this hematuria require any treatment.

Perineal pain during TUHT was reported in 83 (13%) sessions. This pain was mild and did not persist beyond a hyperthermia treatment session. In six (1%) sessions it was a power limiting factor. Of the 74 nonretention patients, 59 (80%) reported an increase in irritative complaints, such as pollakiuria, urgency, and dysuria. These complaints were usually reported following the first few treatments and regressed within 36 h. Following the first TUHT treatment, one of the patients in this study developed symptoms and signs of superficial vein thrombophlebitis of a lower extremity. This problem was successfully managed and did not require a change in TUHT schedule.

Subjective treatment intolerance requiring discontinuation of TUHT was seen in seven (6.7%) patients. Of the 74 nonretention patients, four (5%) had acute retention after the first heat treatment. In three of these patients, a single catheterization resolved the problem, while one patient required temporary suprapubic catheter placement. This catheter was removed near the end of the hyperthermia treatment course and the patient resumed normal voiding.

Urinary tract infection was seen in 12 (12%) patients. In five of these it was an asymptomatic bacteriuria, two had acute prostatitis, two developed orchiepididymitis, two had bacteremia, and one had urosepsis. Nearly all infection problems developed in the 30 patients who presented with urinary retention. All of the seven patients with infection were successfully treated with the appropriate antibiotic therapy.

18.6 Discussion

This study has demonstrated that TUHT is a reasonable treatment alternative in BPH patients who would meet the criteria for surgical treatment except that their poor general condition precludes the safe use of operative management. TUHT is also a good treatment option for patients who refuse surgical treatment for various reasons, such as fear of the operation or fear of postoperative sexual dysfunction.

Treatment tolerance was good in this study in 93% of patients. Acute treatment complications were common but mild and of no clinical importance. Significant complications were seen in seven patients (7%) who developed moderate to severe urinary tract infection (UTI). These complications were seen early in the study. A prophylactic use of antibacterial agents in patients with high risk for developing UTI, such as those presenting with urinary retention, prevented the occurrence of this problem in patients treated later in this study. The most gratifying outcome of this hyperthermia treatment program was the lack of serious late complications such as urethral stricture or incontinence. In fact, serial post-treatment flexible cystoscopies demonstrated normal mucosa without any evidence of injury. These data are similar to the USC experience, where, with a minimum follow-up of 42 months, no late treatment sequelae were seen (Sapozink et al. 1990).

The effect of TUHT was shown to be limited to the immediate periurethral prostate. Histologic changes extended 4–5 cm and 6–8 mm radially (Lauweryns et al. 1991; Baert et al. 1990). Interstitial temperature measurements performed in several patients prior to prostatectomy have shown symmetrical and predictable temperature distributions limited to a cylindrical prostate volume showing histologic changes consistent with those considered to be caused by hyperthermia (Astrahan et al. 1991). This volume was largely confined to lateral lobes, which explains the limited effectiveness of TUHT seen in BPH patients with a predominance of median lobe or median bar involvement (Baert et al. 1991). From the time this observation was made, TUHT was not offered to the patients who, on preliminary flexible cystoscopy, were found to have a prominent median lobe or median bar. Currently, an effort is being made to design a transurethral microwave antenna which will be able to heat preferentially an enlarged median lobe or median bar.

In spite of the demonstrated safety of TUHT and strong evidence of its therapeutic activity, this modality remains investigational. Poor surgical risk BPH patients or those who refuse surgical treatment should be offered TUHT only within the confines of a clinical study (see Chap. 19, 20).

18.7 Summary

During a 15-month period, 104 patients with BPH, including 30 who presented with retention, were treated with 915-MHz transurethral hyperthermia (TUHT). A total of 652 TUHT treatments were given at a temperature controlled on the urethral surface of 45 °C. Follow-up ranged from 6 to 24 months (mean 11 months). Of the 30 retention patients, 57% were catheter-free at 1 year; this included 17.23 patients with lateral lobe hyperplasia versus 0.7 for median lobe or median bar patients. The overall objective response for the 74 nonretention patients was 70% and a major subjective response was obtained in 75% of patients. Of the 104 patients treated, 13 (12.5%) failed TUHT. Surgical treatment was successfully used in 11 and two had permanent suprapubic drainage.

Treatment was well tolerated by the study patients. Acute toxicity was common but clinically insignificant. Significant complications were noted in seven (6.7%) patients who developed infection. Current efforts are directed toward optimization of TUHT for BPH patients.

References

Astrahan MA, Saponzink MD, Cohen D, et al. (1989) Microwave applicator for transurethral hyperthermia of benign prostatic hyperlasia. Int J Hyperthermia 5:283–296

Astrahan MA, Ameye F, Oyen R, et al. (1991a) Interstitial temperature measurements during transurethral microwave hyperthermia. J Urol 145:304–308

Astrahan MA, Imanaka K, Jozsef G, et al. (1991b) Heating characteristics of a helical microwave applicator for transurethral hyperthermia of benign prostatic hyperplasia. Int J Hyperthermia 7:141–145

Baert L, Ameye F, Willemen P, et al. (1990) Transurethral microwave hyperthermia for benign prostatic hyperplasia: preliminary clinical pathological results. J Urol 144:1383–1387

Baert L, Willemen P, Ameye F, et al. (1991) Transurethral microwave hyperthermia: treatment response in different forms of benign prostatic hyperplasia. Prostate 18:315–320

Boyarsky S, Jones G, Paulson DF, et al. (1977) A new look at bladder neck obstruction by the Food and Drug Administration regulators: guidelines for investigation of benign prostatic hypertrophy. Trans Am Assoc Genitourin Surg 68:28–32

Graverson PH, Gasser TC, Wasson JH, et al. (1989) Controversies about indications for transurethral resection of the prostate. J Urol 141:475–481

Lauweryns J, Baert L, Vandehove J, et al. (1991) Histopathology of prostatic tissue after transurethral hyperthermia. Int J Hyperthermia 7:221–230

Lindner A, Braf Z, Lev A, et al. (1990) Local hyperthermia of the prostatic gland for the treatment of benign prostatic hypertrophy and urinary retention. Br J Urol 65:201–203

New Classification of Physical Status (1963) The 1962 House of Delegates of the American Society of Anesthesiologists. Anesthesiol 2: 111

Sapozink MD, Boyd S, Astrahan MA, et al. (1990) Transurethral hyperthermia for benign prostatic hyperplasia with preliminary clinical results. J Urol 143:944–950

Stawarz B, Szmigielski S, Ogrodnik J, et al. (1991) A comparison of transurethral and transrectal microwave hyperthermia in poor surgical risk BPH patients. J Urol 146:353–357

Strohmaier WL, Bichler KH, Fluchter SH, et al. (1990) Local microwave hyperthermia of benign prostatic hyperplasia. J Urol 144:913–917

Yerushalmi A, Fishelovitz Y, Singer D, et al. (1985) Localized deep microwave hyperthermia in the treatment of poor operative risk patients with benign prostatic hyperplasia, J Urol 133:873–876

19 Critical Evaluation of Treatment Modalities in Local Hyperthermia of the Prostate

FILIP AMEYE and LUC BAERT

CONTENTS

19.1 Introduction

Over the past two decades, hyperthermia (HT) in the range of 42°–45 °C has been under intensive study as a treatment for malignant neoplasms. Hyperthermia

FILIP AMEYE, MD, Department of Urology, St. Pieter's Hospital, Catholic University of Leuven, Brusselsestraat 69, 3000 Leuven, Belgium

LUC BAERT, MD, PhD, Professor and Chairman, Department of Urology, St. Pieter's Hospital, Catholic University of Leuven, Brusselsestraat 69, 3000 Leuven, Belgium and Clinical Professor of Urology and Radiation Oncology, University of Southern California School of Medicine, Los Angeles, CA 90033, USA

Petrovich/Baert (Eds.)
Benign Prostatic Hyperplasia

has found its greatest applicability as a potential adjuvant to radiation and chemotherapy.

Recently, microwave HT technology was introduced as a conservative treatment modality for patients with benign prostatic hyperplasia (BPH) who could not be treated surgically. The rationale behind the development of this technique originated in hyperthermic oncology. It assumed that hyperplastic prostatic tissue shrinks in a similar way as neoplastic tissue following the administration of local HT. This shrinking of obstructive tissue results in a subsequent lowering of outflow obstruction.

Microwaves can be delivered to the prostate by transrectal (TRHT) or transurethral (TUHT) techniques. Each treatment modality has its own thermophysical and clinical characteristics. To increase radial power deposition in the prostate and diminish patient intolerance or toxicity, cooling systems have been introduced in all transrectal and some transurethral systems. Finally, two concepts of tissue temperature elevation, applying microwaves, are used. Hyperthermia provides temperatures of up to 45 °C, while thermotherapy (TUMT) is able to reach temperatures of up to 55 °C (see Chap. 13). Focused extracorporeal pyrotherapy (FEP) using focal high-energy ultrasound waves elevates the temperature to 120 °C.

Several HT devices have been developed and are employed in clinical practice, using one of these modalities. Clinical results obtained with each system have been typically reported as excellent or, at least, promising. However, critical review of the literature shows some contradictions. Authors using the same machine or technique have reported broadly different responses. Due to a lack of uniformity in treatment protocols and differences in response evaluation, comparison of the treatment results reported by different groups is very difficult.

Finally, every critical clinician is aware of the difficulty in assessing response patterns of different treatment modalities for BPH. The unpredictable, natural history of BPH has important implications for the interpretation of results from published clinical trials (see Chap. 6). The placebo effects of nonsurgical treatment modalities can strongly influence the treatment outcome. Accurate comparison of pre- and post-treatment objective and subjective parameters is dependent upon the intrinsic absolute value and/or variability of each of these parameters. Severity of symptoms in a given patient may vary substantially from moment to moment without any relation to the applied treatment. Even more problems exist in the assessment of objective urodynamic parameters. Determinations of mean and peak urinary flow rates and residual urine are dependent upon intrinsic factors such as detrusor contractility, voided volume, and the degree of outflow obstruction and α-adrenergic activation. These problems complicate the process of symptom and objective parameter assessment (see Chap. 6).

Interpretation of the thermophysical data for different HT applicators and devices is even more confusing. Specific reports on the physics and techniques of microwave-induced HT for prostatic diseases are very sparse and extrapolated mainly from basic microwave physics as applied to hyperthermic oncology. Manufacturers of the commonly used HT instruments rarely release their scientific data for peer review by microwave engineers and physicists or for evaluation by urologists with a special interest in this field. Results of preclinical testing in phantoms and laboratory animals and/or toxicity studies are not routinely reported or they are incomplete. Occasionally, certain physical features of a hyperthermia device are not correctly reported by the manufacturers.

Consequently practicing urologists face a difficult task in evaluating the physical characteristics of different HT devices and modalities and interpreting the reported clinical data. The goal of this report is to summarize some thermophysical and clinical data in respect of several commonly used HT devices and to present guidelines for preclinical testing of these devices and for the conduct of HT clinical trials. Correlation of the reported data with the proposed guidelines will allow urologists to assess the efficacy of each device. Data were obtained from publications in peer-reviewed scientific journals or from published abstracts containing the data presented at the recent major international meetings. Updated treatment results were also requested from all leading investigators and manufacturers of HT instruments and are included if presented to the author.

19.2 Clinically Applied Hyperthermia Modalities

The modalities of HT can be classified into five groups: whole-body HT, deep regional HT, superficial HT, interstitial HT, and intracavitary HT (Turner and Schaefermeyer 1987).

The theoretical goal of whole-body HT is the elevation of the entire body to a uniformly raised temperature. In practice, however, uniform temperatures are not obtainable. The maximum temperature achievable with this technique is generally considered to be 41.8 °C. At higher temperatures unacceptable toxicity occurs. Interest in the clinical use of whole-body HT is in combining it with systemic chemotherapy. Due to complexity of whole-body HT and potentially severe toxicity, its use is limited to a few major research centers.

Deep regional HT is used in tumors with a depth greater than 5 cm. This technique attempts to heat larger, deep-seated tumors. It is particularly useful, for example, for the treatment of pelvic tumors. Due to technological limitations this hyperthermia modality can be used only in carefully selected patients.

Superficial HT has gained much wider acceptance. This modality involves the heating of tissues from the skin surface to a depth not exceeding 5 cm.

Interstitial HT is also gaining increased acceptance. This treatment modality involves placement of heating devices directly into the tumor. The popularity of this modality has increased as interstitial radiation therapy has become more widely practiced. The use of this technique permits much higher tumor temperatures with lower normal tissue temperatures.

Hyperthermia has also been applied by inserting heating devices into natural body cavities. Transrectal or transurethral hyperthermia is the most common method for application of hyperthermia of the prostrate. The rationale for this modality is similar to that for the interstitial techniques. Even in deep sites, the heating can be localized to the tumor and heating of normal tissues avoided.

19.3 Methods of Prostatic Hyperthermia

19.3.1 Transurethral Hyperthermia

The physical basis for microwave heating of the prostrate has already been extensively described in Chap. 13. The proximity of the prostrate to the naturally accessible cavities overcomes various technological problems to bring the source of energy near the gland. The disadvantage in the use of this technique is its limited radial heat penetration which diminishes with the increase in MW frequency. Using intracavitary devices and frequencies in the range from 433 to 2450 MHz, there are no significant clinical differences in the depth of penetration (see Chap. 13). For practical reasons, 915 MHz is the frequency most commonly used in both TU and TR devices.

19.3.2 Transrectal Versus Transurethral Application

The use of intracavitary HT by the transrectal or transurethral approach has often been the subject of controversy. Each method has its own advantages and disadvantages based on theoretical and clinical considerations.

A major advantage of the intrarectal antenna is the use of a natural body cavity allowing for noninvasive positioning of the applicator immediately adjacent to the prostate. Additionally, this HT application is well tolerated by patients. However, a practical disadvantage of TRHT is the difficulty in assuring exact and reproducible positioning of the antenna against the anterior rectal wall next to the prostate. This difficulty is compounded by the intrinsic applicator design, the width of the rectal ampulla, and the need for patient cooperation. Complicated targeting during this procedure is also needed as microwave power deposition decreases rapidly with the increase in distance from the intracavitary applicator due to geometric dispersion and attenuation. Using a transrectal approach, effective microwave penetration is limited to a depth of 2 cm. Primary deposition of energy therefore occurs in peripheral prostate, while central and adenomatous obstructive tissue is heated to a lesser degree. Consequently, transrectal applicators must operate at high power levels to deliver sufficient energy to central obstructive tissues. Since maximum energy deposition and peak temperature elevations occur immediately adjacent to this applicator, cooling of the anterior rectal wall is required to prevent its overheating. Due to a fear of severe toxicity, target temperatures are generally not higher than 43°–43.5 °C, and multiple treatment sessions are needed.

The transurethral technique is more simple to administer and more reproducible. The inflated Foley balloon, once seated in the trigone, positions the symmetrically radiating antenna and thermometry sensors in the prostatic urethra. The thermal gradient surrounding the applicator is steep enough to confine heating within the prostate yet provides enough penetration to act on the periurethral and central obstructive tissues. This method of antenna positioning and the symmetrical heating pattern make the treatment accuracy independent of patient movement during the treatment. The predictable and symmetrical temperature distribution with these applicators as well as reliable temperature control with nonperturbing thermal sensors also makes the use of invasive thermometry unnecessary. A disadvantage of the use of this technique, however, is the requirement for repeated urethral catheterization.

19.3.3 Transurethral Hyperthermia Versus Thermotherapy

Transurethral hyperthermia applicators do not require urethral surface cooling since the peak temperature occurs in the obstructive tissues immediately adjacent to the applicator, where it can be precisely measured and regulated by the thermosensors. Temperatures of up to 45 °C on the urethral surface have been found to be safe and well tolerated by patients. Higher (> 46 °C) temperatures usually result in patient intolerance and may produce a serious urethral injury. Depending on the device and treatment protocol used, TUHT is usually applied in several 1-h sessions. The optimal number of treatments is not known. Based on our data it appears that five or more treatments are required for high probability of a major response.

Thermotherapy applicators have an incorporated simultaneous conductive cooling system. Urethral surface cooling allows for the application of a greater amount power. This cooling, which limits urethral pain, preserves the integrity of the urethral mucosa. Thermotherapy, defined as a treatment with tissue temperatures between 45° and 55 °C, is capable of causing definite histologic changes in deeper seated normal prostatic tissues. This is achieved by a mechanism of direct necrosis and infarction with preservation of the urethra. These high temperatures can also cause thermal destruction of nontargeted tissues. Precise sonographic targeting and accurate temperature measurements are needed to prevent serious sequelae. An important benefit with the use of this technique is the need for only a single, 60 min treatment session (Harzmann and Weckermann 1991).

19.3.4 Focused Extracorporeal Pyrotherapy

The effect of pyrotherapy is based on the phenomena of a marked and rapid temperature rise (up to 120 °C) and cavitation using focal high-energy ultrasound waves generated by a piezoelectric system. Due to the severe pain resulting from this method, anesthesia during the treatment is required (VALLENCIEN et al. 1992).

19.3.5 Temperature Monitoring

Close monitoring of tissue temperature is required to minimize toxicity and optimize treatment efficacy. At the present time, there is no reliable method of indirect temperature measurements of the prostate during either TRHT or TUHT (see Chap. 13). A major research effort is being directed towards the development of radiometry, which is the most promising method of indirect measurement. Methods utilizing applied power via the antenna are unreliable and should not be used in clinical practice. Power requirements to obtain a specific treatment temperature vary widely during each treatment even in the same patient. The present recommendation is for continuous temperature monitoring using a nonperturbing thermometry system. There should always be one fixed sensor to measure the surface temperature and one movable sensor for thermal mapping. Interstitial temperature measurements are required for each new device evaluation.

19.4 Preclinical Testing Methods of Prostate Hyperthermia Devices

Before an HT device and/or modality is used clinically, a thorough preclinical and premarketing study should be conducted by the manufacturer to evaluate the safety and effectiveness of the device and the applied technique. The United States Food and Drug Administration (USFDA) has recommended a process preceding the clinical use of HT devices for the treatment of BPH. These recommendations are of importance and should be followed. This preclinical testing should consist of a multistep evaluation and safety control of all components of the HT device. The electrical safety, the accuracy of system measurement and control of temperature, the computerized feedback control system, and other important aspects of device safety and performance should be guaranteed before its clinical use. The thermophysical aspects of the antenna should be tested in phantoms to evaluate its heating characteristics. The physical dimensions of an intracavitary applicator may have an important impact on the

Table 19.1. Preclinical testing results of different devices. Overview of reported results of preclinical testing of the currently available hyperthermia devices

	BSD 50	Thermex-II	Prostatron	Prosta thermer	Primus	Prostcare	Microfocus
Phantom studies	+	?	?	?	?	o	?
Antenna evaluation	+	?	?	+	?	o	?
Interstitial temperature	+	?	o	o	+	?	?
Pathological examination	+	+	+	+	o	?	?

+ , Reported in peer-reviewed journals; ?, not published or unknown; o, personal communication or abstract obtained heating patterns. The same may be true in the case of a coaxial cable used in a given treatment session. Knowledge of these important factors will prevent inhomogeneous or hazardous heating during clinical applications. The accuracy of the method and system of temperature monitoring used is of critical importance to prevent the occurrence of major toxicity from overheating. Animal testing of a device represents an important preclinical step to test the device in vivo and allow for evaluation of its safety, toxicity, and biologic effects on the prostate. Prior to large-scale clinical investigation, transperineal temperature measurements in patients are necessary to characterize temperature distributions in human prostatic and periprostatic tissues. Regrettably, some commercial HT devices do not fulfill the above-mentioned criteria or do not provide this information for review (Table 19.1). We first will describe the characteristics of the currently used prostate HT devices and methods. A systematic approach to preclinical testing will be presented and correlated to the reported data for each HT device and/or method.

19.5 Critical Evaluation of Hyperthermia Devices

19.5.1 Available Hyperthermia Devices

Table 19.2 summarizes commonly used and currently available HT devices for the treatment of BPH. It is difficult to compare their technical characteristics since they were designed for different clinical applications. However, a summary and comparison of the features of the currently used devices can be useful in judging the efficiency and reliability of their preclinical testing.

The currently available transurethral devices are the BSD-50, Thermex-II, Prostatron, and Prostcare devices. The *BSD-50 Prostate Machine* uses 915-MHz microwaves, applied in multiple sessions with a mean treatment temperature measured on the urethral surface of 45 °C. This system is designed to operate without urethral cooling. Initially, the number of treatment sessions ranged from five to ten; present protocols call for six sessions of 60 min each, given once or twice a week. Temperature control is obtained with two Bowmann thermosensors. One control thermosensor is located at the center of the helical coil or dipole antennas, where highest temperatures are expected; the second thermosensor allows for thermal mapping along the urethral applicator during treatment (BAERT et al. 1990).

The *Thermex-II* is a device which uses a spectrum of radiofrequency varying between 0.5 and 1 MHz. This system operates without urethral cooling. The treatment consists of one session lasting 3 h, with a mean treatment temperature of 44 °C (VAN DEN BOSSCHE et al. 1991). With new treatment protocols even higher temperatures of up to 48 °C are applied. Temperature mapping is obtained by a multipoint thermal sensor along the transurethral applicator.

Table 19.2 Devices for prostatic hyperthermia and their important characteristics

	BSD 50	Thermex-II	Prostatron	Prostathermer	Primus	Prostcare	Microfocus
Company	BSD	Direx	Technomed	Biodan	Technomatix	Bruker	Breaktrough
Country	USA	Israel	France	Israel	Belgium	France	USA
Method	TUHT	TURF	TUMT	TRHT	TRHT	TUHT/TRHT	TUHT/TRHT
Cooling	No	No	Yes	Yes	Yes	Yes/yes	No/yes
Frequency	915 MHz	50–100 KHz	1300 MHz	915 MHz	915 MHz	915 MHz	915 MHz
Thermometry	TU	TU	TU + TR	TU + TR	TR	Radiometry	TU/TR
Temp. range	43°–45 °C	44.5°–48 °C	45°–55 °C	43 °C	43 °C	45 °C	45 °C
No. of sessions	5–10	1	1	10	10	1/6–10	1/6–10
Duration	60 min	180 min	60 min	60 min	60 min	60 min	60 min

The *Prostatron* applicator uses microwaves up to 1350 MHz with a urethral cooling system incorporated in the urethral microwave catheter (CARTER et al. 1991). The treatment consists of one session of 60 min. Initially, treatment temperatures up to 55 °C were obtained. Higher treatment temperatures up to 70 °C are presently being tested in multiple clinical trials. Due to the high treatment temperatures and related toxicity, a sophisticated temperature control system is provided. The location of the transurethral applicator can be confirmed by transrectal ultrasonography. A fiberoptic thermometry system controls the transurethral and transrectal temperatures.

The current transrectal devices consist of the Prostathermer and Primus systems. The *Prostathermer* employs 915 MHz with a water-cooled transrectal applicator. Treatment consists of ten sessions of 1 h, given once or twice a week, with mean prostatic temperatures of ± 43 °C. Temperature is monitored transrectally and transurethrally. Three thermocouples measure temperatures in the urethra; one is located at the axis of maximum power, and the other two are at each side of this axis. Three thermocouples are in contact with the rectal wall (LINDNER et al. 1990). The *Primus* device has similar characteristics to the Prostathermer, with the exception of a lack of urethral temperature monitoring. Treatment is controlled by direct rectal and calculated urethral temperature monitoring. The urethral temperatures are indirectly monitored with a built-in computer algorithm which calculates temperatures based on the applied power during treatment (VAN ERPS and DENIS 1992).

Two additional devices operate at 915 MHz either transurethrally or transrectally. The *Prostcare* device utilizes a water-cooled transurethral and transrectal applicator, which can be selected separately by the operator. Transurethral treatment consists of one session of 1 h at 45 °C for an average prostate temperature of 45 °C. Patients treated via the rectal applicator receive six or seven sessions of 1 h once or twice a week with an average prostate temperature of 42 °C. Treatment temperature is monitored by following the thermostat-controlled liquid temperature, the applicator surface temperature, the rectal temperature using a rectal probe containing a thermocouple, and temperature measured with a radiometry system. The *Microfocus* applies a similar clinical strategy to that of Prostcare but has a water-cooled transrectal and a noncooled transurethral applicator. The latter applicator is provided in two calibers for small and large prostates. Thermometry is provided by two transurethral and one transrectal thermosensors.

19.5.2 Preclinical Device Testing in Tissue-Equivalent Phantoms

Phantoms are physical models which simulate the characteristics of biologic materials. These phantoms can be used to evaluate the nature and heating patterns of different treatment modalities and to compare the physical (as opposed to clinical) effectiveness of various heating devices.

Static (unperfused) phantoms have to be distinguished from dynamic, liquid-perfused phantoms. Static phantoms can be used only for power deposition studies since the thermal dissipation of tissues is not modeled by phantoms. Various materials have been used in these phantoms for qualitative testing of heating applicators. Although animal tissues and saline solutions of different concentrations were initially used as phantoms, they were not really optimal models of living human tissue. Excised tissues no longer had the same electrical conductivity and dielectric properties as in vivo tissues. Therefore, two kinds of basic phantom material have been developed.

The first represents tissues of high water content, such as muscle and brain. This muscle-equivalent phantom material consists of salt, polyethylene, water, and a gelling material. The second type represents low water content tissues, such as fat or bone. These phantoms are based on mixtures of aluminum powder, acetylene black, and a plasticizer. By appropriately varying the concentration of the constituents, the physical properties of the phantom can be changed to represent tissues of differing water contents, with different intrinsic thermal conductivity and heat capacity. An interesting phantom was described by Astrahan (1979); it consisted of clear gelatin and saline solution. As the phantom was heated to its melting point by a hyperthermia applicator, a liquid zone was formed. By injecting dye into this liquid zone, it was possible to observe through the transparent phantom an isotherm at the liquid–solvent interface.

The use of phantoms permits verification of the characteristics of the applicator with simple laboratory techniques. Phantoms provide a means by which different applicators can be compared. Applicators with the best power deposition patterns can be chosen by such preclinical testing for clinical use. While static phantoms are useful for the study of power deposition patterns in tissue-equivalent materials, they cannot duplicate temperature distributions in vivo since they do not account for the heat exchange due to circulatory perfusion. In order to understand better the effects of blood flow upon the temperature distribution that occurs in vivo, dynamic phantoms become necessary. Dynamic phantoms may help us to understand the contributions of various convective flow processes in vivo. Several attempts have been made to construct such phantoms. An example of a simple dynamic phantom is sponge or other porous medium perfused at different rates with saline solutions.

The goal of developing realistic phantom systems appear to be valid. It would help us to understand not only power deposition in living tissues but also the ultimate temperature patterns obtained in tissues. Phantoms are further useful in that they provide a means of testing and confirming the data obtained through mathematical modeling. The ultimate goal of thermal dosimetry is to predict the temperature distributions that will occur during clinical treatments. Studies with phantoms can help in attaining this goal. In view of the above, every new HT device and/or applicator for treating prostatic disease should undergo strict preclinical evaluation by phantoms.

19.5.3 Dosimetric Hyperthermia Parameters

In testing the characteristics of a new hyperthermia applicator, one of the most important parameters is its iso-SAR pattern. Specific absorption rate (SAR) expresses the rate at which an applicator is capable of increasing the temperature in its surroundings. Testing in static phantoms allows for calculation of SAR, which is expressed in W/kg. In practice, SAR is determined in phantoms by first applying a burst of high power for a short time and subsequently measuring the rate of temperature increase in a specified volume. The heating time has to be short since long heating times and large temperature gradients will produce significant heat conduction. In such situations, temperature patterns will no longer be representative of the power deposition pattern. In order to evaluate the heating ability of a new applicator, it is necessary to provide detailed data on the methodology of the preclinical measurements. Then, the influence of blood flow in the in vivo condition will have to be considered. It is generally accepted that SAR values in the range of the 45–350 W/kg are needed to heat tissues effectively.

In clinical HT applications, means of measuring thermal doses are also needed. Thermal dose should have relevance to a predictable biologic effect(s). The knowledge of temperature during treatment as a function of time, combined with a mathematical description of the time–temperature relationship, permits one to establish the time-equivalent dose (TED). TED is a relatively crude measure to evaluate the biologic effect of heat (LINDNER et al. 1987). It is given in seconds and compares the equivalent time for treatments given at different temperatures to a treatment time given at one predetermined temperature. For example, when $TED_{43.5} = 3600$ s it means that treatment given at various temperatures for different durations gives the same specific effect as if the treatments were carried out for 1 h at 43.5 °C. LINDNER et al. (1987) described a direct correlation between TED (total heat delivery) and the clinical effect obtained.

Every preclinical evaluation of an antenna or device should provide data on these different parameters. The data should then be subjected to a rigorous peer review process. The use of dosimetric parameters will allow us to quantify certain physical characteristics of applicator (SAR) or biologic effectiveness (TED) for different clinical treatments. Comparison of these different parameters will allow scientific evaluation of the various antennas and HT devices available for intracavitary treatment of BPH.

19.5.4 Peer-Reviewed Results of Phantom Studies

19.5.4.1 Introduction

Little information is available in peer-reviewed literature about the physical characteristics of the applicators and/or devices. Data are mostly limited to short communications in abstracts or brief descriptions in commercial information brochures (Table 19.1). Although commercial considerations prohibit the publishing of all technical details and physical characteristics of devices and applicators, this information should be available for official evaluation by USFDA, or similar agencies, prior to their approving the apparatus for clinical use, and to clinicians who want to critically compare and understand the operations of hyperthermia devices. Only this approach can offer us a clinical instrument which will consistently perform with high reliability, safety, and efficacy.

19.5.4.2 Phantom Tests of Transurethral Applicators

Astrahan et al. (1989) reported on the physical characteristics of two types of transurethral antenna. The first antenna consisted of a three-dipole applicator incorporated in a Foley catheter (Astrahan et al. 1989). A newer design consisted of a more flexible helical antenna (Astrahan et al. 1991a). The applicator designs and characteristics were well studied and tested in tissue-equivalent phantoms. Two-dimensional SAR patterns and steady-state temperature distributions in a plane tangent to the applicators were measured. The symmetry of the three-dimensional heating pattern of applicators was studied qualitatively by observing the melting patterns in a transparent, tissue-like gelatin phantom. Electric field measurements were performed by linearly polarized E-field sensors. Evaluations of all these parameters allowed for identification of specific physical characteristics of each applicator and for comparison between the two types of applicator. The heating characteristics of both applicators appeared to be very similar. Both designs had a predominantly axially polarized electric field surrounding the antenna, with a longitudinal heating length of about 4 cm and 0.5 cm effective radial heat deposition. Longitudinal temperature homogeneity was similar, although the hot spot was somewhat broader and better centered for the helical antenna as compared to the three-dipole design of antenna. Radial penetration was slightly better for the dipole array in a plane of maximal phase reinforcement. The steady-state and SAR distributions of the helical antenna suggests a more cylindrical heating pattern compared with the dipoles, but the heating pattern was asymmetrically shifted towards the distal end of the helix. The helical applicator appeared to be well suited for selective heating of a nominally cylindrical volume of about 4 cm length and 0.5 cm radius. Although thermophysically identical, this new design resolved several clinical weaknesses of the dipole array applicator, ensuring simpler operation, smaller size, improved patient comfort, and better mechanical reliability (see Chap. 13).

19.5.4.3 Phantom Test of Combined Transurethral and Transrectal Applicators

Debicki et al. (1992) reported on the physical characteristics of combined transurethral and transrectal antennas. Based on the heating patterns of previously tested transurethral and transrectal applicators, they concluded that neither of these techniques is able to sufficiently heat large volumes of prostate when operating separately. However, when the microwave antennas are used in arrays, the resulting heating pattern can differ significantly from that of the individual antennas due to the interference patterns produced by the microwaves. In regions where the local electric field orientations from the individual antennas are spatially aligned, heating at depth can be selectively enhanced and steered by adjusting the phase relationship between the devices (DEBICKI et al. 1992). This results from the fact that power is proportional to the square of the sum of the electric field vectors from the individual antennas. At the other extreme, in regions where the electric field vectors are directed opposite to one another, the fields cancel, and there is no power deposition. A substantial change in SAR pattern relative to phase shift was predicted by computer modeling. These fundamental predictions were subsequently tested in static phantoms and liquid phantoms, confirming the principle of phase steering. In a particular configuration, mid-plane SAR with the addition of a 240° shifter is about 50 times greater than with a 60° shifter (see Chap. 13).

19.5.4.4 Conclusion

Applicator testing in phantoms permits the study of their hyperthermic characteristics and confirmation of the results of computer simulations. The identification of hot spots is of special importance since it prevents major toxicity. It allows selection of the best applicator design for specific clinical situations and facilitates the planning of further improvements to present designs. Improvements can consist in developing better radial heat deposition patterns in single-antenna systems or improving power deposition in dual-applicator systems through appropriate phase adjustment. Reliable information on the intracavitary applicators is available in peer-reviewed journals. Presentation of applicator characteristics in brief communications or in the form of abstracts is useful as a source of initial information but should be followed by peer-reviewed publications which include critical review of the presented data.

19.5.5 Preclinical Testing in Animal Models

Findings from preclinical phantom testing are not easily extrapolated to animal or human tissues. The major role and impact of changes in blood flow rates during HT treatments cannot be reliably simulated in dynamic phantoms or other studies. Therefore, a device must also be tested in animal models. The obtained data also help to verify the safety of devices, their anticipated performance, and thermal characteristics prior to their use in humans. These tests in animals must include interstitial thermal mapping (including the intraprostatic, periprostatic, and anterior rectal wall tissues) performed in at least five animals. Complete range of power and temperatures planned to be used in the clinic should be tested. The location of the temperature probes must be image verified. Following these detailed measurements, pathologic effects on prostate and periprostatic tissues should be looked for. Preclinical testing should confirm biocompatibility of the urethra-contacting components, electrical safety, accuracy of system measurement and control of temperature, and other important aspects of device safety and performance.

A major problem is to find an optimal animal model for these studies on the prostate. The animal models should closely resemble the human prostate anatomy and histology. Primates may be the best candidates for an animal model because of their close genetic relations to the human species. The cranial and caudal lobes of the rhesus monkey and baboon prostates are probably directly homologous to the human central and peripheral zones. However, most researchers have concluded that the canine represents a good prostate model. It is important to realize that the dog rarely suffers bladder outlet obstruction secondary to enlargement of the prostate. Rather, prostatic hyperplasia is usually secondary to epithelial or glandular proliferation throughout the entire gland, as opposed to the human situation, in which this enlargement is most often limited to the periurethral tissues and is characterized by both glandular and stromal hyperplasia. In addition, the prostate in the dog has a thinner capsule than in the human and it does not develop a median lobe. Anatomically, a retrograde approach to the canine prostatic urethra is difficult due to its intrinsic anatomy. To insert a transurethral catheter, one can perform a perineal urethrostomy or a suprapubic cystostomy. The former technique has the advantage that it simulates more closely this procedure as it is performed in humans. Additionally it allows for cystoscopic evaluation of the external sphincter, verumontanum, and prostatic region pre- and posttreatment. The latter technique facilitates the insertion of the transurethral applicator and direct verification of the position of thermoprobes. However, opening of the bladder and abdominal cavity alters the normal physiologic conditions and intra-abdominal temperatures. The absence of a Denonvilliers' fascia and a loose connection between the posterior base of the prostate and the rectal wall, opposed to the human situations, raises questions about the reliability of the testing of transrectal applicators. Finally, the question arises as to how, exactly, the thermophysical effects can be measured with the interstitial temperature probes. In our experience, it is difficult to insert these probes in a preplanned geometric, reproducible way and to confirm their three-dimensional position by radiographic or ultrasonographic methods. Knowledge of exact probe location is of major importance since the understanding of heating patterns is dependent upon knowledge of the distance between the applicator and temperature measuring points. As an example, 1–2 mm inaccuracy in the measuring position of a thermal sensor may result in a major change in the heating pattern of the applicator beam tested.

19.5.5.1 Animal Studies with Transurethral and Transrectal Applicators

Temperature mapping in canine prostates during TUHT with a three-dipole antenna operating at 915 MHz was reported by Astrahan et al. (1989). Following insertion of the applicator and thermoprobes by cystostomy, radial temperature distributions were measured in the lobes of a normal canine prostate. Longitudinal temperature distributions at the applicator–urethral interface were mapped using a Bowman-type thermistor probe in the thermometry cannula of the applicator. Effective radial heat penetration near the longitudinal center of the applicator was about 0.5 cm with a local gradient of about $-7\,^{\circ}C/cm$ (Astrahan et al. 1989). Roehrborn et al. (1992) reported on thermophysical testings of a transurethral applicator with a helical microwave antenna. Heating was performed with a 915-MHz microwave power generator (Prostek 3000, Clinitherm Corporation, Dallas). Therapeutic temperatures were reached in the periurethral prostate. The radial temperature drop-off in the prostate was about 1 °C per 3-mm distance from the catheter. This would limit the area of effectiveness to a periurethral zone of 1 cm in diameter. No unsafe temperature peaks were noted either intraurethrally or between the prostate and the rectum during the steady-state conditions (Roehrborn et al. 1992). Servadio et al. (1990) evaluated the effects of a transrectal 915-MHz water-cooled skirt-type applicator. Prostatic, urethral, and rectal temperatures were evaluated with copper–constantan thermocouples. They confirmed the previously described characteristic heating profiles of the transrectal, water-cooled antenna. When tissue is not superficially cooled, temperature decreases exponentially, with the maximum temperature being on the rectal mucosal surface. When tissue being heated is cooled superficially, maximum temperatures can be demonstrated inside the prostate (Servadio et al. 1990).

19.5.5.2 Pathologic Changes in Canine Prostates

Roehrborn et al. (1992) observed an intact rectal wall and varying degrees of prostatic inflammation and/or necrosis following the administration of prostatic hyperthermia. Devonec et al. (1991) demonstrated irreversible damage and necrosis in dog prostates with temperatures of 45 °C or higher. The prostates of these dogs were treated for 10–30 min with microwave energy applied transurethrally without cooling, and prostate temperatures of 75 °C. In other dog experiments the treatment was given with the use of a cooling system; severe inflammation was seen, without necrosis of the periurethral region. The urethra, bladder neck, external sphincter, and rectal wall were all normal (Devonec et al. 1991).

After TRHT, Leib et al. (1986) reported specific histologic lesions, which seemed to be time and temperature dependent. The degree of destructive lesions was directly correlated with treatment temperature, its duration, and the number of TRHT sessions. Servadio et al. (1990) studied the pathologic and biochemical effects of different temperatures on a series of dogs. Hyperthermia sessions were given for different lengths of time ranging from 1.5 to 5 h. The prostate temperature was maintained at 42.5 °C or 44.5 °C. The degree of pathologic changes and biochemical alterations (blood counts, liver enzymes) was again directly correlated with temperature and its duration. These observations confirm the importance of heat dose and the necessity of using multiple sessions in prostatic HT treatments.

19.6 Pilot Thermophysical and Clinical Studies

19.6.1 Introduction

Prior to approving a device for a large-scale clinical application, a pilot study consisting of transperineal interstitial temperature measurements should be conducted in BPH patients at the time of the first treatment session. Such a pilot study should monitor complications and characterize the temperature distribution in the prostatic and periprostatic tissues, including that in the rectal wall. Furthermore, this study should demonstrate that unexpectedly high or low temperatures are not being produced within the treated volume of tissue. This information is necessary to ensure that a larger patient population will not be placed at unreasonable risk and that there will be reasonable assurance that the temperatures desired for therapy will be reached and maintained.

After this initial thermophysical pilot study, further clinical studies with transperineal interstitial temperature measurements should be performed on a statistically valid number of patients. These studies are expected to produce a meaningful correlation between the energy applied (or the controlling treatment parameters of the device), the temperature measured, and the clinical results obtained. In contrast to the data obtained from the initial interstitial pilot group, which is primarily intended to examine the temperatures achieved from a safety perspective, these interstitial data should be used to determine the optimal temperatures that need to be achieved in order to yield certain effects. These data may be supplemented by urethral mapping if it is available using the HT applicator or specialized Foley catheter. Although one is aware that interstitial temperature measurements are difficult to perform and potentially painful for the patient, they still should be performed during clinical investigations. Future patients, treated after the device has been made available commercially, will benefit from these tedious measurements through the utilization of fully tested and safe equipment. Thermal dose-response testing has been suggested as an alternative means of demonstrating the correlation between the energy applied and the clinical results obtained, In future clinical studies BPH patients could be randomized to receiving therapy where the target temperature is 42 °C, 43 °C, or 44 °C, given for 45–60 min. This approach has scientific merits but would require significantly larger patient populations to produce meaningful results.

19.6.2 Transperineal Interstitial Temperature Measurements

To obtain the necessary measurements, interstitial thermometry is placed transperineally utilizing 18-gauge needles; at least two catheters for fiberoptic thermal sensors are introduced under local anesthesia and their position is localized.

With the patient in the lithotomy position, transrectal ultrasonography can be used to obtain transverse and sagittal images of the prostate, from which the anatomic landmarks may be identified, including the transition zone and prostatic urethra. Interstitial nonmetallic needles can be placed under digital or sonographic guidance. The location of these needles can be verified and geometrically determined by the use of orthogonal radiographs. Computed tomography can confirm the location of interstitial needles in transverse planes and permit three-dimensional reconstruction (DEBICKI et al. 1992). It is mandatory to obtain the exact three-dimensional distance for each measurement point from the reference point on the applicator surface for later calculations of thermal gradients.

After removing the metallic guides of these nonmetallic needles, thermocouples can be inserted. Thermoprobes used in the measurements should be nonperturbing to avoid interference, which will minimize temperature reading errors. Two types of thermoprobe are currently used: (a) Bowman-type probes with high-resistance leads, consisting of nonmetallic materials impregnated with carbon particles (see Chap. 13); and (b) fiberoptic probes, which comprise glass or plastic optical fibers with low thermal conductivity. These thermoprobes can contain one or more temperature sensors and also allow for thermal mapping during hyperthermic treatments. In transurethral applications, thermal mapping along the applicator can evaluate longitudinal heating patterns of the antenna. A rectal or perirectal thermoprobe can monitor temperatures in the peripheral prostate and its vicinity. In transrectal devices, thermoprobes measure temperatures at the rectum–applicator surface.

Following verification of the location of the probes, temperatures can be measured by changing important HT treatment parameters. These parameters include duration of the session, target temperature, applied power, and cooling temperature. Correlating these temperature data with spatial positions of the thermosensors relative to the applicator(s), one can calculate thermal gradients in tissues. Computer modeling further allows calculation of isothermic regions in prostatic tissues and three-dimensional temperature distributions.

Interstitial temperature measurements provide a very useful technique for evaluating thermophysical treatment efficacy. There are a number of practical problems in performing measurements. The insertion of the needles may be difficult to perform and painful for the patient. The correct positioning of the needles under sonographic guidance is sometimes difficult because of deflection of the needle at the prostatic capsule. Exact localization of the position of the thermoprobes and mapping tracts can be difficult given the inherent inaccuracy of radiologic imaging techniques.

ASTRAHAN et al. (1991a) reported on interstitial temperature measurements during TUHT with a BSD device, using a helical microwave applicator at 915 MHz. The authors demonstrated predictable and symmetrical heating patterns around the prostatic urethra. Clinically relevant heating was limited to the periurethral prostate, with no evidence of hazardous hot spots in the rectal mucosa or outside of the prostate capsule. The effective treatment region was a cylindrically symmetric volume of about 4 cm in length with 0.5 cm effective radial penetration. Maximum temperature elevation occurred in the tissue immediately adjacent to the applicator surface, decreasing at about 6 °C/cm with distance from the applicator surface. Moreover, these findings confirmed the gradients previously observed in phantoms and temperature measurements in canine prostates performed with a similar dipole applicator (ASTRAHAN et al. 1989). The reproducibility of the data from the in vitro and animal studies was a very important indicator of the system stability and predicted safety and efficacy in further clinical treatments.

DEBICKI et al. (1992) reported on interstitial measurements in the prostate using a combined transurethral and transrectal approach. Prostatic temperature profiles were measured in patients treated with TR alone, TU alone, and simultaneous TR and TU heating. In the combined treatments different phase relationships between the antennas were applied. The authors found that a temperature of up to 45 °C could be produced in the center of the prostate. This temperature was higher than on the surface of either applicator and the temperature profiles could be changed by shifting phase (see Chap. 13). Applying the dual-applicator system one could heat the entire prostate well. The results of these measurements were in agreement with the already presented phantom testings and computer simulations (see Chap. 13). This intracavitary HT technique could have an important role in the treatment of patients with locally advanced carcinoma of the prostate in addition to its use in the treatment of BPH.

DEVONEC et al. (1990) reported on interstitial thermokinetics in human prostate using a TUMT applicator. Temperatures of 44 °C were noted at a distance of 15 mm from the urethra. In addition, there was necrosis of tissue in the zone 5–15 mm from the urethra. There was no evidence of rectal injury.

KAPLAN et al. (1992) reported on prostatic and periprostatic interstitial temperature measurements obtained during TRHT using the Primus device and applicator. They observed a maximal prostate temperature of 43.5 °C with a direct relationship between temperature and the distance of the thermocouple from the microwave applicator. The temperature within the first 7 mm from the applicator ranged from 39 °C to 41.7 °C, which did not present a problem of overheating of the anterior rectal wall. Temperature was also measured along the prostatic urethra and it varied between 40° and 43 °C, never exceeding 44 °C. The authors concluded that there was a satisfactory temperature distribution in target tissues without evidence of high temperatures in nontargeted periprostatic tissues.

NEWMANN et al. (1990) reported that intraprostatic temperatures of up to 43 °C corresponded well with the intraurethral temperature readings of the Prostathermer apparatus.

19.6.3 Pathologic Examination of the Prostate

In preliminary phase I studies pathologic examination of prostatic tissues should be performed following the administration of HT, whenever possible. Identification of histologic lesions may indicate dose dependence and may help to establish sound treatment policy. Following the administration of TRHT, interstitial infiltration of mononuclear cells and lymphocytes was seen in the prostate, without signs of tissue necrosis (KAPLAN et al. 1992). The working mechanisms of TRHT was related to heat influence and interaction with α-receptors or hormonal receptors.

After TUHT, LAUWERYNS et al. (1991) described interstitial hemorrhages, complete obliteration of blood vessel lumina due to thrombosis, and further evidence of coagulation and hemorrhagic necrosis in the periurethral prostate. Grossly, the same lesions were seen after TUMT; they were well demarcated up to a depth of 15 mm from an intact urethra (DEVONEC et al. 1991b). Selective shrinking and retraction of the periurethral prostatic parenchyma due to organizing tissue necrosis and cicatrization probably dilates the urethra, reducing or eliminating outflow obstruction (BAERT et al. 1990).

19.7 Evaluation of Clinical Results

Evaluation of clinical results obtained with HT in BPH patients is faced by the common methodological problems of clinical trials which evaluate response to alternative treatments. According to WEIN (1990), an ideal clinical trial for evaluating new treatment modalities for BPH should exhibit an absence of bias, include an adequate number of subjects with sufficient follow-up periods, use appropriate and sensitive methods of evaluation, be conducted under double-blind conditions with a placebo control, and also be statistically valid. Moreover, the well-known unpredictable natural history of BPH should be kept in mind when interpreting clinical data (see Chap. 3).

The elimination of bias is an important factor in the evaluation of any new treatment. Unconscious bias occurs in the assignment of patients to a particular treatment group or in the assessment of responses. A prospective randomized double-blind study helps to eliminate this bias. The study group should be large enough to allow detection of clinically important effects of significant magnitude. Furthermore, this prospective randomized double-blind method is the ideal method to determine the clinical efficacy of any therapeutic intervention.

With an adequate sample size, it ensures that the results obtained are attributable to factors other than sampling variability in the group under consideration. However, it is very difficult to use this double-blind method in studies evaluating new invasive therapeutic techniques such as HT. Patients are mostly aware of the physical characteristics of a given treatment. If HT is administered, they are expecting some sensation of heat; the absence of this sensation can induce patient bias and a suspicion that in fact a sham procedure was performed. Introduction of a transurethral catheter for sham procedures may induce some urethral dilatation, limiting the pure placebo effect. Finally, it is obvious that there are ethical problems in performing sham procedures with an invasive, potentially harmful method.

Appropriate and sensitive methods of evaluation are necessary in order to obtain accurate data on which to base an answer to the primary question under consideration. *Subjective parameters*, including obstructive and irritative symptoms, are difficult to analyze (see Chap. 6). In BPH patients, there is a wide variation in the severity of symptoms and in their combinations. The severity of symptoms in a given patient may vary substantially even between two determinations obtained on two consecutive days. Moreover, symptoms cannot be quantified exactly and it therefore becomes necessary to attach certain grades to the severity of various symptoms by using symptom scores and to analyze pre- to post-treatment changes. Numerous symptom scores have been developed and utilized in practice. The most frequently used symptom score systems are those recommended by Boyarski and by Madsen and Iversen, the Maine Medical Assessment Program score, and the recently developed AUA symptom score (Barry et al. 1992a). This AUA symptom score has been validated in more than 200 BPH patients and in 100 control subjects. It was designed to be self-administered, removing the potential bias of an interview-based questionnaire. A good symptom score system should be sensitive to clinical changes and should meet predetermined criteria. All the above-mentioned scores are predictive of patients' global ratings of degree of bother from the urinary condition. The AUA score discriminates BPH patients from controls significantly better than the Maine Medical Assessment Program score, and equivalently to the Madsen-Iversen and Boyarsky scores. All scores are responsive when BPH patients undergo prostatectomy, although the AUA and Madsen-Iversen scores are significantly more sensitive (Barry et al. 1992b).

Properly chosen urodynamic parameters are important *objective criteria* in the initial evaluation of BPH patients as well as in the assessment of treatment response. The tests considered to be of greatest importance include peak flow rate and the voided volume. However, many factors can influence the accuracy of these tests and induce the well-known variations in peak flow rates in the same patient. Therefore, it is recommended that one should either use flow nomograms or perform flow measurements more than once with recording of the mean volume together with the voided volume. Postvoiding residual volume is another potentially important objective measurement. Although residual urine probably reflects bladder dysfunction, it is difficult to correlate it with either specific prostatic symptomatology or other urodynamic abnormalities. Furthermore, there are wide variations in residual urine volumes in individual patients at different times (BRUSKEWITZ et al. 1982) (Chap. 6).

Statistical validation of the pre- to post-treatment results is necessary to evaluate and compare different treatments and regimens. However, subjective variables are difficult to quantify and statistical analysis of symptom changes has some shortcomings. Determination of statistical significance of changes in objective measures generally is not a problem. However, when considering objective changes, the important concept of clinical versus statistical significance must also be remembered. A post-treatment increase of 2 ml/s in the mean peak flow rate in the study patients may represent a statistically significant change; however, this change may be clinically unimportant. Expressing study results in terms of percent changes rather than presenting the change in absolute values should be avoided. Such data display almost invariably makes treatment effects seem of greater magnitude than they are when the subject of clinical significance is considered. If improvement in symptoms and signs is expressed in percentages of the total number of patients, one should have strict criteria to define in which situations a treatment can be considered successful and what constitutes an improvement.

Subjective and objective study parameters should be standardized. Data collection should be planned in such a way that all possible relevant variables are included. The follow-up period must be long enough to permit evaluation of long-term clinical results. If the study is carried out to determine the therapeutic efficacy of a new method in the treatment of a condition that is generally treated by an operative procedure such as TURP or adenomectomy in BPH, it is of importance to ask whether this new method alters the natural history of the disease as well as the invasive treatment does.

Despite all efforts to optimize evaluation procedures for BPH treatment modalities, the unpredictable natural history of BPH presents an important problem for the interpretation of results from published clinical trials as well as for the design of new clinical studies. Design of clinical trials, investigating new therapeutic modalities, should include a comparison with surgical treatment and should always contain a no-treatment arm.

19.7.1 Recommendation for Clinical Studies

Prior to large-scale clinical application, a controlled randomized placebo-controlled study should be conducted. According to the USFDA recommendations, 100 treatment patients and 30 sham patients may be sufficient to analyze the safety and effectiveness of a particular treatment. The actual size of the treatment and control populations must be statistically based on expected probability of success for the two groups. Without a sham or control group. a much larger study group would be needed to analyze a new treatment. Control patients would not be required to undergo interstitial thermometry.

This sham control is important to assess the placebo effect and the effect of repeated catheterizations by insertion of a transurethral applicator in TUHT or thermosensor in TRHT treatments. A "watchful waiting" group only assesses the natural history of BPH, not the placebo effect or the effects of catheterization. The introduction of sham control, however, presents serious ethical problems since repeated catheterizations may result in infection, and additionally cause substantial patient discomfort. Attempts to compare the HT data with historical TURP data obtained from the literature encounter difficulty in matching TURP patients owing to differences in selection criteria and evaluation methodologies. The use of a concurrent TURP control group undergoing identical evaluation procedures to the HT treatment group should be considered in designing new prospective studies.

Following completion of these extensive thermophysical and clinical studies, further clinical investigation should be limited to a maximum of 150 patients. This clinical study should be conducted on a limited number of medical centers. Safety and effectiveness data on a minimum of 50 patients with at least 3 months' follow-up should be reported. The subject inclusion and exclusion criteria as well as pre- and post-treatment evaluation methods should be clearly defined and consistently used in all HT trials. Only this standardized approach will allow an accurate comparison between different treatment methods.

Data collection and analysis are also important, as is the method of reporting success rates. Objective measures for success must be prospectively established, based on absolute values of improvement in uroflowmetry, residual urine volume, prostate volumes, and symptom scores. Symptom scores should be evaluated and reported to allow an assessment of the obstructive and irritative components and respective post-treatment changes. Treatment results in patients improving in one, two, or all monitored important parameters (uroflow, residual volume, and symptom score) by greater than 75%, 50%, or less than 25% should be presented. These same criteria should also be applied to an evaluation of improvement in just one or two of these parameters. Based on the success criteria established, the number and percent of patients termed successful, improved, unchanged, and failed must be reported. The use of scoring to evaluate the objective data collected is also recommended. Claims for symptomatic relief will be based on improvements in symptom severity. Claims for reduction of obstruction will be based on improvement of objective measurements, such as flow rate, volume, and prostate size. Based on such response criteria, treatment outcome can be reported and the results compared among multiple medical centers. Careful statistical analysis of the treatment outcome is imperative. Finally, a sufficiently long flow-up is needed to determine long-term results and possible late treatment complications.

The duration and magnitude of temperature increase must be documented and assessed. The temperatures achieved and the temperature distributions should be analyzed as a function of treatment session. If possible, treatment response should be correlated with the total amount of energy delivered.

Most of the published reports on hyperthermia clinical trials are based on very limited experience and/or short follow-up. The patient evaluation before and after treatments varies considerably in quality and accuracy, as do the criteria for initial patient selection. Interpretation of reported success rates is frequently very misleading. Users of the same device apply different treatment protocols including differences in controlled temperature and number and duration of treatment sessions. Due to these differences it is very difficult to objectively compare the treatment outcomes and/or to draw conclusions about reported treatment efficacy. A brief discussion on the overall results obtained with the use of several instruments will be presented. The reported results have been compiled from recent peer-reviewed publications, abstracts, or personal communications (Tables 19.3–19.5).

Table 19.3. Clinical results of phase I trials with transurethral devices

Device and study	No.	Follow-up (mos.)	Objective parameters			Subjective parameters	
			%	Peak flow rate (cc/s)	Residual volume decrease	%	Symptom points decrease
TUHT (BSD-50)							
BAERT et al. (1991)	74	12	70	3.0	42	75	5
BOYD et al. (1991)	21	24	81	6.0	90	80.7	6
TURF (Thermex-II)							
VAN DEN BOSSCHE et al. (1991)	50	6	45	2.0	44	51.1	–
MEIER et al. (1992)	65	6	52	0.3	8.8	70	3.4
TUMT (Prostatron)							
CARTER et al. (1991)	50	6	40	6.1	6	80	10.6
LADUC et al. (1992b)	98	6	–	0.9	17.6	–	6

Table 19.4. Clinical results of phase I trials with transurethral devices

Device and study	No.	Follow-up (mos.)	Objective parameters			Subjective parameters	
			%	Peak flow rate (cc/s)	Residual volume decrease	%	Symptom points decrease
TRHT (Primus)							
VAN ERPS and DENIS (1992)	138	12	24	1.8	–[a]	64	4.8
WADA (1991, unpublished)	30	6	53	3.5	28	53	3.3
TRHT (Prostathermer)							
SARANGA et al. (1990)	83	12	42	1.9	74	22	1.3
STROHMAIER et al. (1990)	30	1	7	– 1.1	7	33	1.9
MONTORSI et al. (1992)	132	24	–	1.4	79	–	5.2

[a] –, Not reported

Table 19.5. Clinical results of double-blind placebo-controlled studies

Report	No.	Follow-up (mos.)	Objective parameters			Subjective parameters	
			%	Peak flow rate (cc/s)	Residual volume decrease	%	Symptom points decrease
FABRICIUS et al. (1991) (Primus)							
TRHT group	26	3	20	1.0	40	57	–
Placebo group	25	3	20	1.0	10	32	–
ZERBIB et al. (1992) (Prostathermer)							
TRHT group	38	12	42	1.9	74	68	7.2
Placebo group	30	12	53	2.1	53	33	1.3
BAERT et al. (BSD)							
TUHT group	15	3	–	3.1	3	–	4.8
Placebo group	15	3	–	0.5	– 16	–	3.5
LADUC et al. (1992) (Prostatron)							
TUMT group	23	6	–	3.4	–	–	10.2
Placebo group	23	6	–	1.9	–	–	4.9

[a] –, Not reported

19.7.2 Results of Reported Clinical Trials

19.7.2.1 Results of TUHT with the BSD Apparatus

SAPOZINK et al. (1990) reported on the treatment of 21 BPH patients who had moderate to severe symptoms and signs of urinary outflow obstruction. Each patient received ten TUHT sessions of 60 min each. No late toxicity or sexual dysfunction was noted in these patients with a minimum follow-up of more than 5 years. Major objective improvement was obtained in 81% and major subjective improvement in 71% of the patients. BAERT et al. (1990) conducted a phase 1 trial in 15 severely symptomatic BPH patients. Comparison of post- and pretreatment trial in 15 severely symptomatic BPH patients. Comparison of post- and pretreatment objective and subjective study parameters showed significant major improvement ($P < 0.0002$). The response rates were similar to those reported by SAPOZINK et al. (1990). Treatment was well tolerated and no major toxicity was noted.

The importance of prostate anatomy in TUHT trials was demonstrated in a pilot study of 38 patients by BAERT et al. (1991). The authors found major improvement in the important subjective and objective parameters in 73% of patients with hyperplasia predominantly involving the lateral lobes but only 30% of those with median lobe hyperplasia ($P = 0.018$). This difference in response can be attributed to the thermal characteristics of the transurethral applicator, which was designed to heat lateral lobes only. Median lobe hyperplasia represents an anatomic valve-like obstruction which cannot be effectively treated by TUHT with the present applicator design (BAERT et al. 1991).

These important findings were confirmed in a larger study of 74 patients. An overall objective response was seen in 70% of the 74 nonretention patients. A major subjective response was obtained in 75% of these patients. The best results were again seen in bilobar and trilobar hyperplasia BPH patients. The same findings were observed in a group of 32 patients with urinary retention. Of the 32 patients treated, 25 had predominance of lateral lobes and seven had median lobe hyperplasia. None of the seven median lobe patients resumed and maintained spontaneous voiding while 72% of the 25 lateral lobe hyperplasia patients had spontaneous voiding at 12 months post-TUHT ($P = 0.002$). An additional important finding of this study was an excellent correlation between treatment outcome and applied temperature ($P < 0.001$) (BAERT et al. 1992). BOYD et al. (1991) reported the same success rates in objective and subjective parameters.

A prospective randomized phase II trial comparing three and six sessions was recently reported. A total of 28 BPH patients with moderate to severe signs and symptoms of urinary outflow obstruction were entered in this study. Subjective improvement was recorded in 50% of the patients receiving three sessions (group 1) as compared to 86% of the patients receiving six sessions (group 2). Total symptom score improved by 21.4% in the first group and by 51.1% in the second group ($P < 0.006$). Mean peak flow rate increased by 8.4% in the first group while it increased by 51.1% in the second group ($P < 0.003$). Similar differences existed between the two treatment groups in other important parameters of this study. The authors concluded that six TUHT sessions were more effective in BPH patients than three TUHT sessions (BAERT et al. 1993).

A response to TUHT was examined in BPH patients with smaller (< 50 g) and larger (> 50 g) prostates. A total of 63 poor surgical risk BPH patients were included. Major subjective improvement was obtained in 92% of the patients. There was no difference in the incidence of subjective improvement between the patients with smaller versus larger prostates (NS at $P = 0.75$). Similarly, there was no difference comparing objective study parameters by prostate volume. Failure occurred in 10% of the 40 patients with smaller prostates and 9% of the 23 patients with larger prostates (NS at $P = 0.49$). The authors concluded that the initial prostate volume is not an important predictor of response to TUHT (PETROVICH et al. 1992).

We recently finished a randomized double-blind placebo-controlled study in 30 BPH patients. Preliminary analysis at short follow-up showed significant post-treatment improvement of objective parameters in the TUHT group compared to the sham group. However, a less significant difference in subjective response was seen between the two groups. These data have to be confirmed after longer follow-up periods and statistical validation.

19.7.2.2 Results of TURF Trials with the Thermex II

VAN DEN BOSSCHE et al. (1991) reported on 62 BPH patients who were treated in one single session at temperatures of 44.5 °C. At the 4-month follow-up, 57% of the patients showed subjective improvement. Objective improvement, defined as an increase of 50% in maximum flow rate and a decrease of 50% in residual urine, was observed in 43% of the patients. There was a twofold increase in PSA levels at 1 day after treatment, but values returned to normal after 1 month. No changes in prostatic volume were observed. Among the group of 17 patients showing retention, eight regained spontaneous voiding with acceptable peak flow rate and minimal residual urine. The same investigators compared the efficacy of TURF at 44.5 °C and 47°–48 °C. At 44.5 °C, 60% of the patients were subjectively improved, while 71% were improved at 47°–48 °C. Objective improvement was not dependent upon applied temperature (personal communication). MEIER et al. (1992) reported objective and subjective improvements in 52% and 70% of patients respectively. In a subgroup of patients with peak flow rates lower than 10 ml/s, objective and subjective improvement was seen in 70% and 67% of the patients respectively.

19.7.2.3 Results of TUMT with the Prostatron

CARTER et al. (1991) reported the results of TUMT with the temperature controlled at 45.5 °C in 50 BPH patients. Seventy-five percent of the patients with outflow obstruction before treatment had a substantial improvement in symptom score, which was reduced from 12 to 2.8 points. Peak flow rates improved from 8.2 ml/s to 14.3 ml/s at the 3-month follow-up. Of the 19 patients in retention, eight regained spontaneous voiding. The only side-effects were self-limited urethral bleeding and short-term obstruction apparently secondary to urethral edema. Such improvements in objective and subjective parameters were not confirmed by LADUC et al. (1992b). The authors reported improvements in peak flow rate and symptom score of only 0.9 ml/s and 6 points respectively. TUMT causes significant PSA elevations, suggesting major tissue necrosis, but no changes in prostate volume (LADUC et al. 1992a). The same group of investigators reported subjective improvement in both placebo- and TUMT-treated patients. There was a slight objective improvement in the placebo group compared to a moderately good improvement in the TUMT group (personal communication). In a multicenter retrospective analysis of more than 1100 patients, with a mean follow-up of 78 months, symptom score improved from 13.2 to 5 points and peak flow rate increased from 9.0 to 12.9 ml/s respectively (LADUC et al. 1992b).

19.7.2.4 Results of TRHT with the Prostathermer

SERVADIO (1992) reported on the treatment of 312 patients with a 4-year follow-up. He indicated that only 36% patients required surgery; all other patients had sufficient objective and subjective improvement to preclude prostatectomy. Significant improvement was noted in maximal peak flow rates, with 34% showing > 3 ml/s flow rate increase at the end of the first year of follow-up and 46% at the end of the second year. In a group of 72 patients with complete retention, all carrying a permanent indwelling catheter, 50% resumed spontaneous voiding after HT and 40% remained catheter-free at 1 year (LINDNER et al. 1990).

However, STROHMAIER et al. (1990) reported only 7% objective improvement in 30 BPH patients treated with TRHT. SARANGA et al. (1990) reported on a study of 83 patients with severe obstructive symptoms. Although some improvement was found in the scoring of both subjective and objective parameters, the number of patients benefiting was small, with only 28% showing improvement in both parameters. Approximately 50% reported subjective improvement, which was significant in only 25%. In 42% of patients there was objective evidence of improvement. In an extensive report on 192 patients with a 2-year follow-up period, MONTORSI et al. (1992) reported only a minor amelioration of urinary flow rates and subjective symptoms. According to maximum flow nomograms all patients were still obstructed post-treatment.

ZERBIB et al. (1992) conducted a double-blind placebo-controlled study on 68 patients. The authors demonstrated a greater objective improvement in the treatment group than in the sham group (53% vs 13%). Subjective improvement was similarly higher in the treatment group (68% vs 33%). A statistically significant subjective improvement was seen in the sham group (33%) which was not accompanied by any significant objective improvement.

19.7.2.5 Results of TRHT with the Primus

VAN ERPS and DENIS (1992) reported on treatment of 138 patients with symptomatic BPH given TRHT. The mean follow-up period was 3 months. Substantial symptom relief, especially in the irritative category, was noted in 64% of the patients. Symptom score ranged from 8.4 to 3.6 points post-treatment. Only 24% of the patients showed an increase in peak flow rate of > 50%. Of the initial subjective responders, 72% remain stable, not requiring additional treatments. WADA reported objective and subjective improvement in 53% of patients (personal communication). FABRICIUS et al. (1991) conducted a double-blind placebo-controlled study. The authors reported subjective improvement in 57% of TRHT-treated patients as opposed to 32% in the sham group. Objective results were poor in both groups, with improvement seen in 20% of the patients.

19.7.2.6 Comparative Studies Evaluating Different Hyperthermia Systems

In a retrospective study, using the same patient selection and evaluation methodology, STAWARZ et al. (1991) reported a statistically significant difference in the treatment outcome in TUHT-treated patients as compared to those treated with TRHT. In a prospective study comparing the two TRHT devices and the Thermex II, WATSON et al. (1991) reported the best results with the Prostathermer. In a prospective randomized trial, PETERSSON (1993, unpublished data) obtained good results after TUMT, compared to TURP. These results were analyzed at 12 months post-treatment. Treatment results were similar for both treatment groups, with virtually identical flow rates, residual urine, and symptom scores.

19.8 Conclusion

Analysis of the available clinical data shows variable treatment outcomes with the use of the same and different instruments to deliver hyperthermia. The precise role of HT in the conservative treatment of BPH has not yet been well defined. The published results of clinical studies utilizing several different treatment methods and different HT devices are faced with a lot of methodological problems. Conducting multicenter, well-controlled prospective randomized studies should permit objective assessment of the therapeutic efficacy of prostatic HT.

The HT devices have to be reliable and permit safe and accurate treatment delivery. Applicator characteristics have to be studied in the laboratory and in vivo. More accurate systems for indirect temperature measurements have to be developed. Pilot clinical studies must adhere to a strict protocol of inclusion and evaluation criteria and be reported with a sufficient follow-up. Until these criteria have been fulfilled, and studies have been subjected to a peer review process and reported in scientific journals, HT has to be considered an investigational treatment modality.

References

Astrahan MA (1979) Concerning hyperthermia phantom. Med Phys. 63:235–232

Astrahan MA, Sapozink MD, Cohen D, Luxton G, Kampp TD, Boyd S, Petrovich Z (1989) Microwave applicator for transurethral hyperthermia of benign prostatic hyperplasia. In J Hyperthermia 5:283–296

Astrahan MA, Imanaka K, Jozsef G, et al. (1991a) Heating characteristics of a helical microwave applicator for transurethral hyperthermia of benign prostatic hyperplasia. Int J Hyperthermia 7:141–155

Astrahan MA, Ameye F, Oyen R, Willemen P, Baert L, Petrovich Z (1991b) Interstitial temperature measurements during transurethral microwave hyperthermia. J Urol 145:304–308

Baert L, Ameye F, Oyen R, et al. (1990) Transurethral microwave hyperthermia for benign prostatic hyperplasia: preliminary clinical and pathological results. J Urol 144:1383–1387

Baert L, Willemen P, Ameye F, Petrovich Z (1991) Treatment response with transurethral microwave hyperthermia in different forms of benign prostatic hyperplasia: a preliminary report. Prostate 18:315–320

Baert L, Ameye F, Pike M, Willemen P, Astrahan MA, Petrovich Z (1992) Transurethral hyperthermia for BPH patients with retention. J Urol 147:1558–1561

Baert L, Ameye F, Astrahan M, Petrovich Z (1993a) Transurethral microwave hyperthermia for benign prostatic hyperplasia: the Leuven clinical experience. J Endourol 7:61–69

Baert L, Ameye F, Pike M, Petrovich Z (1993b) Optimization of transurethral hyperthermia: number of treatments. Urology (in press)

Barry MJ, Fowler FJ, O'Leary MP, Bruskewitz RC, Holtgrewe HL, Mebust WK, Cockett AT and the Measurement Committee of the American Urological Association (1992a) The American Urological Association symptom index for benign prostatic hyperplasia. J Urol 148:1549–1557

Barry MJ, Fowler FJ, O'Leary MP, Bruskewitz RC, Holtgrewe HL, Mebust WK, and the Measurement Committee of the American Urological Association (1992b) Correlation of the American Urological Association Symptom index with self-administered versions of the Madsen-Iversen, Boyarski and Maine Medical Assessment Program symptom indexes. J Urol 148:1558–1563

Boyd SD, Sapozink MD, Astrahan MA (1991) Microwave hyperthermia for the treatment of benign prostatic hyperplasia. Probl Urol 5:441–448

Bruskewitz RC, Iverson P, Madsen PO (1982) Value of postvoid residual urine determination in evaluation of prostatism. Urology 20:602–607

Carter SS, Patel A, Reddy P, Royer P, Ramsay JW (1991) Single-session transurethral microwave thermotherapy for the treatment of benign prostatic obstruction. J Endourol 5:137–144

Debicki P, Astrahan MA, Ameye F, Oyen R, Baert L, Haczewski A, Petrovich Z (1992) Temperature steering in prostate by simultaneous transurethral and transrectal hyperthermia. Urology 40:300–307

Devonec M, Cathaud M, Carter S, Berger N, Perrin P (1990) Transurethral microwave application. Temperature sensation and thermokinetics of the human prostate. J Urol 143:414A

Devonec M, Berger N, Perrin B (1991a) Transurethral microwave heating of the prostate – or from hyperthermia to thermotherapy. J Endourol 146:1128–1135

Devonec M, Berger N, Bringeon G, Carter S, Perrin P (1991b) Short and long term histological effects of TUMT on benign prostatic hypertrophy. J Urol 145:363A

Fabricius PG, Schäfer J, Schmeller N, Chaussy C (1991) Efficacy of transrectal hyperthermia for benign prostatic hyperplasia: a placebo-controlled study. J Urol 145:363A

Harzmann R, Weckermann D (1991) Lokale hyperthermie bei prostataerkran-kungen. Aktuel Urol 22:10–14

Kaplan SA, Shabsigh R, Soldo KA, Olsson CA (1992) Prostatic and periprostatic interstitial temperature measurements in patients treated with transrectal thermal therapy (local intracavitary microwave hyperthermia) J Urol 147:1562–1565

Laduc R, Bloem FA, Debruyne FM (1992a) Transurethral microwave thermotherapy in benign prostatic hyperplasia. J Urol 147:344A

Laduc R, Bloem FA, Debruyne FM (1992b) Trnasurethral microwave thermotherapy (TUMT) in the treatment of patients with benign prostatic hyperplasia. Eur Urol Update Series 1(6):42–47

Lauweryns J, Baert L, Vandenhove J, Petrovich Z (1991) Histopathology of prostatic tissue after transurethral hyperthermia. Int J Hyperthermia 7:221–230

Leib Z, Rothem A, Lev A, Servadio C (1986) Histopathological observations in the canine prostate treated by local microwave hyperthermia. Prostate 8:93–102

Lindner A, Golomb J, Siegel Y, Lev A (1987) Local hyperthermia of the prostate gland for the treatment of benign prostatic hypertrophy and urinary retention: a preliminary report. Br J Urol 60:567–571

Lindner A, Braf Z, Lev A, Golomb J, Leib Z, Siegel Y, Servadio C (1990) Local hyperthermia of the prostate gland for the treatment of benign prostatic hypertrophy and urinary retention. Br J Urol 65:201–203

Meier AH, Weil EJ, van Waalwijk van Doorn ES, Verhaegh GT, Janknegt RA (1992) Transurethral radofrequency heating or thermotherapy for benign prostatic hypertrophy. Eur Urol (in press)

Monotorsi F, Galli L, Guazzoni G, et al. (1992) Transrectal microwave hyperthermia for benign prostatic hyperplasia: long term clinical, pathological and ultrastructural patterns. J Urol 148:321–325

Newman D, Knapp P (1990) Interstitial temperature mapping in the human prostate during transrectal hyperthermia treatment for BPH. J Endourol 4 (Suppl 1): 135

Petrovich Z, Ameye F, Pike M, Boyd S, Baert L (1992) Relationship of response to transurethral hyperthermia and prostate volume in BPH patients. Urology 40:317–321

Roehrborn CG, Krongrad A, McConnell JD (1992) Temperature mapping in the canine prostate during transurethrally-applied local microwave hyperthermia. Prostate 20:97–104

Sapozink MD, Boyd SD, Astrahan MA, Jozsef G, Petrovich Z (1990) Transurethral hyperthermia for benign prostatic hyperplasia: preliminary clinical results. J Urol 143:944–950

Saranga R, Matzkin H, Braf Z (1990) Local microwave hyperthermia in the treatment of benign prostatic hypertrophy. Br J Urol 65:349–353

Servadio C (1992) The use of hyperthermia for benign prostatic hyperplasia. Curr Opin Urol 2:12–17

Servadio C, Lindner A, Lev A, Leib Z, Siegel Y, Braf Z (1989) Further observations on the effect of local hyperthermia on benign enlargement of the prostate. World J Urol 6:204–208

Servadio C, Leib Z, Lev A (1990) Local hyperthermia to canine prostate. Urology 15:156–163

Stawarz B, Szmigielski S, Ogrodnik J, Astrahan M, Petrovich Z (1991) A comparison of transurethral and transrectal microwave hyperthermia in poor surgical risk benign prostatic hyperplasia patients. J Urol 146:353–357

Strohmaier W, Bichler KH, Fluchter SH, Wilbert DM (1990) Local microwave hyperthermia of benign prostatic hyperplasia. J Urol 144:913–917

Turner PF Schaefermeyer T (1987) Technical aspects of hyperthermia. In: Issels RD, Wilmanns W (eds) Application of hyperthermia in the treatment of cancer. Springer, Berlin Heidelberg New York (Recent results in cancer research, vol 107, pp 76–86)

Vallencien G, Chartier-Kastler E, Chopin D, Veillon B, Brisset JM, André-Bougaran J (1992) Focused extracorporeal pyrotherapy: experimental results. Eur Urol (in press)

van den Bossche M, Noel JC, Schulman CC (1991) Transurethral hyperthermia for benign prostatic hypertrophy. World J Urol 9:2–6

Van Erps P, Denis LJ (1992) Transrectal hyperthermia treatment in benign prostatic hyperplasia. Eur Urol (in press)

Watson G, Permutter A, Shah T, Barnes D (1991) Heat treatment for severe symptomatic prostatic outflow obstruction. World J Urol 9:7–11

Wein AJ (1990) Evaluation of treatment response to drugs in benign prostatic hyperplasia. Urol Clin North Am 17:631–640

Zerbib M, Steg A, Conqui S, Martinache PR, Flam TA, Debre B (1992) Localized hyperthermia versus the sham procedure in obstructive benign hyperplasia of the prostate: a prospective randomized study. J Urol 147:1048–1052

20 Optimization of Treatment for Benign Prostatic Hyperplasia: Outcome of Clinical Trails and Future Directions

ZBIGNIEW PETROVICH, FILIP AMEYE, and LUC BAERT

CONTENTS

20.1 Introduction

It has been estimated that 800 000 American males present annually with symptoms and signs of benign prostatic hyperplasia (BPH) requiring some therapy. Of these 800 000 patients, 400 000 are treated surgically each year (RUTKOW 1986). The annual cost of treatment of BPH was estimated in the United States in 1990 to be approximately 4.0 billion dollars (COTTON 1991). In spite of a large number of patients being treated for BPH, the indications for the treatment are not well defined. It has been suggested that less than 25% of surgically treated patients have "solid" indications for this treatment. Wide geographic variations in the incidence of prostatectomy have been reported. In

ZBIGNIEW PETROVICH, MD, Professor and Chairman, Department of Radiation Oncology, University of Southern California, Kenneth Norris Jr. Cancer Center, 1441 Eastlake Avenue, Los Angeles, CA 90033, USA
FILIP AMEYE, MD, Department of Urology, St. Pieter's Hospital, Catholic University of Leuven, Brusselsestraat 69, 3000 Leuven, Belgium
LUC BAERT, MD, PhD, Professor and Chairman, Department of Urology, St. Pieter's Hospital, Catholic University of Leuven, Brusselsestraat 69, 3000 Leuven, Belgium and Clinical Professor of Radiology and Radiation Oncology, University of Southern California School of Medicine, Los Angeles, CA 90033, USA

Petrovich/Baert (Eds.)
Benign Prostatic Hyperplasia

an interesting study comparing the incidence of common surgical procedures between New England, Norway, and the West Midlands District of England, the incidence of prostatectomy per 100000 population was 264, 236, and 132, respectively (MCPHERSON et al. 1982). If the current incidence of prostatectomy does not change, nearly 30% of American males will have undergone this procedure by the age of 80 (GLYNN et al. 1985).

In the past 15 years, there has been major interest in applications of less invasive treatment for BPH patients. The alternative treatments which appear most promising include laser prostatectomy, endoprostheses, pharmacologic therapy, and hyperthermia. Unfortunately, the indications for the use of these alternative treatments are also not well defined and treatment outcomes are frequently not reported in an objective fashion.

It is imperative that future studies will include important pretreatment subjective and objective parameters, provide detailed data on treatment methodology, and provide detailed data on treatment outcomes as defined in Chap. 6.

It would be very helpful for the analysis of data on treatment outcome in BPH patients if peer-reviewed scientific journals would adopt a uniform policy on a minimum requirement for data reporting of clinical trials. The American Urological Association (AUA) has provided the leadership in this area by recommending uniformity in the evaluation of symptom scores (BARRY et al. 1992). The AUA-recommended symptom score, which has recently been validated, should replace the most commonly used Boyarsky and Madsen symptom scores for all new clinical trials on patients with BPH.

20.2 Outcome of Surgical Treatment

In spite of the large number of BPH patients treated with surgery there is a relative paucity of reported data on treatment outcome (GRAVERSON et al. 1989; LEPOR and RIGAUD 1990). It is generally believed that transurethral prostatectomy (TURP) results in good to excellent improvement in more than 80% of treated patients (Chap. 8). The remaining 15%–20% of patients either have minimal improvement or no improvement following TURP. Additionally, 2% of patients treated with prostatectomy, who initially show good response to treatment, present annually with treatment failure and require more surgery (ROOS and RAMSEY 1987). Otherwise, the response to TURP is durable (BRUSKEWITZ et al. 1986).

Treatment complications of importance have been reported in approximately 20% of surgically treated patients (MELCHIOR et al. 1974; ROOS and RAMSEY 1987; ROOS et al. 1989; MEBUST et al. 1989). An additional problem, which has been relatively poorly documented, is sexual dysfunction in patients following prostatectomy (BRUSKEWITZ et al. 1986; LIBMAN and FICHTEN 1987).

Surgical treatment is a safe and effective therapy for patients with symptoms and signs of BPH. Surgery remains the gold standard against which all new treatment modalities have to be compared for efficacy. There is a need, however, to establish better criteria for applying surgical treatment for the majority (75%) of symptomatic BPH patients, in whom treatment indications have not been well defined. It is unrealistic to expect a prospective randomized trial comparing surgery with observation only in those 75% BPH patients who may not have well-defined indications for therapeutic intervention. In the absence of randomized trials, careful reporting of important pretreatment parameters, as well as reporting of details on treatment outcome, will help to define treatment indications in these patients. In scientific reports, more attention should also be paid to short- and long-term effects of surgical and other therapy for BPH on patients' quality of life (Fowler et al. 1988).

20.2.1 Newer Surgical Techniques

Newer surgical techniques for the treatment of BPH patients include balloon dilation, prostatic stents, and laser prostatectomy.

20.2.1.1 Balloon Dilation

Balloon dilation of the prostate has been under investigation for the past several years. The early reports on nonrandomized trials showed its effectiveness in BPH patients, which subsequently led to the Food and Drug Administration's approval of some catheter designs. In a recently reported prospective randomized double-blind trial comparing the effectiveness of balloon dilation and standard cystoscopy, these early reports were questioned (Lepor et al. 1992a). There was no difference in the effectiveness of balloon dilation and simple cystoscopy in terms of improvement in mean symptom score and lack of improvement in mean peak flow rates. Based on this prospective randomized trial, balloon dilation appears of no value in the management of symptomatic BPH patients.

20.2.1.2 Urethral Stents

Urethral stents offer an interesting, simple surgical technique which is particularly useful in poor surgical risk patients who are not suitable candidates for prostatectomy. This technique, however, is still evolving and only a few reports with long-term results are available for review (Baert et al. 1993a). The place of endoprostheses in the management of symptomatic BPH patients will be defined following the results of prospective randomized trials.

20.2.1.3 *Laser Prostatectomy*

Laser prostatectomy is a new surgical technique which appears to have effectiveness in the treatment of symptomatic BPH patients. At the present time, only results of phase I studies are available for review, and long-term follow-up data are lacking (Chap. 11). The main advantage of the use of laser prostatectomy over traditional prostatectomy is in its shorter postoperative recovery period, resulting in a shorter hospital stay. In a recently published report of a prospective randomized trial in 25 BPH patients comparing laser prostatectomy and standard TURP, the treatment effectiveness was equal in both groups (KABALIN 1993). There were, however, fewer acute complications in the laser-treated patients as compared to those treated with TURP. More data from prospective randomized trials are necessary for the evaluation of usefulness of this technique in the treatment of BPH patients.

20.3 Outcome of Pharmacologic Treatment

The most effective pharmacologic agents in the treatment of BPH have been α-blockers. Early trials with these drugs have demonstrated their effectiveness but also presented problems with their toxicity (Chap. 12). Recently developed agents with selective α_1-blocker action showed good effectiveness with a much lower incidence of side-effects in comparison to a nonselective drug such as phenoxybenzamine. The primary mode of action of α_1-blockers is to reduce the dynamic component of outflow obstruction caused by BPH. They have no effect in reducing the static component of this obstruction.

A number of clinical trials with terazosin and prazosin have been reported and claimed therapeutic efficacy in symptomatic BPH patients. Objective evaluation of these trials, however, was difficult due to flaws in their design or flaws in outcome evaluation or both. An important prospective randomized phase III study in 314 BPH patients has recently been reported (LEPOR et al. 1992a). The patients were assigned to placebo or terazosin and given a single daily dose of 2, 5, and 10 mg. This study demonstrated a significant improvement in important pretreatment subjective and objective parameters in the terazosin group as compared to the placebo group. There was also evidence of greater improvement with the increase of terazosin dose from 2 to 10 mg daily. Toxicity of this terazosin therapy was of no major clinical significance. More follow-up data will be necessary for complete evaluation of this important trial.

In order to reduce the static component of obstruction, hormonal manipulations have been studied. The outcome of reported prospective trials have been disappointing. A recent report of outcome of a multicenter prospective, placebo-controlled randomized trial was likewise disappointing (GORMLEY et al. 1992). This study compared the use of 1 and 5 mg finasteride (inhibitor of 5α-reductase) with a placebo in 895 BPH patients. The treatment was given daily for a period of 12 months. Although statistically significant improvement in symptoms and signs of obstruction in patients receiving 5 mg finasteride over the placebo group was reported, these differences were of questionable clinical significance.

It is apparent that more work needs to be done to evaluate the effectiveness of pharmacologic agents in BPH patients. Patients treated with modern α_1-blockers have consistently demonstrated up to 70% improvement. The BPH patients who were entered into the α_1-blocker studies, however, had only mild symptoms of prostatism. A major problem with α_1-blockers is the need for their continued use for an indefinite period of time. At this time, an effort is being made to develop new and more selective agents with a higher degree of efficacy and lower toxicity. Present clinical trials are directed toward combination therapy to simultaneously reduce the static and dynamic components of outflow obstruction caused by BPH.

20.4 Outcome of Hyperthermia Trials

Application of hyperthermia (HT) for patients with BPH is a development of the past 15 years. HT was first used transrectally (TRHT) and subsequently transurethrally (TUHT). Related to the HT treatment mode is transurethral microwave thermotherapy (TUMT) (see Chaps. 13, 14, and 19).

20.4.1 Transrectal Hyperthermia

The use of TRHT in 29 patients with severe symptoms of BPH was reported by Yerushalmi et al. (1985). Of the 18 nonretention patients, three (17%) had more than 50% improvement in symptom score, nine (50%) had 30%–50% improvement, and six (33%) had less than 30% improvement. Of the 11 retention patients, eight (73%) resumed and maintained spontaneous voiding following the course of treatment. TRHT was given on an outpatient basis without sedation or anesthesia, and was well tolerated by the study patients who were in poor general condition and could not be treated surgically. A major weakness of this report was the lack of temperature data and the lack of data on important objective parameters, such as flow rates.

An important study on the use of TRHT in 72 BPH patients in retention was reported by Lindner et al. (1990a). Of the 72 study patients, 36 (50%) had spontaneous voiding 1 month post-treatment and 29 (40%) maintained spontaneous voiding 12 months post-treatment. TRHT was well tolerated by these patients. Of the 435 patients treated with TRHT, 27 (6%) developed complications. Only 3 of the 27 patients with complications required emergency prostatectomy to control hematuria. The remaining patients responded well to conservative management (Lindner et al. 1990).

In a prospective randomized trial, 68 BPH patients were assigned to receive TRHT or sham treatment ($n = 30$) (ZERBIB et al. 1992). The treatment group demonstrated subjective response in 68% of patients and objective response in 53%. This compared with 33% subjective response and no objective response in the 30 sham group patients. The authors concluded that "treatment had a definite therapeutic effect in BPH in excess of placebo." One would question, however, the clinical importance of an improvement in the mean peak flow rate from the initial 7.6 cc/s to the post-treatment result of 9.6 cc/s.

In contrast to these good results obtained with TRHT, STROHMAIER et al. (1990), in a study of 30 BPH patients, showed the treatment benefit in only two (7%) patients. SARANGA et al. (1990) reported treatment results in 114 BPH patients. Of the 83 nonretention patients, an improvement in objective and subjective parameters was seen in only 28%, while of the 31 retention patients 61% resumed spontaneous voiding.

A comparison of TRHT and TUHT in a group of 36 BPH patients showed statistically significant and clinically important better subjective and objective results in 14 TUHT patients versus those managed with TRHT (STAWARZ et al. 1991). In view of the above variable results reported in patients treated with TRHT, it was of interest to see a report on interstitial temperature measurements in 15 BPH patients (KAPLAN et al. 1992). T_{max} of $> 43\,^{\circ}C$ was recorded in the prostate in up to 2 cm from the rectal antenna.

Histologic studies in patients treated with TRHT showed edema and white cell infiltrates but no tissue necrosis (MONTORSI et al. 1992; STROHMAIER et al. 1990). The mechanism of action of TRHT in BPH patients does not have a satisfactory explanation. It has been postulated that TRHT acts in a similar fashion to α-blockers (Chaps. 14 and 16).

20.4.2 Transurethral Hyperthermia

Transurethral hyperthermia is a simple and reproducible treatment technique which was developed in 1985 for the management of BPH patients (Chaps. 13, 14, and 19). The first phase I study used ten 1-h HT sessions in 21 patients with moderate to severe signs and symptoms of BPH (SAPOZINK et al. 1990). Treatment tolerance was excellent and mild toxicity was common but of no clinical significance. This toxicity consisted of bladder spasms (26%), mild hematuria (23%), and dysuria (9%). A mean urethral surface temperature more than 43 °C was easy to obtain and easy to maintain. Good or excellent subjective and objective improvement was reported in 71% and 81% of patients, respectively. Of the 21 patients treated, 17 (81%) had major improvement. An additional patient, who was initially tabulated as a treatment failure, demonstrated late response which was maintained for 7 years of follow-up. It is of interest to note that with a follow-up of more than 5 years, three additional patients developed recurrence of their symptoms of prostatism and required prostatic resection. Therefore, of a total of 21 patients treated, 15 (71%) maintained their response for at least 5 years (unpublished data). No late treatment complications were noted.

These good treatment results were confirmed in a phase I study of 15 patients reported by the group from the University of Leuven (BAERT et al. 1990). Detailed histologic studies of resected prostates following TUHT performed in several patients showed changes limited to a cylindrical volume of periurethral prostate. These changes consisted of edema, interstitial hemorrhages, and a well-defined zone of tissue necrosis. All the above changes were limited to a volume of periurethral prostate of 4 cm in length and 6 mm radially. The severity of histologic changes had increased and they were seen further away from the urethra with each subsequent treatment (BAERT et al. 1990; LAUWERYNS et al. 1991). Healing, resulting in fibrosis, produced retraction of the urethra, thus relieving the static component of outflow obstruction. Detailed interstitial temperature measurements performed during TUHT in patients and in multiple canines demonstrated hyperthermic temperatures (> 42 °C) only in a well-defined periurethral zone (ASTRAHAN et al. 1991; DEBICKI et al. 1992; STAWARZ et al. 1991).

In several phase II studies, the optimal anatomic configuration of the prostate, the optimal treatment temperature, the number of TUHT treatments, and the importance of prostate volume were defined. In a study of 32 poor surgical risk patients presenting in retention and treated with TUHT, 72% of bilobar and trilobar hyperplasia patients were catheter-free at 1 year post-treatment, while of the seven median lobe or median bar patients, only one had temporary (4 months) response (BAERT et al. 1992). This study has also demonstrated a strong correlation between treatment temperature and response ($P = 0.002$).

In a larger study of 72 patients, bilobar and trilobar hyperplasia patients had more than twice the response rate of the median lobe or median bar patients (BAERT et al. 1991). Based on the above data, we feel that patients with median lobe and median bar should not be considered for TUHT. In another phase II study of 63 poor surgical risk BPH patients, treatment response was found to be independent of prostate volume (PETROVICH et al. 1992). Finally, in a prospective phase II randomized trial, six TUHT sessions were shown to be superior in terms of treatment response to three TUHT sessions ($P = 0.01$) (BAERT et al. 1993).

A new and interesting development in prostatic HT was the simultaneous use of transurethral and transrectal antennas applied with phase steering (DEBICKI et al. 1992; PETROVICH et al. 1993). This antenna array was capable of heating the entire prostate to hyperthermic temperatures (> 42 °C). Currently, a prospective randomized trial is underway comparing TUHT with TURP or open prostatectomy and observation only (Fig. 20.1). Hopefully, in several years, this study will help to define the place of TUHT in the management of patients with BPH. Additionally, it may provide important data on the natural history of this disease.

In any clinical study employing TRHT or TUHT, it is mandatory to continuously monitor the temperature (Chaps. 13, 14, and 19). HT systems

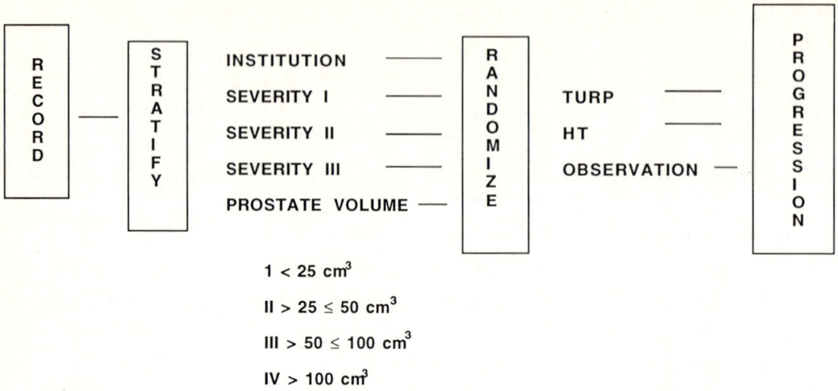

Fig. 20.1. A schema of a phase III prospective randomized trial comparing TUHT with prostatectomy (open and endoscopic) versus observation only

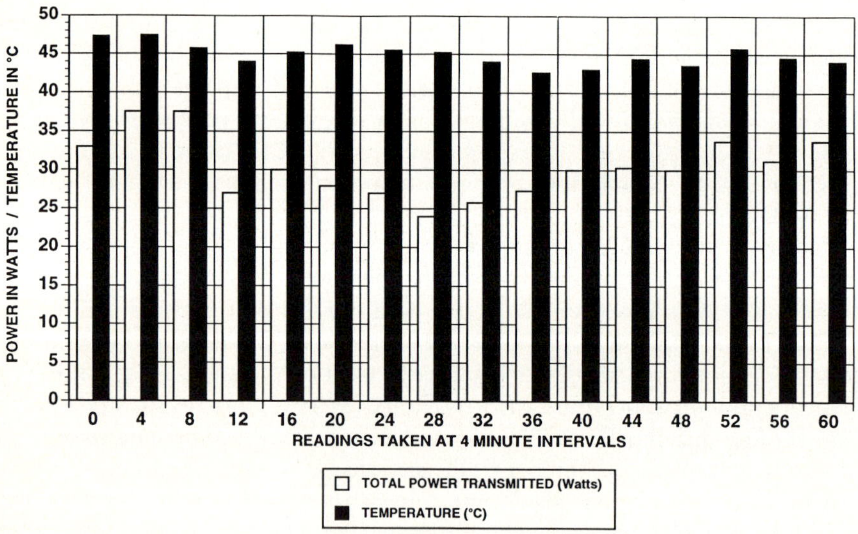

TOTAL POWER TRANSMITTED (Watts)	33	37.5	37.5	27	30	27.9	27	24	25.8	27.3	30	30.3	30	33.75	31.2	33.75
TEMPERATURE (°C)	47.25	47.4	45.7	44	45.2	46.2	45.5	45.2	44	42.6	43	44.4	43.5	45.7	44.5	44

a

Fig. 20.2a–c. Total transmitted power required to maintain urethral surface temperature at 45 °C. The measurements were obtained in a BPH patient treated at USC with TUHT at weekly intervals. Note the wide power variations to maintain the same temperature

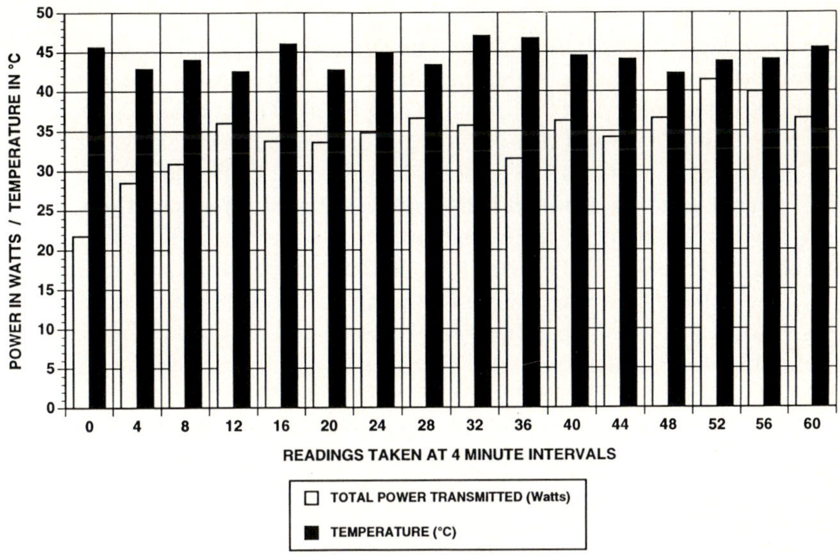

TOTAL POWER TRANSMITTED (Watts)	21.75	28.5	30.9	36	33.75	33.6	34.8	36.6	35.7	31.5	36.3	34.2	36.6	41.4	39.9	36.6
TEMPERATURE (°C)	45.6	42.8	44	42.5	46	42.7	44.8	43.3	47	46.7	44.5	44	42.2	43.75	44	45.5

b

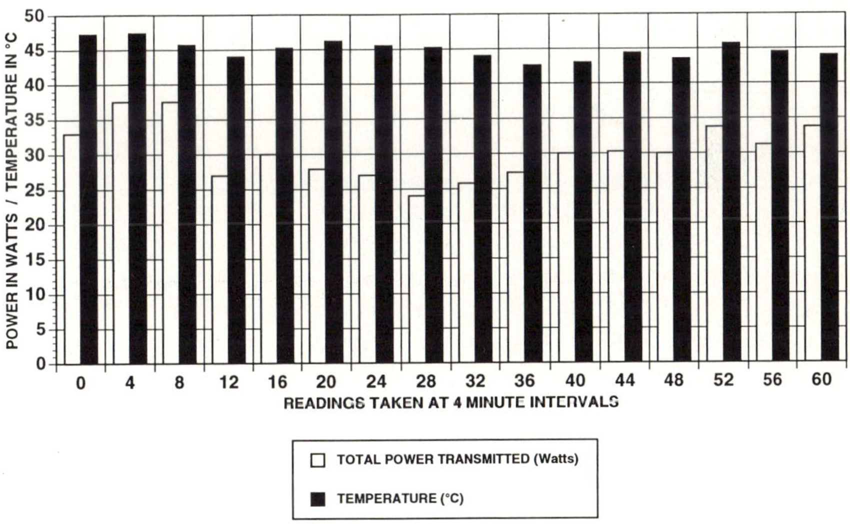

TOTAL POWER TRANSMITTED (Watts)	33	37.5	37.5	27	30	27.9	27	24	25.8	27.3	30	30.3	30	33.75	31.2	33.75
TEMPERATURE (°C)	47.25	47.4	45.7	44	45.2	46.2	45.5	45.2	44	42.6	43	44.4	43.5	45.7	44.5	44

c

Fig. 20.2b, c.

utilizing various algorithms based on applied power instead of temperature measurements are grossly inaccurate and should not be used in clinical practice. The authors performed a series of interstitial temperature measurements in patients treated with TRHT (unpublished data). The measured temperatures were from a few to several degrees centigrade different from the value predicted with the use of algorithms based on applied power. Fortunately, the measured temperatures were always lower than the one based on calculations.

A similar problem exists in patients treated with TUHT. In a study of patients treated with TUHT, urethral surface temperature was maintained at 45°C. The applied power to obtain this temperature was widely variable during each treatment in the same patient and between different treatments in the same patient. Figure 20.2 demonstrates this problem. The measurements were obtained using the USC TU applicator with three dipole antennas (Chap. 13). The power requirement (total power for three-antenna array) to maintain urethral temperature at 45°C ranged from a low of 22 W to a high of 40 W (Fig. 20.2).

20.4.3 Transurethral Thermotherapy

Transurethral thermotherapy is the newest addition to prostate heating modalities (Chaps. 13, 14, 17, and 19). Recent reports showed a low incidence of complications and high response rates in patients with prostatism (DEVONEC et al. 1991, 1993; BLUTE et al. 1992).

In a study presented at the AUA Meeting in 1992, 49 BPH patients were randomized to receive TUMT or TURP (PETTERSSON et al. 1992). In the 25 TUMT patients, mean peak flow rates increased from 7.1 cc/s before the treatment to 13.5 cc/s 6 months following the treatment ($P < 0.01$). The symptom score on the Madsen scale decreased from the initial 10.8 to 3.3 6 months following TUMT ($P < 0.01$) (PETTERSSON et al. 1992). Of the 25 TUMT patients, eight (32%) developed urinary retention following their treatment. Similar excellent treatment results were obtained in the 24 TURP patients.

OGDEN et al. (1993) reported a randomized comparison of TUMT with a sham treatment in 43 BPH patients. In the 21 sham patients, there was no change in subjective and objective study parameters. In the 22 TUMT patients at 3 months' follow-up, there was a decrease in the mean Madsen score from the initial 14.5 to the post-treatment score of 4.3 (70% change). The mean peak flow rate changed from 8.5 cc/s to 13.0 cc/s (53% improvement) and PRV was reduced from a mean of 147 cc to a mean of 12 cc (92% decrease). Acute retention developed in 22%of TUMT patients. One patient failed TUMT and required prostatectomy (OGDEN et al. 1993).

No correlation between patients, pretreatment symptoms or signs, and the treatment outcome was noted in a large retrospective study (BERG et al. 1993). There was a correlation, however, between response and applied power during TUMT. Clinical results appeared durable with a longer follow-up period (DEVONEC et al. 1993).

20.5 Conclusion

Based on the available evidence, less invasive forms of therapy for symptomatic BPH patients are in the process of evolution. Prospective phase III randomized trials are needed to define the role of each new treatment modality in the management of BPH patients. Each new modality should be compared against "the gold standard" which is prostatectomy and each study should contain a no-treatment arm. The no-treatment arm is of critical importance to define indications for therapeutic intervention and to allow for a better understanding of the natural history of this common disease.

Uniform standards in treatment monitoring and in evaluation of treatment outcome should be carefully followed and the findings reported in peer-reviewed journals.

References

Astrahan MA, Ameye F, Oyen R, et al. (1991) Interstitial temperature measurements during transurethral hyperthermia. J Urol 145: 304–308

Baert L, Ameye F, Willemen P, et al. (1990) Transurethral microwave hyperthermia for benign prostatic hyperplasia: preliminary clinical results. J. Urol 144: 1383–1387

Baert L, Willemen P, Ameye F, Petrovich Z (1991) Transurethral microwave hyperthermia: treatment response in different forms of benign prostatic hyperplasia. Prostate 18: 315–320

Baert L, Ameye F, Pile M, et al. (1992) Transurethral hyperthermia for BPH patients with retention. J Urol 147: 1558–1561

Baert L, Verhamme L, Van Poppel H, et al. (1993a) Long term consequences of urethral stents. Br J Urol 68: 604–607

Baert L, Ameye F, Pike M, Petrovich Z (1993b) Optimization of transurethral hyperthermia: number of treatments. Urology (in press)

Barry MJ, Fowler FJ Jr, O'Leary MP, et al. (1992) The Measurement Committee of the American Urological Association's Symptom Index for Benign Prostatic Hyperplasia. J Urol 148: 1549–1557

Berg C, Choi N, Colombeau P, et al. (1993) Responders versus non-responders to thermotherapy in BPH: a multicenter retrospective analysis of patients and treatment profiles. J Urol (in press)

Blute ML, Tomera KM, Hellerstein DK, et al. (1992) Transurethral microwave thermotherapy for prostatism: early Mayo Foundation experience. Mayo Clin Proc 67: 417–421

Bruskewitz RC, Larsen EH, Madsen PO, Dorflinger T (1986) 3 year follow-up of urinary symptoms after transurethral resection of the prostate. J Urol 136: 613–615

Cotton P (1991) Case for prostate therapy wanes despite more treatment options. JAMA 266: 459–460

Debicki P, Astrahan MA, Ameye F, et al. (1992) Temperature steering in prostate by simultaneous transurethral and transrectal hyperthermia. Urology 40: 300–306

Devonec M, Berger N, Perrin P (1991) Transurethral microwave heating of the prostate: from hyperthermia to thermotherapy. J Endourol 5: 129–135

Devonec M, Fendler JP, Jouver P, et al. (1993) Thermotherapy in benign prostatic hypertrophy: an update of clinical results and latest developments. J Endourol (in press)

Fowler FJ, Wennberg JE, Timothy RP, et al. (1988) Symptom status and quality of life following prostatectomy. JAMA 259: 3018–3022

Glynn RJ, Campion EW, Bouchard GR, et al. (1985) The development of benign prostatic hyperplasia among volunteers in the Normative Aging Study. Am J Epidemiol 121:78–90

Gormley GJ, Stoner E, Bruskewitz RC, et al. and Finasteride Study Group (1992) The effect of finasteride in men with benign prostatic hyperplasia. N Engl J Med 327:1185–1191

Graversen PH, Gasser TC, Wasson JH, et al. (1989) Controversies about indications for transurethral resection of the prostate. J Urol 141:475–481

Kabalin JN (1993) Laser prostatectomy performed with a right angle firing neodymium:Yag laser fiber at 40 watts power setting. J Urol 150:95–99

Kaplan SA, Shabsigh R, Soldo KA, Olsson CA (1992) Prostatic and periprostatic temperature measurements in patients treated with transrectal thermal therapy (local intracavitary microwave hyperthermia). J Urol 147:1562–1565Lauweryns J, Baert L, Vandenhove J, Petrovich Z (1991) Histopathology of prostatic tissue after transurethral hyperthermia. Int J Hyperthermia 7:221–230

Lepor H, Rigaud G (1990) The efficacy of the transurethral resection of the prostate in men with moderate symptoms of prostatism. J Urol 143:533–537

Lepor H, Sypherd D, Machi G, Derus J (1992a) Randomized double-blind study comparing the effectiveness of balloon dilation of the prostatic hyperplasia. J Urol 147:639–644

Lepor H, Auerbach S, Puras-Baez A, et al. (1992b) A randomized, placebo-controlled multicenter study of the efficacy and safety of terazosin in the treatment of benign prostatic hyperplasia. J Urol 148:1467–1474

Libman E, Fichten CS (1987) Prostatectomy and sexual function. Urology 29:467–478

Lindner A, Braf Z, Lev A, et al. (1990a) Local hyperthermia of the prostate gland for the treatment of benign prostatic hypertrophy and urinary retention. Br J Urol 65:201–203

Lindner A, Siegel YI, Sarange R, et al. (1990b) Complications in hyperthermia treatment of benign prostatic hyperplasia. J Urol 144:1390–1392

McPherson K, Wennberg JE, Hovind OB, Clifford P (1982) Small area variations in the use of common surgical procedures: an international comparison of New England, England and Norway. N Engl J Med 307:1310–1314

Mebust WK, Holtgrewe HL, Cockett ATK, Peters PC and Writing Committee (1989) Transurethral prostatectomy: immediate and postoperative complications. A cooperative study of 13 participating institutions evaluating 3,885 patients. J Urol 141:243–246

Melchior J, Valk WL, Foret JD, Mebust WK (1974) Transurethral prostatectomy: computerized analysis of 2,223 consecutive cases. J Urol 112:634–642

Montorsi F, Galli L, Guazzoni G, et al. (1992) Transrectal microwave hyperthermia for benign prostatic hyperplasia: long term clinical, pathological and ultrastructural patterns. J Urol 148:321–325

Ogden CW, Reddy P, Johnson H, et al. (1993) Sham versus transurethral microwave thermotherapy in patients with symptoms of benign prostatic bladder outflow obstruction. Lancet 341:14–17

Petrovich Z, Ameye F, Pike M, et al. (1992) Relationship of response to transurethral hyperthermia and prostate volume in BPH patients. Urology 40:317–321

Petrovich Z, Ameye F, Baert L, et al. (1993) New trends in the treatment of benign prostatic hyperplasia and carcinoma of the prostate. Am J Clin Oncol 16:187–200

Pettersson S, Dahlstrand C, Fall M, et al. (1992) Transurethral microwave thermotheraphy versus transurethral resection for benign prostatic hyperplasia: preliminary results of a randomized study (abstract). J Urol 147A:305A

Roos NP, Ramsey EW (1987) A population based study of prostatectomy: outcomes associated with differing surgical approaches. J Urol 137:1184–1188

Roos NP, Wenneberg JE, Malenka DJ, et al. (1989) Mortality and reoperation after open and transurethral resection of the prostate for benign prostatic hyperplasia. N Engl J Med 32:1120–1124

Rutkow IM (1986) Urological operations in the United States: 1979–1984. J Urol 135:1206–1208

Sapozink MD, Boyd SD, Astrahan MA, et al. (1990) Transurethral hyperthermia for benign prostatic hyperplasia: preliminary clinical results. J Urol 143:944–950

Saranga R, Matzkin H, Braf Z (1990) Local microwave hyperthermia in the treatment of benign prostatic hypertrophy. Br J Urol 65:349–353

Stawarz B, Szmigielski S, Ogrodnik J, et al. (1991) A comparison of transurethral and transrectal microwave hyperthermia in poor surgical risk benign prostatic hyperplasia patients. J Urol 146:353–357

Strohmaier WL, Bichler KH, Fluchter SH, Wilbert DM (1990) Local microwave hyperthermia of benign prostatic hyperplasia. J Urol 144:913–917

Yerushalmi A, Fishelovitz Y, Singer D, et al. (1985) Localized deep microwave hyperthermia in the treatment of poor operative risk patients with benign prostatic hyperplasia. J Urol 133:873–876

Zerbib M, Steg A, Conquy S, et al. (1992) Localized hyperthermia versus the sham procedure in obstructive benign hyperplasia of the prostate: a prospective randomized study. J Urol 147:1048–1052

Subject Index

List of Contributors

FILIP AMEYE, MD
Department of Urology, St. Pieter's Hospital, Catholic University of Leuven, Brusselsestraat 69, 3000 Leuven, Belgium

KEN ANSON, MD, FRCS
Research Registrar in Urology, Department of Urology and Minimally Invasive Therapy, Whittington Hospital, Highgate Hill London N19 5NF, United Kingdom

MELVIN A. ASTRAHAN, PhD
Associate Professor, Department of Radiation Oncology, University of Southern California, School of Medicine, 1441 Eastlake Avenue, Los Angeles, CA 90033, USA

LUC BAERT, MD, PhD
Professor and Chairman, Department of Urology, St. Pieter's Hospital, Catholic University of Leuven, Brusselsestraat 69, 3000 Leuven, Belgium

and

Clinical Professor of Urology and Radiation Oncology, University of Southern California, School of Medicine, Los Angeles, CA 90033, USA

KARL-HORST BICHLER, MD, PhD
Professor and Chairman, Department of Urology, Eberhard-Karls-University, Hoppe-Seyler-Straße 3, 72076 Tübingen, Germany

STUART D. BOYD, MD
Associate Professor, Department of Urology, University of Southern California, School of Medicine, 1200 North State Street, # 5900, Los Angeles, CA 90033, USA

LUTHER W. BRADY, MD
Professor and Chairman, Department of Radiation Oncology and Nuclear Medicine, Hahnemann University, Broad and Vine Streets, Philadelphia, PA 19102-1192, USA

Reginald C. Bruskewitz, MD
Professor of Surgery, Division of Urology, University of Wisconsin, Clinical Sciences Center, 600 Highland Avenue, Madison, WI 53792, USA

Paola Dal Cin, PhD
Center for Human Genetics, University of Leuven, Herestraat 49, 3000 Leuven, Belgium

Piotr S. Debicki, PhD
Department of Radiation Oncology, University of Southern California, School of Medicine, 1441 Eastlake Avenue, Los Angeles, CA 90033, USA

M. Devonec, MD, PhD
Professor, Department of Urology, Antiquaille Hospital, Claude Bernard University, 69321 Lyon, France

Christopher M. Dixon, MD
Assistant Professor, Department of Urology, New York University, 550 First Avenue New York, NY 10016, USA

J.P. Fendler, MD, PhD
Department of Urology, Antiquaille Hospital, Claude Bernard University, 69321 Lyon, France

Eef Hoeben
Doctorate Student, Department of Developmental Biology, Laboratory for Experimental Medicine and Endocrinology, Catholic University of Leuven, 3000 Leuven, Belgium

P. Joubert, MD
Department of Urology, Antiquaille Hospital, Claude Bernard University, 69321 Lyon, France

Joan Keit, MD
Chief Resident, Department of Radiation Oncology and Nuclear Medicine, Hahnemann University, Broad and Vine Streets, Philadelphia, PA 19102, USA

Herbert Lepor, MD, FACS
Professor of Urology, Department of Urology, New York University, School of Medicine New York, NY 10016, USA

W. Mattauch, MD
Department of Urology, Eberhard-Karls-University, Hoppe-Seyler-Straße 3, 72076 Tübingen, Germany

Glenn B. Mieszkalski, MD
Chief Resident, Department of Radiation Oncology and Nuclear Medicine, Hahnemann University, Broad and Vine Streets, Philadelphia, PA 19102, USA

Raymond H. Oyen, MD
Adjunct Clinic Head, Department of Radiology, Catholic University of Leuven, Herestraat 49, 3000 Leuven, Belgium

P. Perrin, MD, PhD
Professor and Chairman, Department of Urology, Antiquaille Hospital, Claude Bernard University, 69321 Lyon, France

Zbigniew Petrovich, MD, FACR
Professor and Chairman, Department of Radiation Oncology, University of Southern California, Kenneth Norris Jr. Cancer Center, 1441 Eastlake Avenue, Los Angeles, CA 90033, USA

Malcolm C. Pike, PhD
Professor and Chairman, Department of Preventive Medicine, University of Southern California, School of Medicine, 1420 San Pablo Street, PMB A-201, Los Angeles, CA 90033-9987, USA

Morten Riehmann, MD
Research Fellow, Department of Surgery, Division of Urology, University of Wisconsin, Clinical Sciences Center, 600 Highland Avenue, Madison, WI 53792, USA

Ellen Shapiro, MD, FACS, FAAP
Professor of Urology, Department of Urology, New York University, School of Medicine New York, NY 10016, USA

Donald G. Skinner, MD
Professor and Chairman, Department of Urology, University of Southern California, School of Medicine, 1200 N. State Street, Suite 5900, Los Angeles, CA 90033, USA

Bronislaw Stawarz, MD, PhD
Professor and Chairman, Department of Urology, MMA Postgraduate Medical School, ul. Listopada 15-10, 03-446 Warsaw, Poland

W.L. Strohmaier, MD, PhD
Department of Urology, Eberhard-Karls-University, Hoppe-Seyler-Straße 3, 72076 Tübingen, Germany

STANISLAW SZMIGIELSKI, MD, PhD
Professor, Center for Radiobiology and Radiation Safety, MMA Postgraduate Medical School, 11/3 Pulawska, 02-515 Warsaw, Poland

GISKE URSIN, MD, PhD
Post-doctoral Fellow, Department of Preventive Medicine, University of Southern California, School of Medicine, 1420 San Pablo Street, Los Angeles, CA 90033-9987, USA

HERMAN VAN DEN BERGHE, PhD
Professor and Chairman, Department of Human Genetics and Head of Center for Human Genetics, University of Leuven, Herestraat 49, 3000 Leuven, Belgium

HENDRIK VANDEURSEN, MD, PhD
Professor, Department of Urology, St. Pieter's Hospital, Catholic University of Leuven, Brusselsestraat 69, 3000 Leuven, Belgium

HEIN VAN POPPEL, MD, PhD
Professor, Department of Urology, St. Pieter's Hospital, Catholic University of Leuven, Brusselsestraat 69, 3000 Leuven, Belgium

GUIDO VERHOEVEN, PhD
Professor of Pathophysiology, Laboratory for Experimental Medicine and Endocrinology, Chairman, Department of Developmental Biology, Catholic University of Leuven, 3000 Leuven, Belgium

GRAHAM WATSON, MD, FRCS (Urol)
Consultant Urologist, Department of Urology and Minimally Invasive Therapy, Whittington Hospital, Highgate Hill, London N19 5NF, United Kingdom

and

Senior Lecturer, Institute of Urology, London, United Kingdom

Springer-Verlag and the Environment

We at Springer-Verlag firmly believe that an international science publisher has a special obligation to the environment, and our corporate policies consistently reflect this conviction.

We also expect our business partners – paper mills, printers, packaging manufacturers, etc. – to commit themselves to using environmentally friendly materials and production processes.

The paper in this book is made from low- or no-chlorine pulp and is acid free, in conformance with international standards for paper permanency.